Cost-Benefit and Cost-Effectiveness Analysis in Health Care

Principles, Practice, and Potential

health
administration
press

Cost-Benefit and Cost-Effectiveness Analysis in Health Care

Principles, Practice, and Potential

Kenneth E. Warner
Bryan R. Luce

Health Administration Press
Ann Arbor, Michigan
1982

Library of Congress Cataloging in Publication Data

Warner, Kenneth E., 1947-
 Cost-benefit and cost-effectiveness analysis in health care.

 Bibliography: p.
 Includes index.
 1. Medical care—Cost effectiveness. 2. Medical care—United States—Cost effectiveness. 3. Medical economics—United States. I. Luce, Bryan R. II. Title.
 RA410.5.W29   362.1'068'1   81-30165
 ISBN 0-914904-81-7   AACR2

Health Administration Press
A Division of the Foundation of the
American College of Healthcare Executives
1021 East Huron
Ann Arbor, Michigan 48104
(313) 764-1380

Contents

List of Tables and Figures

FIGURES

Foreword

Many health care professionals approach cost-benefit and cost-effectiveness analysis (CBA-CEA) with something akin to what Sir James Fraser described as "the awe and dread with which the untutored savage contemplates his mother-in-law." This is unwise and unnecessary. Greater familiarity with the objectives and methods of CBA-CEA and with its strengths and weaknesses will make it abundantly clear that this new and rapidly growing analytical technique is neither a purgative nor a panacea nor a placebo.

This book by Kenneth Warner and Bryan Luce is an excellent way for health care professionals to obtain that familiarity. The authors build on their valuable contributions to the Office of Technology Assessment's review of CBA-CEA in order to produce a text-treatise that is notable for its readability, thoroughness, and balance.

By virtue of their candor in discussing difficult issues, their ability to eschew jargon, and their clear sense of priorities, the authors have made a complex subject readily accessible to a wide audience. Health care students and practitioners, administrators, planners and policymakers will all find that a careful reading of this book will equip them with a good understanding of the principles, practice and potential of CBA-CEA. It will not, and does not intend to, provide the technical training necessary to become a practitioner of the technique.

Although the style and content of the book make it eminently suitable as an introduction to the subject, the authors have not skimped in their substantive coverage of applications to health care. On the contrary, their review and analysis of the relevant literature is extremely thorough, making this volume an important reference work for any serious scholar or practitioner of CBA-CEA.

The third major strength of the book is its balance. The CBA-CEA approach has been hailed as the salvation of medical care by some writers and deplored as an immoral, impossible activity by others. Warner and Luce take a hardheaded look at the actual, real-world applications of CBA-CEA (rather limited, to date), analyze the circumstances which limit its application (both inherent problems and particular features of the current political-economic environment), and define its potential usefulness (both as a process and as an applied analytical tool).

Although I recommend the book with enthusiasm, I must caution the reader against being overly influenced by the authors' forceful delineation of the weaknesses and limitations of CBA-CEA. It is important to appraise these weaknesses and limitations in light of alternative ways of allocating scarce resources. In my opinion, the interest in and use of CBA-CEA stem from a growing realization that we live in a world of scarce resources and that the fundamental economic problem of society is to allocate these resources in a way that will best satisfy human wants. Health is a basic human want, perhaps the most basic, but it is still only one of many competing wants. Neither this society nor any other can allocate to health all the resources that physicians and other health professionals believe might benefit their patients. What, then, is to be done? Given the wide range of potential choices in the use of health-care facilities, personnel, and technologies, decision-makers clearly need a better understanding of the consequences of the alternatives. That is precisely what CBA-CEA is designed to do.

This book is skeptical of the idea that CBA-CEA in itself will be effective in controlling health care costs or in correcting the misallocation of health care resources. To be sure! There must be a will to do this, and there must also be financial and organizational mechanisms to implement that will. Given the will and the mechanisms, however, CBA-CEA offers the most rational, humane basis for effective, efficient allocation. Health care professionals should not fear such efforts but should welcome and cooperate actively in them. Mounting pressures from taxpayers, business firms, and labor unions to control expenditures make some constraints inevitable. It is in the best interests of patients and professionals for these constraints to be derived from careful study of costs and benefits rather than from capricious budget ceilings and regulatory roulette. When constraints on health care are imposed without regard to costs and benefits, the nation's health suffers more than is necessary.

When CBA-CEA is applied it will be important to insulate the individual practitioner from explicit involvement on a day-to-day basis because of potential conflict with the commitment to do what is best for each patient. Ordinarily, the appropriate time for evaluations and trade-offs is when decisions are made about construction of facilities, authorization of new technologies, training of personnel, and setting of standards and procedures. It is not important for every health care professional to be able to perform CBA-CEA, but it is essential for them to understand how and why these analyses are performed. This book provides a major contribution toward that end.

Victor R. Fuchs
Stanford University and
National Bureau of Economic Research

Preface

No one needs an education in economics to know that the costs of personal health care are high and growing rapidly. Charges on hospital bills, the price of medical insurance, and the magnitude of medical care tax dollars make this vividly clear to health professional and consumer alike. The issue of what to do about the costs of care has become a frequent theme of deliberations in both professional and policymaking circles.

While the existence of the problem is obvious, one may need an education in economics to appreciate its underlying causes and proposed solutions. This book is intended to address this need, with particular focus on a tool of economic analysis which is receiving much attention in the health policy community: cost-benefit and cost-effectiveness analysis (CBA and CEA, respectively). Both government agencies and private organizations have been calling for intensified activity in CBA-CEA, with an eye toward applying the findings to medical resource allocation. The literature on health care CBA-CEA has burgeoned in recent years, and the term "cost-effective" has become mandatory in describing desirable health care services. Yet despite this newfound prominence, CBA and CEA mystify most health care professionals. Even many scholars and policymakers conversant in the jargon of health services research have a distorted perception of the true value and limitations of CBA and CEA. In a world in which these labels are invoked with increasing frequency, an appreciation of the meaning and potential usefulness of the techniques seems essential.

Thus, a principal purpose of this book is to demystify CBA-CEA. By describing the techniques of CBA-CEA in plain English, we hope to make the literature, and perhaps even the techniques, accessible to a wide spectrum of health care professionals, including physicians, medical students, nurses, administrators, and health planners and policymakers. We hope to clarify the strengths and weaknesses of analysis and thereby distinguish appropriate from inappropriate uses of CBA-CEA. Furthermore, by examining the political and economic environments in which health care professionals function, we hope to stimulate some thought on the potential usefulness of CBA-CEA in a variety of institutional settings. All of the professional groups mentioned above have a vested interest in cost-effective care, but their interests are not perfectly congruent; occasionally, they may be directly in conflict with one another.

This book is intended primarily for the CBA-CEA novice, although several aspects should be of interest to knowledgeable analysts. Our review of the literature includes two features not found in previous studies. First, as described in Appendix A, we have developed a CBA-CEA bibliography that includes hundreds of contributions not covered in other bibliographies of health care CBA-CEA. The obscurity of these contributions often results from where they were published (for example, a medical specialty journal). In fact, these contributions to the CBA-CEA literature are the first contact numerous health care professionals have with CBA-CEA; as such, these articles and books are worthy of attention. They are included with more well-known articles in Appendix C, which lists most items in the bibliography by topic. Appendix D includes abstracts of more than fifty studies.

The second feature unique to our book is that we categorized CBA-CEA publications by date of publication, type of publication, medical function, and so on. This categorization permits one to analyze empirically the growth of the literature, both in terms of its magnitude and its nature. Presented in text discussion and in Appendix B, this analysis suggests important qualitative aspects of the growth of interest in health care CBA-CEA.

Most of our discussion of CBA-CEA methodology, intended for the novice, will be familiar to the experienced analyst. Nevertheless, our presentation includes some unpublished ideas that we believe reflect the emerging state of the art. We have also taken pains to identify common analytical errors; these should be relevant to novice and expert alike.

The substance and structure of the text follow the book's title: principles, practice, and potential. Before addressing the three Ps, however, we offer some introductory material in the first two chapters. Chapter 1 provides background on the nature, magnitude, and causes of the health care cost problem, concluding with a discussion of cost containment ideas and activities in both the public and private sectors. The chapter is intended to serve as a "primer" on medical economics. Chapter 2 introduces the reader to CBA-CEA, discussing the concept of cost-effective medical care, defining CBA and CEA, and presenting historical background on the application of these techniques to health care and nonhealth care problems. The chapter closes with some recent developments indicating the current intensity of interest in CBA-CEA in both health professional and policy circles.

Chapter 3, on principles, presents the methodology of CBA-CEA. Chapter 4, on practice, examines the health care CBA-CEA literature by presenting our empirical analysis of trends in the growth and character of the literature, identifying substantive topics of interest, reviewing publications that have conveyed principles and practice to the health care community, and assessing the quality of the literature. Chapter 5, on potential, evaluates the health policy uses and future usefulness of CBA-CEA. In this chapter we consider the spectrum of influences that CBA-CEA might have on health care resource allocation in general. We then explore the past uses and potential usefulness of analysis in the context of four categories of possible users: individual providers of care, institutional providers, organizations financing care, and organizations involved in monitoring or otherwise regulating the quality of care. The chapter closes with a discussion of general considerations, both technical and "environmental" (for example, political and economic), which define the potential usefulness of CBA-CEA. In the concluding chapter, Chapter 6, we summarize the main points related to principles, practice, and potential and offer some ideas on an agenda for research directed toward improving the state of the art in CBA-CEA and in the effectiveness with which it is applied to health policy problems.

The breadth of this book is considerable. Nevertheless, its substantive focus is narrow. Almost all of the CBA-CEA principles presented herein can be applied to a wide variety of social problems, such as education, criminal justice, and national defense. Unlike the principles, however, the application of analysis does not always generalize across substantive areas. Thus, our discussion of the practice of CBA-CEA in health care should not be construed as characterizing the application of CBA-CEA in general. Similarly, the policy potential of analysis is largely a function of a constellation of political and economic factors which vary from one organizational or professional setting to another. Consequently, the potential of CBA-CEA in health care policy can differ significantly from its potential in other areas. In particular, we note that both the practice and potential of CBA-CEA in nonmedical health areas—such as individual health behaviors and environmental pollution—differ from those we will explore. We concentrate on personal health care services because they are central to current health care policy and because we want to set boundaries to an already sizable topic.

Thus, our aim is not to create a new cohort of analysts. Rather, we hope to leave readers with a sufficient knowledge to discern the wheat in a study and discard the analytical chaff. As the health care cost-containment debate intensifies and diversifies, we hope that our efforts will help health care professionals to become effective, informed participants in the search for solutions.

This book grew out of work undertaken in support of a two-year study, entitled "The Implications of Cost-Effectiveness Analysis of Medical Technology," conducted by the Congressional Office of Technology Assessment (OTA). The review of literature and general exploration of the policy potential of CBA-CEA were initiated by Warner in his capacity as a consultant to OTA. Luce, then a senior analyst at OTA, was responsible for describing CBA-CEA methodology for the OTA report and for examining the uses and usefulness of analysis in health planning. Our written contributions to the OTA study constituted a first working draft of this book. Revisions since then have been extensive, both in terms of organization and content. However, this book's origins explain why we owe a debt of gratitude to all of the people connected with the OTA project, including OTA staff, members of the study's advisory panel, authors of case studies, and numerous expert reviewers of drafts of the OTA report. In revising our book, we have borrowed liberally from the general insights of all these people, as well as from specific reactions to drafts of the OTA report.

The assistance of two OTA analysts deserves special recognition. As project director for the OTA study, Clyde Behney read and criticized all of our early drafts and offered guidance and encouragement during and after the OTA study. On more than one occasion, he substituted his eloquence and wisdom for our dry, occasionally naive prose. The contributions of David Banta, Assistant Director of OTA, have been both direct, in reviewing our drafts, and indirect, reflecting several years of stimulating interaction with us on the subject of medical technology assessment.

Both Behney and Banta helped us fit our academic knowledge into a policymaking framework.

Early in our research, over two dozen health services researchers offered their comments on the value and limitations of CBA-CEA in a variety of policy contexts. As with the reviewers of the OTA drafts, their numbers preclude our listing them all here. Nevertheless, we extend our sincere appreciation for their thoughts and suggestions, many of which are incorporated in the text.

Later chapter drafts benefited from the suggestions of Paul Feldstein, Robert Grosse, Harold Luft, Richard Scheffler, and Jack Wheeler. James Bush devoted considerable effort to educating us about health status indexes.

Each of us owes his own special debt of gratitude: Warner's understanding of both the technical and philosophical issues in CBA-CEA has benefited immensely from working with Robert Grosse at The University of Michigan; Grosse is one of the pioneers in the application of cost analysis and CBA-CEA to health care problems. Luce owes much to the years of productive interaction he spent with Stuart Schweitzer and Shan Cretin of the UCLA School of Public Health.

A final group of important contributors to Warner's appreciation of CBA-CEA is the Public Health students he has had in the last nine years. Several of their insights, often corrections of Warner's errors generously conveyed as questions, have greatly expanded his perspective on the uses and meaning of analysis.

The technical aspects of our research and of producing the book were accomplished with the assistance of an unusually competent staff. Rebecca Hutton compiled the bibliography and assisted in categorizing the publications for our empirical analysis of the growth of the literature. The intelligence, imagination, and energy she devoted to these tasks are also reflected in her abstracts of dozens of CBA-CEA studies, many of which are included in Appendix D. Hillary Murt assisted in updating the bibliography and topics lists (Appendix C). Claire Brant and Laura Stephens combined secretarial and computer skills in using textedit to put the bibliography into the computer. Kerry Brittain Kempf and Virginia Cwalina edited the bibliography in its later stages. Blair Potter wielded a tough but effective pencil in editing the entire manuscript. Marjorie Blough typed the manuscript more times than she would care to remember, but each time combining cheerfulness with her extraordinary speed and accuracy.

Our families provided the kind of support that makes an undertaking like this one bearable. Further, by sharing her hands-on experience in health care administration, Warner's wife, Patricia, has provided him with a vivid, if vicarious, insight into the real world of health care resource allocation.

Much that is of value in this book we owe directly to the input of these individuals. We are grateful for all of their assistance.

Kenneth E. Warner
Bryan R. Luce

Costs of Health Care: Dollars and Sense

THE LITANY OF health care cost problems has become familiar to virtually everyone. As we entered the decade of the 1980s, health care expenditures in the United States exceeded $240 billion per year, or almost $1,100 for every man, woman, and child in the country (Freeland et al., 1980). The typical American must work more than a month each year simply to pay medical bills: the insurance premiums, taxes, and out-of-pocket costs that finance our personal health care system.

While the magnitude of health care costs may be the consumer's principal worry, health care policymakers and analysts regard with greater concern a second dimension of the problem—the rate of growth of costs. Expenditures have more than doubled in the last six years; they have quadrupled since the late 1960s. Even adjusting for general inflation, the growth in costs has been sufficient to boost health care expenditures from 7.6 percent to 9.5 percent of the gross national product (GNP)[1] in the last decade. If such differentials in the rates of GNP and health expenditure growth persist until the turn of the century, health expenditures will account for approximately 15 percent of the GNP.

A third dimension of the cost problem, at least as it is perceived in Washington, is the distribution of the burden between the private and public sectors. In the mid-1960s, government bore a quarter of that burden. Today, government's share is 40 percent. Thus, while the overall costs of care have been rising rapidly, government's obligations have accelerated even more rapidly. In an era of tight money in government, the implications of this largely nondiscretionary budgetary growth are obvious.

Concern about the high and rising costs of care has prompted a wide variety of cost-containment efforts among numerous, diverse groups in both the public and private sectors. Underlying these efforts is the search for an appropriate balance between the costs of care and the amount and quality of care. The challenge is to determine which medical interventions are effective, and under what circumstances, and then to compare their costs in order to assess their relative cost-effectiveness. The task is a monumental one—determining effectiveness is itself immensely difficult (U.S. Congress, Office of Technology Assessment, 1978a)—but explicitly or implicitly it is a goal of most of these groups and their programs.

With the desire to control inflation has come the need to identify, and to understand what is meant by, cost-effective medical interventions. Two closely related evaluative techniques, cost-benefit and cost-effectiveness analysis (CBA and CEA, respectively), are being used to meet this need. Interest in these techniques and in their findings has grown exponentially through the past decade, as measured by contributions to the professional health care literature. The perceived policy utility of CBA-CEA, both in health and in other areas, is reflected in the fact that more than sixty-five bills introduced in the 94th and 95th Congresses required various agencies to incorporate CBA, CEA, and related techniques into their formal decision-making procedures (U.S. Congress, Office of Technology Assessment, 1980a). A reading of both proposed legislation and the professional literature, combined with discussions at professional meetings, suggests, however, that the enthusiasm for CBA-CEA is matched by confusion about the procedures, meaning, and usefulness of these techniques.

In this chapter, we examine the health care cost problem, further exploring its empirical dimensions, explaining its causes, and identifying public and private sector efforts to grapple with it.

THE HEALTH CARE COST PROBLEM: NATURE AND CAUSES

QUANTITATIVE DIMENSIONS

Table 1.1 provides data indicating both the "stock" and the "flow" problems—that is, the magnitude and rate of growth—of health care costs. National expenditures on health care exceeded $200 billion in 1979 and equaled nearly $1,100 per person in 1980. Their

Table 1.1: National Expenditures on Health Care

Year	Total Expenditures ($ Billions)	Annual Increase (%)	Total Expenditures as Share of GNP (%)	Expenditures per Capita ($)
1950	12.7	—	4.5	81.86
1955	17.7	6.9	4.4	105.38
1960	26.9	8.7	5.3	146.30
1965	43.0	9.8	6.2	217.42
1966	47.3	10.0	6.3	236.51
1967	52.7	11.4	6.6	260.35
1968	58.9	11.8	6.8	288.17
1969	66.2	12.4	7.1	320.70
1970	74.7	12.8	7.6	358.63
1971	82.8	10.8	7.8	393.09
1972	92.7	12.0	7.9	436.47
1973	102.3	10.4	7.8	478.38
1974	115.6	13.0	8.2	535.99
1975	131.5	13.8	8.6	604.57
1976	148.9	13.2	8.8	678.79
1977	170.0	14.2	9.0	768.77
1978*	192.4	13.2	9.1	863.01
1979*	216.9	12.7	9.3	970.51
1980*	244.6	12.8	9.5	1,078.00

Sources: U.S. Department of Health, Education, and Welfare, 1980, table 64; Freeland et al., 1980.
*Estimates.

9.5 percent share of the GNP means that, out of every $10 of goods and services, $.95 is devoted to medical care.

The rapid rate of growth can be seen in the annual percentage increase in expenditures and the increasing share of the GNP allocated to health care. The latter serves as a more significant index of the cost inflation problem because general price inflation accounts for much of the annual increases in expenditures. In particular, note that the health expenditure share of the GNP has more than doubled over the last quarter of a century. Thus, compared to the $.95 out of each $10 we are now spending on health care, in 1955 we spent only $.44.

Table 1.2 illustrates the third health cost problem: the dramatic increase in the federal government's share of health care expenditures since the mid-1960s. Indeed, growth in the federal government's burden accounts for all of the relative shift in financing

Table 1.2:   Distribution of Personal Health Care
Expenditures by Source of Payment

	Public Sector (%)			Private Sector (%)
Year	Federal Government	State and Local Government	Total	
1950	10.4	12.0	22.4	77.6
1955	10.5	12.5	23.0	77.0
1960	9.3	12.5	21.8	78.2
1965	10.5	11.4	21.9	78.1
1970	22.3	12.1	34.4	65.6
1971	23.3	12.2	35.5	64.5
1972	23.7	12.3	36.0	64.0
1973	23.8	12.3	36.2	63.8
1974	25.6	12.6	38.2	61.8
1975	27.1	12.6	39.7	60.3
1976	27.6	11.6	39.2	60.8
1977	27.8	11.5	39.3	60.7
1978	28.0	11.8	39.9	60.1
1979	28.3	12.0	40.3	59.7

Source: U.S. Department of Health and Human Services, 1981, table 67.

from the private to the public sector. In the mid-1960s, the federal share of expenditures stood at 10.5 percent, actually slightly less than the share of state and local governments. Within a few years of the advent of Medicare and Medicaid, however, the federal portion more than doubled, while that of state and local governments did not change. From 1965 until the end of the 1970s, the total public sector share of the national health care bill nearly doubled, reaching 40 percent of the total; the federal share almost tripled, from a relatively insignificant 10 percent to well over a quarter of the national total. This translates into a budgetary obligation of more than $50 billion in 1979, up from less than $4 billion in 1965. Even adjusting for general inflation over the period, federal expenditures on personal health care were six times greater in 1979 than they were in pre-Medicare 1965.

CAUSES OF THE HEALTH CARE COST PROBLEM

While it is exceedingly difficult to disentangle the myriad causes of increasing health care costs and to determine their relative importance, principal causes can and should be identified. An appreciation of what these causes are and how they contribute to increasing health costs is the first step toward bringing the costs under control.

Although the notion of increasing costs has a universally negative connotation, not all cost growth is undesirable. Total health care costs result from the prices of medical goods and services and the quantities of goods and services consumed. Increases in either of these variables—price or quantity—can represent desirable phenomena. Rising prices can accompany improvements in the quality of the goods and services, while increasing quantities can reflect greater access to needed health care.

Use of the word "can" implies "might not," however. Clearly, much of the recent growth in health care prices and quantities does not reflect socially desirable developments; such growth is the appropriate target for cost-containment policies and the subject of most of the ensuing discussion. But first we should acknowledge the legitimate (that is, acceptable) sources of growth in health care costs. For example, to the extent that rising prices accompany new or improved services of at least comparable social value, the price increases should be welcomed. The price of treating childhood leukemia has risen markedly over the past three decades, but a diagnosis of acute leukemia need no longer spell death. Similarly, many adult victims of heart disease, stroke, advanced osteoarthritis, and other diseases can look forward to longer, higher quality lives thanks to technological improvements in diagnosis and therapy—improvements that have distinctly higher price tags.

Factors Affecting the Demand for Health Care

The demand for health care services has increased significantly and persistently over the last several decades. The reasons for increases in demand are numerous and varied. Two factors typically influence the demand for most goods and services. One is that demand rises as incomes rise. For many goods and services, including medical care, demand rises more rapidly than income, simply indicating that people choose to spend proportionately more of their additional income on such goods and services. Thus, as the U.S. population has grown richer over the years, it has chosen to devote proportionately more of its resources to the provision of health services. This historical phenomenon within our country has a parallel across countries at the present time: the percentage of a country's resources spent on personal health care tends to be greater in countries with higher GNPs per capita. This conventional demand factor accounts for much of the historic growth in the health care sector of the United States. In the most recent years, however, its explanatory value is limited, since real personal income has not been rising.

The other factor typically increasing demand is that, when consumers perceive that the quality of a product has improved, they want more of it. While the quality of much of health care clearly has improved significantly over the years, it is the consumers' perception, rather than actual improvement, which defines demand.

A third factor in rising demand for health care reflects the changing demographics of the U.S. population: we are aging. In 1950, 8 percent of Americans were 65 years of age or older. Today, that figure has grown to 11 percent, and it is projected to exceed 12 percent by the turn of the century. The elderly consume more health services, and hence incur more costs, than other age groups. For example, in 1977, per capita personal health care expenditures for the elderly totaled $1,745, or 3.4 times as much as the $514 per capita attributable to the nonelderly population. Thus, while the elderly constitute a relatively small proportion of the population, they account for nearly 30 percent of total national expenditures on personal health services. As the population continues to age, the growing proportion of elderly will exert additional pressure on health care expenditures. Clearly, however, this source of health cost growth should not necessarily be viewed negatively, since it often affords the elderly an opportunity to live longer, fuller lives.

The Role of Insurance

Probably the principal factor in the growth of demand for medical care services has been the increased breadth and depth of health insurance in both the public and private sectors. Larger proportions of the population have become covered by health insurance, and the insurance packages are covering more and more services. Public programs, principally Medicare and Medicaid, have added demand directly and intentionally. The growth in private insurance has added demand indirectly by divorcing much of the consumption of resources from direct financial liability; that is, it has channeled payment through third-party payers (insurers) and spread the costs of care among a large number of purchasers of the insurance. Unlike the preceding influences on growth of demand, which are common to many goods and services, the extent of the reduction in direct payment for health care services is unique to the medical care marketplace.

The direct and intentional growth of demand brought about by Medicare and Medicaid resulted from the perception that there was a financial barrier between significant segments of our population and the health care services they needed. The explicit purpose of these social programs was to remove that barrier. Thus some of the quantity component of increased public sector costs for health services represents a desired outcome. Although the financial barrier to access has not been completely eliminated, it has been reduced sufficiently to have significantly increased access to care for many of the poor and elderly. Indeed, the poorest segment of the population now accounts for more physician visits per year than the most affluent.[2] This subsidized increase in the demand for care accounts for much of the government's fiscal burden in health services. In the first decade following introduction of the social insurance programs, government's medical care expenditures for the elderly rose from $3 billion to over $18 billion, while its expenditures for the nonelderly poor increased from $2 billion to $16 billion.

While much of Medicare- and Medicaid-induced demand has been desirable, these programs have shared with private health insurance a tendency to increase demand to the point where total costs of services exceed perceived benefits. Insured consumers compare the benefits of services with the out-of-pocket costs they will incur directly, whereas the true costs of the services are the out-of-pocket charges *plus* charges covered by insurance. In effect, the insured consumers' understandable failure to consider insured costs results in demand for services for which total social costs exceed the benefit received. Patients stay in hospitals longer than the social cost-benefit calculus would recommend, physicians order more laboratory tests and X-rays, and so on. As a consequence, health care prices and costs are pushed unnecessarily high.

Theory. We will explore some of the dimensions of such socially excessive demand more fully below. First, however, the theoretical basis for the phenomenon will be explained using some elementary economic analysis. Figure 1.1 presents a simplified characterization of a medical care marketplace. In this case, we will call it the market for physician visits. S, indicating supply, shows how many visits physicians will supply at each of several fees or prices per visit. D, demand, indicates the number of visits consumers desire at each of the prices. S and D exhibit standard supply and demand relationships: suppliers (physicians) will offer more services if they can get a higher price—hence the positive slope of S—while con-

Figure 1.1:   Hypothetical Market for Physician Visits

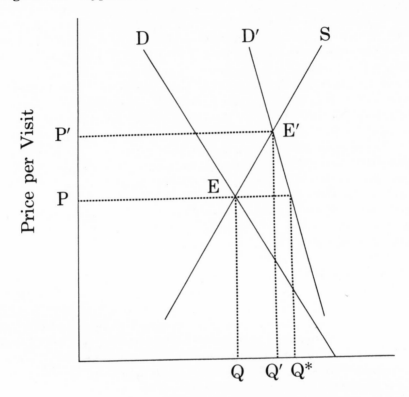

sumers (patients) will demand more services at lower prices—hence the negative slope of *D*. Point *E*, equilibrium, represents the only market price at which suppliers and demanders want the same number of services. At a higher price than *P*, suppliers would find consumers unwilling to purchase all of the units of service they offered to the market. The suppliers would be forced to reduce their prices, which would decrease the number of services they wanted to provide but increase the number consumers wanted to purchase. The price reduction process would continue until price reached *P*, at which point consumers would demand precisely the number of services suppliers wished to provide (*Q*). Similarly, at a price less than *P*, consumers would demand many more units of service than suppliers would be willing to provide. Hence consumers would bid against each other for the inadequate supply of services. This bidding would drive the price up, causing some consumers to drop out of the market and some suppliers to offer more services. This price (and hence supply and demand) movement would persist until price reached P, at which point all demand would be precisely satisfied (Q).

Suppose that S, D, and E represented the situation in 1965, the year before the introduction of Medicare and Medicaid. Implementation of these social programs had the effect of increasing demand. That is, at every physician visit price, the number of visits demanded was greater than before, reflecting the addition of subsidized Medicare and Medicaid demand. The locus of new price-quantity points—the new demand curve—represents a shift to the right, to D'. Thus at the old equilibrium price, P, consumers would now desire Q^* visits; but physicians have not changed the number of visits they wish to provide (Q). At P, the addition of Medicare-Medicaid demand has created excess demand. As before, consumers must bid against each other for the inadequate supply of services. The price is bid up, some consumers drop out of the market, and the higher price induces physicians to offer more services. As price rises, excess demand diminishes. The new equilibrium is attained at point E'. The equilibrium fee for a visit has risen from P to P', and the number of visits has increased from Q to Q'. (Note that Q' is lower than the number of visits the now-increased number of consumers would have liked to have had at the old equilibrium price, P.)

The relative amounts of price and quantity change are measures of the responsiveness to price changes of the quantity supplied or demanded. The price elasticity of demand (or supply) is defined as the percentage change in quantity demanded (supplied) that is induced by a 1 percent change in market price. Demand (supply) is called elastic (responsive) if the quantity demanded (supplied) changes by more than 1 percent in response to a 1 percent change in price. If quantity changes by less than 1 percent, demand (supply) is called inelastic. In Figure 1.1, if supply were less elastic than S—that is, if physicians' supply of visits were less responsive to price changes and therefore S were steeper—an increase in demand would drive price up still higher than P' and would fail to induce an increase in the number of visits equal to Q'. In the extreme, if physicians intended to provide only a fixed number of visits (say, Q), regardless of price, the supply curve would be vertical (perfectly inelastic) and all demand subsidization would simply drive up the fee for a visit. No increase in the quantity of services consumed would be realized, although different people might now be consuming the fixed quantity (for example, with Medicare, the elderly might have captured a larger share of the available physician visits). This would be the most inflationary outcome in terms of price and the least desirable outcome in terms of policy. At the other extreme, a flat, or horizontal, supply curve (perfectly elastic) would translate increases in demand entirely into additional services. This noninflationary price outcome is the policy ideal. Reality lies somewhere in between.

Obviously, the above analysis is a gross oversimplification of the real medical care marketplace, but the basic phenomenon—the market's rationing mechanism—is applicable and the qualitative results are a reasonable characterization of the effects of adding demand to the market. That is, the introduction of Medicare and Medicaid produced the theoretically expected results: consumption of personal health services increased, and the price of those services also rose.

Empirical Dimensions of Insurance. The growth in the depth and breadth of private insurance is both cause and effect in increasing health care costs. The high and rising costs of care have induced many individuals and groups to seek greater protection. This has been accomplished by many uninsured individuals' acquiring coverage and by covered individuals' increasing their coverage. A few employee groups have achieved first-dollar coverage: their insurance programs pay all of their medical bills. Members of such groups experience virtually no out-of-pocket costs for the medical services they receive.

The increase in insurance coverage throughout the nation is shown in table 1.3. Private insurance coverage was virtually nonexistent before World War II. It grew rapidly during the 1950s, accounting for less than 10 percent of all personal health care expenditures in 1950 but over 20 percent by 1960. The share of private insurance has grown gradually but persistently since then. Note, however, the relationship between direct (out-of-pocket) payments and those covered by third parties under private insurance programs: in 1950, 88 percent of the costs of health care paid by private individuals were paid directly; in 1979 that amount had dropped to 54 percent.

The increase in third-party financial liability increases demand for care through a phenomenon known as "moral hazard"

Table 1.3: Distribution of Direct versus Third-Party Payment

| Year | Direct Payment (%) | Third-Party Payment (%) | | | | Direct Payment as Share of Total Private Payment* (%) |
		Private Health Insurance	Government	Philanthropy and Industry	Total	
1940	81.3	—	16.1	2.6	18.7	100.0
1950	65.5	9.1	22.4	2.9	34.5	87.8
1955	58.1	16.1	23.0	2.8	41.9	78.3
1960	54.9	21.1	21.8	2.3	45.1	72.2
1965	51.6	24.2	21.9	2.2	48.4	68.1
1970	40.0	24.1	34.4	1.6	60.0	62.4
1975	32.4	26.7	39.6	1.3	67.6	54.8
1979	31.8	26.7	40.2	1.3	68.2	54.4

Source: U.S. Department of Health and Human Services, 1981, table 67.
*Total Private Payment is the sum of Direct Payment and Private Health Insurance.

(Pauly, 1968). Demand increases because the financial burden of an insured service is no longer borne directly by consumers; it is paid by the third-party insurer, thereby diffusing the burden to thousands of policyholders. Thus, the direct (out-of-pocket) cost of the service to the insured—the cost influencing their demand for the service—is considerably less than the total cost of the service. In essence, the consumers' perception of the price of the service leads them to demand more services than they would demand were they bearing the full financial burden. Hence at every market price (fee-for-service), quantity demanded is greater than it would be in the absence of insurance. The effect of the insurance is similar to that depicted in figure 1.1: demand shifts from D to D'. As a consequence, the market price rises along with the quantity of services consumed. Thus a response to the rising costs of care—acquisition of insurance coverage—has contributed to the continuing escalation in health care costs. Again, the elasticities of supply and demand will determine the relative growth in price and quantity.

Social programs, primarily Medicare and Medicaid, have added directly to the demand for health care. Even in the absence of moral hazard, this added demand would have applied pressure to the prices of health care services. However, combining private and public sector insurance coverage, we find that the new demand has been added primarily through third-party liability. In 1940, over

$.80 of each health care dollar came directly out of consumers' pockets (see table 1.3). A decade later, the ratio of direct payment to third-party payment was 2 to 1. Now less than a third of each health care dollar is paid directly by the consumers of the services.

There is nothing inherently wrong with insurance. Clearly, the major social insurance programs have accomplished much of their intended goal: to remove the financial barrier between medical indigents and services. Even the nonindigent may benefit if they seek health-promoting care they avoided before having insurance. And certainly it seems desirable that everyone have a measure of insulation from the overwhelming costs of catastrophic illness. Nevertheless, the price of this desirable protection and expansion of opportunity is inflation of health care costs, the phenomenon reflecting consumption of more and more services at higher and higher prices.

Tax Policy and Insurance. Tax policy exacerbates the demand problem. The personal income tax subsidizes both the purchase of health insurance (taxpayers who itemize deductions can include half of premium payments up to $150) and the direct expenditures of those taxpayers with unusually large medical expenses (expenses in excess of 3 percent of adjusted gross income can also be itemized). More important, both employers and employee groups have tax incentives to use health insurance as a form of compensation: for the employee, employer-paid insurance premiums are not taxable as personal income; for both employer and employee, benefits like insurance do not enter the Social Security tax base. Thus from the perspective of an employee, a dollar of nonwage compensation buys a dollar's worth of insurance; after taxes, a dollar of wage income buys only, say, $.65 of insurance or other goods and services.[3] However the insurance market might equilibrate in the absence of these tax incentives, their existence assures more widespread, deeper insurance coverage—and with it, more moral hazard.[4]

Effects of Insurance on Hospital Care. To this point, the general demand-based explanation of health cost inflation has said little about specific components of cost increases. However, a moment's reflection on the nature of insurance coverage can suggest some: consumers first insure themselves against those occurrences that are infrequent, unpredictable, and very costly. For instance, whereas the majority of expenditures on physicians' services come directly out of consumers' pockets, almost all Americans have some form of hospitalization insurance coverage; over 90 percent of all hospital costs are paid by third parties. This has had two important effects: first, there appear to be excess hospitalization and excess use of ancillary services. Regarding the former, some patients are hospitalized for problems that could be taken care of less expensively—but at greater direct cost to them—in ambulatory care. Also, some patients may remain hospitalized longer than necessary for rest or for a sense of security. The important point is that the value of the bed rest or of the security probably would not be sufficient to induce the same patients to remain hospitalized if they had to pay the additional costs. Similarly, ancillary hospital services tend to be overutilized. For example, an X-ray or a laboratory test that would provide minimal additional information may be ordered since neither the physician nor the insured patient will have to bear the cost. In fact, not only is there no incentive not to use such services, there are actually financial incentives to use them, since guaranteed third-party reimbursement provides additional revenues to the hospital. From the physicians' and patients' points of view, the deciding variable is benefit, not cost. However, these costs mount up and are ultimately borne by society as a whole. As insurance coverage grows, one would expect the intensity of care—the inputs per case or day—to grow also.

The second effect, which has occurred partially as a result of the above, is that the costs of hospital care have escalated more rapidly than other components of health care costs. Table 1.4 shows that hospital expenditures have risen from 30 percent of total expenditures in 1950 to 40 percent at present. Table 1.5 demonstrates that, since 1950, the rate of growth of hospital expenditures has exceeded that of all other major expenditure categories, with the exception of nursing home care. Note, however, the reduction in this trend between 1975 and 1979.

Aggravating the volume and price effects of insurance is the technical reimbursement system itself. Initially, both private and public third-party payers simply reimbursed hospitals for charges. The inflationary potential of such a system is obvious. Over time, Medicare and state Medicaid programs, as well as Blue Cross and other private insurers, insisted on paying only "legitimate" costs. The obvious problems in establishing what constitutes legitimate costs have created a long-standing controversy and myriad associated accounting problems. To date, the basic reimbursement mechanisms have not proven very effective in constraining cost increases. Traditionally it has not been difficult, and indeed often

Table 1.4:   Distribution of National Health Care Expenditures

Expenditure Category	Percent of Total Expenditures					
	1950	1960	1965	1970	1975	1979
Hospital Care	30.4	33.8	33.1	37.1	39.5	40.2
Physician Services	21.7	21.1	20.2	19.1	18.9	19.1
Dentist Services	7.6	7.4	6.7	6.3	6.2	6.4
Nursing Home Care	1.5	2.0	4.9	6.3	7.6	8.4
Other Professional Services	3.1	3.2	2.5	2.1	2.0	2.2
Drugs and Drug Sundries	13.6	13.6	12.4	11.0	8.9	8.0
Eyeglasses and Appliances	3.9	2.9	2.9	2.6	2.3	2.1
Government Public Health Activities	2.9	1.5	1.9	1.9	2.4	2.9
Research	0.9	2.5	3.4	2.5	2.5	2.2
Construction	6.7	3.9	4.8	4.6	3.8	2.5
Other	7.7	8.1	7.2	6.5	5.9	6.0

Source: U.S. Department of Health and Human Services, 1981, table 68.

Table 1.5:   Average Annual Increase in National Health Care Expenditures

Expenditure Category	Increase (%)					
	1950-79	1950-60	1960-65	1965-70	1970-75	1975-79
Hospital Care	11.3	9.0	8.8	14.9	13.4	13.1
Physician Services	9.7	7.5	8.3	11.1	11.7	13.0
Dentist Services	9.6	7.5	7.3	11.1	11.6	13.4
Nursing Home Care	17.0	10.9	31.5	17.8	16.6	15.2
Other Professional Services	8.9	8.1	3.7	9.1	10.4	15.7
Drugs and Drug Sundries	8.2	7.8	7.3	9.5	7.6	9.5
Eyeglasses and Appliances	7.8	4.7	9.3	9.7	9.1	9.9
Government Public Health Activities	10.2	1.4	14.7	11.8	17.3	17.6
Research	13.5	18.9	16.9	5.5	11.4	9.3
Construction	6.5	2.2	13.8	11.4	8.1	1.0

Source: U.S. Department of Health and Human Services, 1981, table 69.

not necessary, to justify capital improvements, salary increases, or added staff. As we discuss later, however, several recent cost-containment efforts are aimed at challenging the legitimacy of many such expenditures, especially those for capital equipment and improvements.

While the majority of hospitals are classified as nonprofit, several objectives of hospital decision-makers pressure them to undertake cost-increasing, and hence revenue-increasing, activities. The goal of offering patients high quality medical care is shared by hospital boards, administrators, and medical staff. The acquisition and maintenance of modern, sophisticated plant and facilities are commonly viewed as essential in competing with other hospitals for physicians, and hence patients. Such endeavors are inevitably accompanied by substantial price tags. The predominant reimbursement mechanisms make such expenses recoverable.

All of the above combine to produce the notion that we overutilize hospitals. Experience with health maintenance organizations (HMOs), which provide comprehensive care on a prepayment basis, provides empirical evidence to support the notion. With HMOs, there is no "insurance difference" between ambulatory and inpatient care: enrollees are insured fully against all costs by virtue of their membership premiums. Furthermore, there is no fee charged for each service provided, so neither the hospital nor the physician has a financial incentive to induce overutilization of services. On the contrary, the incentive is to conserve resources, to use only those services that are necessary and "worth the cost." In this setting, hospitalization rates tend to be substantially lower— often 50 percent lower—than those in the predominant fee-for-service setting. Rates of ambulatory care services are higher. Total costs of HMO care run 10 to 40 percent below those of fee-for-service care. While some detractors have argued that the quality of HMO care is inferior, the limited evidence available on patient types and health outcomes does not support this argument (Luft, 1980).

Several years ago, Martin Feldstein developed data that provide a perspective on the profundity of changes in the financing of hospital care. Between 1950 and 1968, average cost per patient day, adjusted for general inflation, rose a dramatic 172 percent, from $18.64 to $50.64 (in 1957–59 dollars). However, given the rapid growth in private and public insurance, direct consumer expenditures actually *fell* by 16 percent, from $9.06 to $7.60. As Feldstein said, "This means that, because of the growth of third-party payments, the 'average' patient at the time of his illness had to forego less of other goods and services in 1968 to buy a day of hospital care than he did in 1950. It is not surprising that patients' demands for more and better hospital services have increased," since the direct costs are those which "influence patients' demands for hospital care at the time that they decide to purchase." Furthermore, Feldstein observed that the growth in real wages over the period meant that workers had to work fewer hours in 1968 than in 1950 to pay those direct costs of a day of care (Feldstein, 1971*b*, p. 15).

Insuring hospital care also increases the intensity of care—

that is, the number of services provided per patient day of care. A growing body of evidence indicates that increasing intensity is serving more to inflate the costs of care than to increase the quality of care. Scitovsky and McCall (1976) studied the inputs used, and the costs associated with them, in treating several common ailments in 1951, 1964, and 1971. Overall, they found significant increases in intensity, particularly in diagnostic testing, for conditions whose prognosis had not changed fundamentally. For example, the authors found that the number of laboratory tests run per case of perforated appendix had risen from 5.3 in 1951 to 31.0 in 1971, with total costs of treating the illness rising from $516 to $2,062. Controlling for general inflation, this represented a 156 percent increase in the cost of treatment.

Other analysts also have found rapidly escalating use of diagnostic tests. Fineberg (1979) observed that in the first half of the 1970s, the number of laboratory tests increased at an annual rate of over 14 percent. In 1977, some 5 billion tests, individually inexpensive, accounted for approximately $11 billion in expenditures. Clinical chemistries alone totaled about $3 billion that year. Redisch (1974) believes that "explosive growth" in a handful of physician-controlled services[5] accounted for 40 percent of the increase in hospital operating costs in the early Medicare period of 1968 through 1971. Supporting the hypothesis that many of these tests may be of marginal value, several analysts have documented significant variability in diagnostic test utilization among physicians treating homogeneous patient populations. For example, Schroeder et al. (1973) found a seventeenfold variation in laboratory use among internists dealing with a clinic population.

The aggregate importance of the intensity factor is indicated in table 1.6, in which proportionate responsibility for recent years' health expenditure growth is assigned to prices, population, and intensity. Clearly, price increases have been the dominant influence in the growth of health costs over the last decade. Increases in the size, and changes in the composition, of the population explain 7 percent of the growth. From a quarter to a third of increases in health costs are attributable to increasing intensity. Thus, while intensity is not the principal cause of health expenditure growth, it is clearly a significant one.

Along with the less expensive diagnostic tests, increasing intensity includes the use of expensive, capital-embodied technologies. Several of these have captured the public's (and the profession's) fancy in recent years—the CT (computerized tomo-

Table 1.6:   Source of Growth in Personal Health Care Expenditures

| Year | Source of Growth (%) | | | Total (%) |
	Prices	Population	Intensity	
1970	54	8	38	100
1971	65	11	24	100
1972	42	8	50	100
1973	43	7	50	100
1974	71	6	23	100
1975	80	5	15	100
1976	71	7	22	100
1977	68	7	25	100
1978	68	7	25	100
Total 1969–78	63	7	30	100

Source: U.S. Department of Health, Education, and Welfare, 1980, table 65.

graphy) scanner being the most notable example from the 1970s. In some analysts' minds, these technologies are the villain in the health cost drama (Altman and Blendon, 1979). Policy attention has focused on the capital costs of such technologies (relevant cost-containment efforts are discussed below), but the weight of the evidence suggests that these costs are not as significant as many have feared (Maloney and Rogers, 1979; Warner, 1979a). One case study of hospitals in the Boston area found that acquisition of expensive technologies accounted for less than 10 percent of hospital cost growth. The authors of the study noted that, although equipment expenditures had been rising rapidly and thus might become a more significant contributor to cost inflation in the future, at present, if such equipment does contribute significantly to cost inflation, it must be because of the additional labor and supplies needed to monitor and operate it (Cromwell et al., 1975). It certainly has not been established that such technology invariably contributes significantly to inflation. In the case of the CT scanner, much maligned in the mid-1970s, recent thinking suggests that scanning can be a highly cost-effective diagnostic tool, replacing expensive, invasive diagnostic procedures. The degree to which such potential is realized is a function of the appropriateness of use, itself a function of reimbursement practices. Thus, it seems probable that numerous scans are performed, at a charge of $150 to $250 each, with only very limited expectation of useful findings. The procedure's noninvasiveness may encourage this, along with the patient's protection from financial liability. In addition, reimbursement practices serve to recover the initial capital investment more quickly as the number of services provided increases.

In summary, all technologies—big and small, sophisticated and simple, expensive and cheap—are candidates for excessive use in an environment in which consumption decision-making and financial liability are divorced.

> [A]s third-party payment has increased over the years, the benefit required to justify a [technology use] decision in the eyes of doctors and patients has declined. This has led to increased use of resources in all sorts of ways—including the introduction of technologies that otherwise might not have been adopted at all and, more often, the more rapid and extensive diffusion of technologies that had already been adopted to some extent (Russell, 1977, p. 3).

This need not imply sinister or selfish motivation on the part of anyone. To be sure, in some instances providers stand to profit by additional, possibly unnecessary utilization of services, but excess use is also observed in settings devoid of a direct profit motive, such as when providers are salaried. This behavior is often wholly rational and consistent with the economic environment: if the patient will not bear the financial burden of resource consumption, the physician, looking after the patient's best interests, is correct in providing all services that may benefit the patient, regardless of their cost. "In short, when those making the decisions pay none of the cost, resources are used as though they cost nothing" (Russell, 1976, p. 3). The fault lies in the incentive system, not in providers' responses to it.

Health Care Price Inflation

Whereas table 1.6 depicted the dominant role of price inflation in health cost growth, table 1.7 is included to help explain the parameters of health care price inflation. In part, of course, health care price increases simply reflect general inflation. But as the data show, health prices have risen consistently more rapidly than the general rate of inflation, and even more rapidly than the prices of other services (which have increased faster than the prices of goods). From 1950 to 1979, medical prices more than quadrupled, while the general price level tripled.

In theory, the consumer price index (CPI) reflects the cost of constant-quality goods and services. In practice, particularly for components like medical care, quality changes often are hard to

Table 1.7:   Average Annual Change in the Consumer Price
Index and Some of Its Medical Care Components

Period	All Items (%)	All Services (%)	All Medical Care (%)	Semiprivate Hospital Room (%)	Physician Fees (%)	Prescriptions (%)
1950–55	2.2	3.8	3.8	6.9	3.4	1.9
1955–60	2.0	3.3	4.1	6.3	3.3	2.6
1960–65	1.3	2.0	2.5	5.8	2.8	-2.4
1965–70	4.2	5.7	6.1	13.9	6.6	-0.2
1970–75	6.7	6.5	6.9	10.2	6.9	1.6
1975–78	6.6	8.2	9.2	12.0	9.6	6.5
1978–79	11.5	11.2	9.4	11.0	9.2	7.9

Source: U.S. Department of Health and Human Services, 1981, table 64.

detect and, if detected, to account for. Some of the medical care price rise undoubtedly reflects improvements in the quality of medical goods and services. To the extent that this is true, the medical care component of the CPI overstates pure price inflation. Nevertheless, it is certain that substantial price inflation has occurred.

Medicine is labor-intensive, although growth of sophisticated technology and other nonlabor inputs has been reducing that intensity somewhat. In the general economy, the cost of labor has been rising more rapidly than the cost of other inputs. For several years, health care prices were affected further by a wage catch-up phenomenon, in which relatively underpaid hospital workers experienced wage growth in excess of that of similar, nonhospital employees (Fuchs, 1976). Much of this growth has been related to the unionization of nurses and allied health workers.

Table 1.8 breaks hospital inpatient expenses into payroll and nonpayroll. The data show the dominance of wage costs over nonwage costs, although the proportion of total costs attributable to payroll has been declining steadily. Table 1.9 lends additional insight into the components of hospital cost growth. It shows that increased wage rates have paced the price side of the cost equation (cost equals prices times quantities), while nonlabor inputs have consistently risen more rapidly than the number of employees.

Although the costs of hospital care have grown rapidly and have increased their position of preeminence in the health-cost hierarchy (table 1.4), nursing home care has experienced the most rapid cost growth of any of the components of the health care system. Since 1950, expenditures on nursing home care have increased 17 percent a year, one and a half times as rapidly as

Table 1.8: Hospital Payroll and Nonpayroll Expenses per Inpatient Day

Year and Period	Payroll*	Nonpayroll	Total	Payroll Costs as Share of Total (%)
	Adjusted Expenses per Inpatient Day ($)			
1971	53.10	30.33	83.43	63.6
1972	59.24	35.37	94.61	62.6
1973	62.86	38.92	101.78	61.8
1974	68.76	44.45	113.21	60.7
1975	79.00	54.08	133.08	59.4
1976	88.08	64.16	152.24	57.9
1977	99.63	73.62	173.25	57.5
1978	110.82	82.99	193.81	57.2
	Average Annual Change (%)			
1971–72	11.6	16.6	13.4	—
1972–73	6.1	10.0	7.6	—
1973–74	9.4	14.2	11.2	—
1974–75	14.9	21.7	17.6	—
1975–76	11.5	18.6	14.4	—
1976–77	13.1	14.7	13.8	—
1977–78	11.2	12.7	11.9	—
Total, 1971–78	11.1	15.5	12.8	—

Source: U.S. Department of Health and Human Services, 1981, table 70.
*Includes employee benefits.

Table 1.9: Average Annual Increases in Average Hospital Expenses per Patient Day, According to Contributing Factors

Period	Price Increases (%)			Quantity Increases (%)			Total Increases (%)
	Wages	Nonlabor	Total	Employees	Nonlabor	Total	
1960–65	4.8	1.3	3.5	1.7	5.8	3.2	6.7
1965–68	6.6	3.4	5.3	3.4	9.8	5.9	11.2
1968–71	10.1	5.4	8.2	3.3	10.2	6.1	14.3
1971–74	7.0	7.0	7.1	2.0	6.6	3.7	10.7
1974–76	10.6	7.8	9.5	2.5	12.4	6.5	16.0
1976–78	8.9	7.2	8.2	3.3	6.4	4.6	12.8

Source: U.S. Department of Health and Human Services, 1981, table 71.

hospital costs (see table 1.5). As a result, nursing home expenditures have grown from a relatively inconsequential 1.5 percent of national health care expenditures in 1950 to 8.4 percent in 1979 (see table 1.4). Clearly, social insurance coverage has played a major role in this growth. Once again we see the positive and negative sides of social insurance programs: access to needed services is greatly enhanced, but so are costs.[6]

Factors Affecting the Supply of Health Care

No discussion of health care costs can ignore the supply side. For years it was assumed that the restriction of the supply of physicians through various professional and legal mechanisms (such as licensure and the limited number of slots in medical schools and residencies) served to inflate professional fees and restrict the availability of services (Friedman, 1962). This would be the effect of supply restriction in a conventional market, as illustrated in figure 1.2. Free enterprise supply (S) and demand (D) would produce market equilibration at point E, implying price (fee) P and quantity of services Q. Artificial restriction of supply would push S back to S'. Market equilibrium would move up the demand curve to point E', where the market-clearing price, P', would be higher and the quantity of services consumed, Q', lower than those that would obtain in a free market.[7] Conversely, should supply be increased, represented by the shift in the supply curve to S'', the conventional workings of the marketplace would lead to more services being consumed (Q'') at a lower price (P'').

The logic of this argument is sound, and in an earlier era, when patients paid most of their health care bills directly, reality may well have mirrored the theory. Recent experience, however, suggests that this classic supply-demand relationship may no longer hold for physicians' services. For instance, since the mid-1960s there has been a deliberate federal government policy to increase the number of physicians in this country. Table 1.10 shows how successful this program has been to date and how it is expected to affect the future supply of physicians. Notice that, not only has the number of physicians risen dramatically, the physician-to-population ratio has also increased steadily. However, as the supply of physicians has increased, fees have not dropped, as the simple theory would have predicted. On the contrary, physician fees have escalated: since 1960, the physician fee index in the medical care component of the CPI has consistently outpaced growth in the

Figure 1.2: The Effect of Restricting Supply in a Conventional
            Market

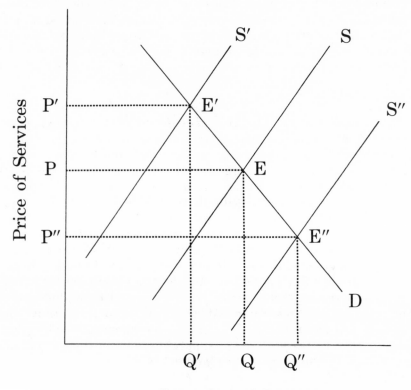

Quantity of Services

overall CPI and in the services-only share of the CPI (see table 1.7).
Indeed, there is reason to suspect that average *effective* physician
fees have risen even more rapidly than the physician fee index
indicates. This is demonstrated in figure 1.3. The top line traces the
growth in what physicians have identified as their usual and
customary fees; this is what the CPI physician fee index measures.
Years ago, however, the absence of public funding of medical
services made charity care far more common than it is today.
Physicians offered services to medical indigents at fees below what
was usual and customary; in some cases, services were provided
free of charge. Since the mid-1960s, however, the need for charity
care has diminished substantially. Physicians charge almost all of
their patients the full usual and customary fee. Consequently, the

Table 1.10:   Professionally Active
Physicians (M.D.'s and D.O.'s) in the
United States and Outlying U.S. Areas

Year*	Physicians (No.)	Professionally Active Physicians per 10,000 Population (No.)
1950	219,900	14.2
1960	259,500	14.2
1970	323,200	15.5
1971	334,100	15.9
1972	345,000	16.3
1973	350,100	16.4
1974	362,500	16.8
1975	378,600	17.4
1976	390,600	17.9
1977	395,200	17.9
1978	419,520	18.8
1979	433,600	19.3
1980	444,000	19.7
1985	519,000	21.9
1990	594,000	23.9

Source: U.S. Department of Health and Human Services,
1981, table 47.
*Figures for 1950 to 1979 are estimates; 1980–90 are
projections.

gap between the usual and customary fee and the average actual
fee has diminished. Growth in the latter is depicted in the lower
line. As its greater slope suggests, actual average fees have increased more rapidly than usual and customary fees, the basis of
the CPI measure.

Of course, this increase in supply has not been occurring in a
vacuum. As we emphasized above, during this same period demand
for physicians' services also increased substantially. Consequently, theory would describe a tug-of-war, in which increasing demand
is pulling price up while increasing supply is pulling it down. Since
price has risen steadily, it would appear that the demand forces are
stronger than the supply forces. But the economics of health care
does not always conform to theory. For one thing, the pervasiveness of third-party payment has shifted the demand curve.
Demand as suppliers see it (at full price) deviates from demand as
consumers see it (price as out-of-pocket cost only). Furthermore,

Figure 1.3: Growth in Usual and Customary and in Average
Actual Physician Fees

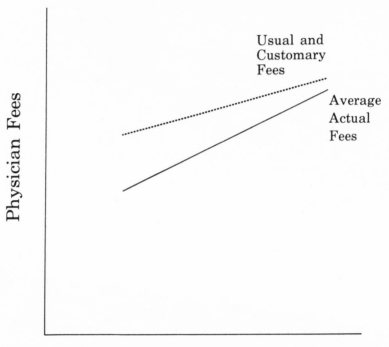

increases in physician fees in the face of growing supply have led to
the notion that physicians can create some of the demand for their
services, a reasonable idea to the layperson—after all, physicians
possess the relevant expertise and generally define case management. But the notion of suppliers creating their own demand runs
contrary to the logic of conventional market economists. Many
health economists, however, find the idea plausible, and both
theoretical and empirical research, particularly regarding the demand for surgery, is beginning to lend credibility to it (Fuchs, 1978;
Green, 1978; Sweeney, 1980). Indeed, the idea of the supplier
creating demand has contributed to a prominent health economist's characterization of every additional physician as representing a claim on hundreds of thousands of dollars of society's
resources (Reinhardt, 1975).

The significance of the supply-creating-demand theory is
heightened when one contemplates past federal policies to increase

the availability of institutional care. Beginning in 1946, when the Hill-Burton Act was passed, federal monies fueled a 30-year hospital modernization and bed expansion program that more than doubled the nation's hospital beds and that increased the bed-to-population ratio from 3.2 per thousand in 1940 to 4.6 per thousand in 1977. Likewise, due largely to the demand-stimulating effect of Medicare and Medicaid, the number of nursing home beds increased from fewer than 570,000 in 1963 to 1.4 million in 1977. Adding to this growing supply of beds has been an ambitious Veterans Administration (VA) program, which has increased both short-term and long-term beds for veterans.

The notion of physicians creating demand is not without conceptual flaws. If physicians can create demand, what stops them from creating still more demand and hence increasing their incomes by even greater amounts? Similarly, if they can set their own fees, what keeps them from raising them still higher? A number of responses can be posited, though none without reservation. Several responses relate to the target income hypothesis, which suggests that physicians have a level of income that they feel is appropriate. They will juggle the quantity of services provided and fees charged to achieve their target incomes. Thus, in the absence of the ability to actually create demand—for example, in an area having an excess of surgeons—physicians will raise their fees to compensate for the reduced per-surgeon workload. If physicians can create demand, they will perform in the aggregate more surgical procedures.

Factors constraining the escalation of fees, demand, or both could include "objective" limits—for example, a patient might tolerate two computerized tomography (CT) scans in a given week but balk at a third—and "subjective" limits—an unwillingness on the part of physicians to deviate more than a certain amount from what they perceive to be optimal medical care. That is, in exchange for increased income, they may tolerate some psychological discomfort associated with providing what they view to be unnecessary services; but beyond some quantity of such services, the discomfort will weigh more heavily than the value to them of the additional income. Restriction of fee escalation undoubtedly reflects some market forces, as well as regulatory constraints; it might also represent a collective professional consciousness that, if health care costs climb too rapidly, the amount of governmental intervention into the medical care marketplace could be greatly increased.

Concern about governmental intervention may motivate a lot

of professional behavior that is difficult to explain otherwise. An analysis of the political economy of professionalism allows for collective behavior oriented toward the long-term economic interests of members, but with spokespersons generally couching positions in terms of protecting the public's interest (P. Feldstein, 1977). For example, the threat in the late 1970s of federal legislation to contain hospital costs led various elements of the health care industry to band together to mount a Voluntary Effort to control hospital costs. Presented as the industry's demonstrating leadership in attacking a social problem, the Voluntary Effort was clearly motivated directly by the fear of specific federal legislation and indirectly by concern about further governmental incursions into the industry's territory.

CONCLUSION

A note on the aggregate statistics of health care economics in the last few years seems an appropriate way to close this discussion of health cost inflation. Growth in both hospital and total health care costs in the late 1970s and into 1980 was held to approximately the general rate of inflation, thus stalling the seemingly inexorable tightening of the health sector's grip on the economy's resources. The directors of the Voluntary Effort were quick to claim credit for this relative restraint, though in fairness to a wide variety of related actors and activities (discussed in the next section), it is difficult to apportion credit. The optimistic view of this short-term success was that it represented the dawning of an era of awareness of the economic and political scarcity of health care resources. In this view, the concerted efforts of a variety of health care professionals, plus a general heightened sensitivity among practitioners to the need for cost containment, would combine to moderate health cost growth in the future. The cynical view was that the success was purely short-term, the industry's pragmatic response to the "clear and present danger" of increased governmental presence in health care. As cost containment faded from the political agenda, the pessimists argued, the vigor of the Voluntary Effort would dissipate and cost inflation would reemerge with renewed intensity. Unfortunately, preliminary data for 1981 support the pessimistic view. Health cost growth exceeded general inflation in 1981 by one of the largest amounts ever.

   Even if private sector desire to contain costs remains alive, the difficulty of doing so may increase. One can argue that recent success was easy, because years of relatively unconstrained budgets have padded the health system with fat. Cost containment circa 1980 simply involved trimming some of that fat. Containing inflation in the long run will become increasingly more difficult as the cost containment scalpel approaches the lean of health services. Of particular importance is the economic environment of the delivery of personal health care services. The incentives in the predominant system of reimbursement are antithetical to cost containment. Barring significant changes in this basic economic environment, the guardians of the public's health care dollars will find these incentives a formidable and persistent opponent.[8]

COST-CONTAINMENT IDEAS AND ACTIVITIES

The health care cost problem derives in part from both public and private sector efforts to address inequities in the availability and cost of care. Success in these endeavors has gone a long way toward solving one social problem—barriers to access to care—but in the process has contributed to the social cost problem. The gains in access to health care made in the last fifteen years should be inviolable, at least to a significant degree. Thus we seek to reverse the inflationary impact of increasing demand without infringing on access to care. The magnitude of the health care cost problem and the government's response to it have engendered a wide and evolving variety of proposals and programs to contain the costs of care. Cost containment is perhaps the central focus of today's federal and state health policymakers. It is also a significant concern of numerous groups in the private sector, ranging from the providers of care—physicians and other health professionals, hospitals, HMOs, and so on—to those who pay the bills—consumers and third-party payers.

It is useful here to determine what importance the assessment of the cost-effectiveness of medical technologies and procedures may have for efforts at containing costs. While we defer defining cost-effectiveness until the next chapter, it should become clear that the majority of ongoing cost-containment efforts emphasize the attainment of economic efficiency in the use of individual technologies and procedures, a striving toward "value for money," the avoidance of unnecessary use of resources, and the realization of desired medical outcomes at reasonable cost.

Most cost-containment efforts fall into the piecemeal, or incremental, category, which emphasizes individual inefficiencies in medical care delivery. At the heart of this approach is the preservation of the basic elements of the health care delivery system as it now stands. Thus, the incremental approach is in direct contrast to systemic efforts to solve the cost problem. The systemic approach— for example, fundamentally revising the reimbursement mechanism—views one or more of the basic elements of the current health care system as the source of the cost problem. By definition, this approach represents a more radical deviation from the status quo delivery system, as it entails a direct assault on the perceived institutional source of the problem. It is our belief, or perhaps bias, that a systemic approach would have a much higher probability of containing health care costs. At the same time, however, a major variation from the status quo might impose other costs on society, whereas significant costs resulting from disruption seem unlikely from the incremental approaches.

In the remaining pages of this chapter we chronicle the major cost-containment efforts since the mid-1960s. Early efforts generally fell into the incremental category. The limited success of these efforts has turned attention in recent years toward more systemic changes. We have organized our presentation by the locus of the efforts: the public sector (state and federal governments) and the private sector.[9]

PUBLIC SECTOR

The federal government's prominence in the cost-containment arena is a reflection of the magnitude of its involvement in health care, both as a major purchaser of health care services and as a major factor in the evolution of the system in which the cost inflation problem has arisen. Among the federal policies that have contributed to the cost problem are a national hospital expansion program, dating from 1946; a national program to increase the supply of physicians and other health professionals, since the mid-1960s; a national program to finance health care for the needy, since 1965; and a tax-incentive program to subsidize private health insurance. It is interesting to note that the original Medicare law insisted that the law not be used to interfere with the existing organizational practice of medicine. Nevertheless, because it was clear from the beginning that increasing costs would accompany the increasing demand, the original legislation did require hospitals to institute hospital utilization review programs for the federal beneficiaries.

The first attempts to "rationalize" the health system in the Medicare era were billed as voluntary programs, with the federal government supplying monies as a catalyst for health facilities and health programs to cooperate among themselves. The 1965 Regional Medical Program (RMP) amendments to the Social Security Act provided funds to coordinate research and health service delivery efforts to combat heart disease, cancer, and stroke. Although RMP was not intended as a cost-containment program, it represented an attempt to spend money more efficiently. The next year, however, Congress passed the Partnership for Health Act, which established a network of local and state Comprehensive Health Planning (CHP) agencies mandated to act as the catalyst to coordinate the health care system within a geographic area. Although the law was all carrot and no stick, and was not effective in containing costs, it established a base upon which future state and federal legislation has been built. For instance, throughout the late 1960s and early 1970s, increasing numbers of states passed certificate of need laws, which required hospitals to obtain planning agency approval before investing in new facilities or expensive technologies. The certificate-of-need process is clearly a tool designed to contain costs. Although early efforts were aimed at slowing the increase in beds, later efforts have concentrated on major capital equipment such as CT scanners. This has brought to the forefront the need for methodologies to balance the costs of a technology's acquisition with its potential benefits, and to do so in some sort of rational and generally acceptable manner. Since the certificate-of-need process applies individually to expensive technologies and facilities, it is a classic example of the piecemeal approach to cost containment.[10]

While the states were adding regulatory teeth to the weak federal planning legislation, many states were also retrenching on liberal Medicaid programs by decreasing benefits and increasing eligibility requirements. The federal government, too, tightened up Medicare reimbursement requirements in the 1968 and 1972 amendments. Included in the latter was legislation establishing and funding a network of local Professional Standards Review Organizations (PSROs), groups of physicians intended to "promote the effective, efficient, and economical delivery of health care services of proper quality for which payment may be made under the Act." Funded by the Department of Health and Human Services, PSROs were expected to establish local standards for institutionalized health care and to monitor the appropriateness of care received by federal beneficiaries. The PSRO program was billed primarily as a quality control effort, but most knowledgeable observers agree that the primary intent of the legislation, as well as the thrust of subsequent efforts, was cost containment. Analysis has suggested that PSRO efforts have reduced the number of Medicare hospital days by about 2 percent; but the value of this reduction, compared with the cost of achieving it, remains controversial. A recent analysis by the Health Care Financing Administration estimated that the monetary benefits of the program, regarding Medicare patients, exceeded costs by 10 percent. This savings amounted to less than 0.1 percent of relevant Medicare expenditures. Reanalysis of the data by the Congressional Budget Office concluded that program savings fell short of costs by 30 percent (U.S. Congress, Congressional Budget Office, 1979). Evaluation of effects on the quality of care is hindered by the general problems involved in measuring quality, as well as difficulties specific to the program. The debate on the relative merits of PSROs continues, but by all assessments undertaken to date, the program cannot be considered a major force promoting cost containment.

The first truly systemic approach to cost containment was embodied in the 1973 HMO Act, which provided federal monies to stimulate the growth of the HMO movement. It was believed that the incentives of a prepaid capitation system would not only provide more efficient health care to individual beneficiaries, but also effectively compete with the fee-for-service sector and thus help drive down the costs of the entire system. To enhance competition, the law required employers to offer federally qualified HMOs as an option to their employees. The ambitious objectives of this legislation went largely unrealized, partly because the law required such comprehensive services to qualify that many HMOs found themselves unable to compete with the traditional insurance system. Thus, it has been argued that the restrictive letter of the law defeated its spirit (Starr, 1976). A striking example of the restrictiveness is that Kaiser Permanente did not qualify under the original law's definition.

In 1974 Congress passed a major piece of legislation in the tradition of trying to contain health care costs through the regulatory—or incremental—approach: the National Health Planning and Resources Development Act. This legislation strengthened the planning process by replacing CHP agencies with a stronger network of Health Systems Agencies (HSAs), by calling for national health planning guidelines to be developed, and by requiring all states that received federal Medicaid monies to implement a certificate-of-need program. In addition to carrying out certificate-of-need review, HSAs were empowered to review existing facilities for appropriateness and to review and comment on the use of federal funds for specific health programs (for example, family planning clinics). The 1974 legislation gave regulatory muscle to a previously weak national planning system, but the accomplishments of the HSAs in containing costs and, more generally, in rationalizing the allocation of health care resources have been limited. We believe this is attributable partly to the piecemeal approach implicit in HSA activities and partly to the political complexity of the planning task.

In 1976 Congress passed the landmark Health Manpower Bill, which called for a halt to the increase in medical school enrollments. The law states that: "Congress finds and declares that there is no longer an insufficient number of physicians and surgeons in the United States and that there is no longer further need for affording preference to alien physicians and surgeons in admission to the United States." The law's intent, at least in part, was to contain costs, based on the premise that physicians can and do induce demand beyond some optimal level. The irony of attempting to contain costs by slowing the physician supply is that part of the original rationale given to increasing the number of physicians was to break the monopoly on supply which, it was claimed, organized medicine had used to keep physician incomes high. The 1976 law also called for increased numbers of physician assistants and nurse practitioners, an approach to cost containment envisioning a more efficient mix of health professionals through health manpower substitution.

The most recent legislative effort to contain costs through the incremental approach is the 1978 amendments establishing the National Center for Health Care Technology. The technology center was charged with coordinating federal health technology assessment activities and with advising the Health Care Financing Administration (HCFA) on Medicare reimbursement decisions for individual technologies. The linkage to HCFA created a mechanism whereby cost containment objectives could be sought.

Notwithstanding the 1976 manpower and 1978 technology legislation, most federal efforts since the 1974 HSA planning law have leaned toward a systemic approach to cost containment. A major, multipronged—but certainly not coordinated—thrust has been to increase competition in the health sector. First were amendments passed in 1976 and 1979 designed to strengthen the

1973 HMO Act by allowing more flexibility in coverage requirements. The intention was to make it easier for HMOs to qualify for federal funding and, therefore, to compete more effectively with the fee-for-service insurance industry. Furthermore, the 1979 HMO amendments barred HSAs from denying a certificate-of-need if an HMO could demonstrate that the investment was beneficial to its subscribers and that the investment was more efficient for the HMO than other investments. Such a provision is in direct and intentional conflict with the assumption that the health care system is inherently immune to traditional market forces.

Second, there have been even more explicit attempts to stimulate competitive forces. For instance, the same 1979 amendments required HSAs to strengthen "competitive forces in the health services industry whenever competition and consumer choice can constructively serve ... to advance the purposes of quality assurance, cost-effectiveness, and access." In addition, the Federal Trade Commission (FTC) has been increasingly active in combating anticompetitive industry practices; for example, it has worked to prevent professional societies from barring advertising by their members. The FTC has brought suit against the Michigan State Medical Society, which allegedly has interfered with Blue Cross-Blue Shield cost-containment efforts, and against the American Medical Association for antitrust violations. In addition, the FTC has investigated state medical societies' participation in and possible control of open-panel medical prepayment plans.

Third, there is increasing congressional interest in using market incentives within a national health insurance context. More than a decade ago, Martin Feldstein (1971a) proposed a form of national catastrophic illness insurance, called major risk insurance, which attempted to direct national health insurance toward the true insurance function—protecting the consumer against large, unforeseen expenses—while promoting equity by tying consumers' out-of-pocket expense limits to their incomes. Given the protection of major risk insurance, Feldstein asserted, consumers would not insure against the remaining, actuarially expected costs of care. Hence, they would be sensitive to physician fees and other charges for the majority of their health care events, and conventional market forces would constrain demand and restrict the ability of providers to inflate their fees. Feldstein's insurance idea was never embodied directly in major national health insurance bills, but proposed legislation on catastrophic insurance has contained several of its principles.

The competition approach to national health insurance received a boost when then-Secretary of Health, Education, and Welfare (HEW) Joseph Califano commissioned Stanford economist Alain Enthoven to develop an insurance proposal incorporating competitive market influences. Enthoven's proposal (1978), which he called "consumer-choice health plan," relied on consumers using vouchers to select among competing health care delivery organizations. The proposal placed a lot of weight on the further development of HMOs. Enthoven's proposal was not formalized into a Carter administration proposal, but the 96th Congress saw three procompetition national health insurance bills introduced by members of both major political parties. Similar bills received even more attention in the conservative 97th Congress.

Another recent systemic approach to cost containment was embodied in the Carter administration's foray into hospital cost containment. Although Congress did not pass the administration's hospital cost-containment bills, the very existence of the bills and the force with which they were presented created an environment in which the private sector felt compelled to mount a Voluntary Effort to contain costs. The basic principle of the administration's plan was to place a ceiling on hospitals' revenues, in essence imposing a budget constraint, and allow institutional decision-makers (primarily physicians and administrators) to decide how available resources should be allocated. The plan had certain technical flaws [for example, it permitted certain costs to leak outside the hospital and thereby escape being included in the ceiling (Hughes et al., 1978; Warner, 1978)] and it was watered down for political reasons (for example, exempting wage increases from the ceiling), but it did identify the need for a budget constraint and acknowledged the desirability of allowing experts within the institutions to determine the allocation of resources.

Several states have been quite active in devising mechanisms to contain the costs of hospital care. Indeed, for those states that are constitutionally required to balance their budgets, health costs pose a more immediate problem than for the federal government. The most common state effort, other than certificate-of-need activities (or simply curtailing benefits), is hospital rate review. Although there is a variety of approaches to hospital rate-setting, all seem to focus on reimbursing the facilities on a prospective basis. This usually entails careful budgetary review, facility by facility— a time-consuming and complex process. Evidence from a recent study indicates that, from 1975 to 1978, states with comprehensive rate review programs were moderately successful in containing costs (U.S. Department of Health, Education, and Welfare, Health Care Financing Administration, 1980). Other analysis is currently under way to confirm or reject this finding.

Another, more recent state approach to cost containment is to reimburse hospitals on the basis of case mix. That is, instead of a fee for each service or for each day of hospitalization, the hospital is paid a predetermined amount for each case, based on the average costs incurred in treating patients with that particular diagnosis. Such a system is being tested in twenty-six New Jersey hospitals. All commercial insurers, Blue Cross, state Medicaid, and federal Medicare programs are participating. The New Jersey experiment has identified 383 separate diagnostic-related groups (DRGs), each of which is reimbursable. Each admission is given a DRG classification, and one fee is paid, regardless of whether the patient is discharged the next day or the next month. The DRG system represents another attempt to change the fundamental economic incentives of the health care system at the institutional level, in this case by rewarding short, low-intensity hospital stays (Reiss, 1980).

PRIVATE SECTOR

Private sector organizations involved in health care cost containment span the spectrum of health care interests; they include consumers, individual and institutional providers of care, and third-party payers. We shall merely identify prominent examples of efforts in each of these areas, emphasizing activities in provider groups.

Consumer involvement in cost containment has been more recent and limited than either provider or payer involvement. In part, this undoubtedly reflects the lack of organizational vehicles for most consumers. However, it probably also represents a relative lack of appreciation of the magnitude of the cost escalation problem. While health care prices have risen, the consumer has become progressively more isolated from them because of the rapid growth of insurance coverage. Because much of this coverage is provided publicly or privately through employee benefits, consumers are further isolated from an awareness of what their coverage costs.

The costs of health insurance have made institutional consumers vividly aware of the cost inflation problem. In recent years, both employers and employee groups have realized that insurance premiums are progressively eating into employee benefits and driving up business costs. The federal tax treatment of employer-paid premiums—exemption from the Social Security and personal income tax bases—insulates both management and labor from the true costs of care, but the sheer magnitude of costs is correcting this tax-created myopia. As a consequence, several labor and management teams are exploring alternative delivery mechanisms, including HMOs, and seeking innovative insurance programs. Clearly, consumers have the ability to exert substantial pressure on providers and insurers to develop cost-containing alternatives to the present system.

The private insurance system is an obvious instrument for injecting competition (and with it, cost containment) into health care delivery. Clark Havighurst, an articulate proponent of "private cost containment," has identified several steps insurers could take, some in cooperation with providers, to foster cost-consciousness within the system. He points to such devices as coverage limitations and indemnity plans as simple means of achieving the desired end. In addition, Havighurst calls for strong antitrust action. Barriers to significant innovation in private insurance coverage include the federal tax law's incentives, provider opposition, market control, and the apparent intransigence of private insurance companies (Havighurst, 1979).

As a group, private sector third-party payers have not demonstrated much enthusiasm for promoting cost containment. Most active have been several Blue Cross-Blue Shield plans that have attempted two types of cost-control mechanisms: (1) a variety of hospital reimbursement innovations, such as prospective reimbursement (a systemic approach), and (2) individual nonreimbursement practices (an incremental approach). As an example of the latter, some plans refused to reimburse for CT body scans in the early days of scanning, before their effectiveness had been demonstrated. Consequently, rates of body scans in areas where they were not reimbursable decreased considerably in relation to those in areas where Blue Cross-Blue Shield reimbursed the cost. In 1979 the national Blue Cross-Blue Shield Association recommended to member plans that they no longer automatically reimburse hospitals for entry batteries of laboratory tests. This recommendation derived from the perception that the yield from such batteries was insufficient to justify their cost. Representatives of Blue Cross-Blue Shield, as well as commercial insurers, have expressed a desire for sound cost-effectiveness information on which they could base reimbursement decisions.

In many respects, the principal private sector organizations attempting to grapple with cost inflation represent provider groups, both individual (for example, physicians) and institutional (for example, hospitals). Among the latter, the most visibly active has been the American Hospital Association (AHA). Acting in concert with several other organizations, including the American Medical Association (AMA), the AHA mounted the Voluntary Effort to control hospital costs. As we noted above, the Voluntary Effort was a direct response to the threat of governmental regulation of hospital cost containment. Proponents of the Voluntary Effort have argued that the industry can control itself more efficiently than could government. Its pleas for an attempt to demonstrate its sincerity reached sympathetic ears in Congress, which agreed to withhold federal legislation to give the industry a chance. Organizers of the Voluntary Effort were quick to claim credit for the contained growth in hospital costs in the years immediately following initiation of the effort, but the multiplicity of cost-containment efforts makes it difficult, perhaps impossible, to attribute containment to any one source. Furthermore, the true test of the Voluntary Effort, indeed of all cost-containment efforts, lies in the future. The costs of health care will be contained when their growth is consistent with that of other service activities, not greater.

Among institutional providers, HMOs stand out as the only organizations exhibiting a long-term commitment to cost containment: cost containment is one of the major features of HMOs. Their prepayment plan encourages efficiency among providers, many of whom have a direct profit-sharing stake in their organization's aggregate efficiency. HMOs have not been significantly more involved than other providers in formally assessing the cost-effectiveness of medical technologies and practices, though the informal assessment prompted by the payment mechanism undoubtedly affects behavior (see Chapter 5). It is interesting to note that, while the cost of HMO care does tend to be lower than that of fee-for-service care, the rate of cost increase has been similar for the two delivery systems (Luft, 1980).

The health care cost problem has often been blamed on the physician. Expenditures on physician services per se account for only 19 percent of the total spent on personal health care, but the physician has considerable influence on, and often direct control of, the utilization of other health care resources. Decisions on hospitalization and the use of hospital services, the most expensive component of health care, reside primarily with physicians. Physicians determine when patients are to be hospitalized, what diagnostic testing and treatment will be done, and how long they will stay. They also decide on the dispensing of prescriptions. Thus physicians' influence on health care costs vastly exceeds their personal share of these costs (Fuchs, 1974). Nevertheless, influence and control must be distinguished from culpability for cost inflation. As we emphasized earlier in this chapter, if blame must be placed, we would point our fingers at the incentive system. Often the physician "responsible" for an enormous hospital bill has acted responsibly in looking out for the well-insured patient's best interests.

Because of their central role in health care resource utilization, it is desirable that physicians become integrally involved in the attempt to contain inflation. Physicians should not necessarily be the final arbiters of cost-effectiveness, but they do hold a monopoly on half of the equation: clearly they are the principal force in determining the effectiveness of the weapons in the medical arsenal. And as the captains of the health care team, they are in a unique position to implement cost-effective alternatives to current medical practice.

In recent years, numerous physician organizations have become concerned with cost containment. Many physicians have been attracted to the cause by a genuine appreciation of the parameters of the problem and the need to do something about it. Cynics charge that physicians have been motivated primarily by the desire to preserve control over the system, to keep the tentacles of government from further violating the boundaries of their turf. Regardless of motivation, however, the fact of physician awareness of and involvement in the cost-containment debate represents an important development, one which should influence the shape of the debate for years to come.

There are several prominent physician-based cost-containment activities. The PSRO program is one such effort, but since it is mandated by law, we discussed it as a public cost-containment initiative.

The magnitude and nature of the health care cost problem have been studied recently by a national commission established by the AMA. The commission incorporated wide-ranging expertise, including that of health economists. The findings of the group were released in the *Report of the National Commission on the Cost of Medical Care* (American Medical Association, 1978). The AMA has sponsored other, related activities. The same year, the Resident

Physicians Section of the AMA produced a report intended to explain and promote cost-effective medical practices. In the spirit of "physician, heal thyself," the hope was that fostering cost-consciousness in the new generation of practitioners would serve the national goal of cost containment (Kridel and Winston, 1978).

Several state medical associations have studied their own states' health care cost problems and alternative local approaches to cost containment. While these efforts understandably have achieved less visibility nationally than the work of the AMA, several of them represent thoughtful, comprehensive assessments. In some instances, the associations have developed detailed blueprints for state programs to combat health care cost inflation. For example, the Minnesota Medical Association's Commission on Health Care Costs produced forty-one recommendations covering such diverse areas as the promotion of competitive market forces in health care delivery; encouragement of health promotion activities by physicians, industry, and third-party payers; improvement of utilization review and implementation of physician feedback mechanisms; reduction of excess hospital bed capacity; teaching medical students and practicing physicians to be sensitive to cost-effective medical practices; encouragement of appropriate self-care by consumers; and improvement in the cost-effectiveness of government regulation of care (Minnesota Medical Association, 1979).

Education seems to be the means medical leaders prefer in attacking the health care cost problem. Programs designed to make physicians sensitive to costs are being developed at all levels of the education-practice continuum. Health economics is joining anatomy and physiology in the curriculums of some of the nation's medical schools. In 1977, a survey by the American Association of Medical Colleges found 19 percent of the schools offering coursework related to cost containment, with another 15 percent developing or planning such instruction (Hudson and Braslow, 1979). The emphasis on cost containment in the intervening years may well have increased these numbers substantially.

Several hands-on experiences have been put into operation to teach cost-effective provision of care. Residents at a few teaching hospitals receive direct training in cost-effective case management, while residents and postgraduate practitioners at other institutions receive indirect training. For example, several institutions have experimented with attaching cost data to ordering forms or reporting cost profiles (an analysis of costs generated by each physician) to staff physicians (Grossman, 1981). Believing that "cost-effective medicine is effective medicine," the American College of Physicians has launched an educational effort related to appropriate diagnostic testing to promote economic efficiency in physician behavior.

In the face of inconsistent and even contradictory market incentives, the ability of education to significantly contribute to cost containment is problematic at best. Nevertheless it must be recognized that many critics of the American medical system attribute a share of the blame for cost inflation to medical education. These critics argue that medical students and young physicians have been taught to use the entire medical armamentarium to diagnose or treat illness, paying little or no attention to the cost implications of their decisions. To the extent that this perception of past medical education is accurate, injection of cost-consciousness into current and future education seems a worthwhile endeavor.

CONCLUSION

The high and rising costs of health care do not constitute a new problem. Indeed, the persistence of the problem is the major reason we have avoided the overworked descriptor "crisis." Of course, the longer the problem persists, the greater it becomes. And as the data in the first half of this chapter indicated, the rate of growth is such that rather dramatic increases in the magnitude of health care costs can occur, and have occurred, in a very few years.

Two features of the health care scene differentiate today's fiscal situation from that of fifty years ago. First, the increasing divergence between consumption of care and direct payment for care has created an economic environment in which the principal constraints on the costs of care are the state of the art of medical technology, health care politics, and medical judgments regarding appropriate amounts and types of care. Conventional market constraints are rapidly disappearing, increasing the risk of continuing cost inflation. However, perhaps because of growing awareness of the implications of the deterioration of the conventional marketplace, interest in introducing competitive forces has arisen in both professional and policy circles.

The second feature, not independent of the first, is that significant segments of the health care industry, particularly health care professionals, have acknowledged the existence of the problem and have volunteered to seek its resolution. Whether their motivation is to minimize governmental intrusion or simply to practice more efficient medicine, the involvement of health care professionals and organizations fundamentally alters the character of the cost-containment drama. In particular, it makes these groups the writers and directors of the drama rather than merely the actors or the props.

The extent of physician concern about cost containment is difficult to gauge, and the impact on costs of increasing physician concern is virtually impossible to assess. Regarding the former, a survey by the American College of Physicians of its 15,000 members suggests that interest levels are high: 45 percent of the membership responded to a questionnaire on the cost-of-care issue; the usual rate of response is about 15 percent. Physician interest and involvement can be expected to ebb and flow with the position of health cost containment on the social agenda.

As our glimpse at both public and private health sector activities suggested, a focus on the incremental approach to cost containment implies an allegiance to procedure-specific cost-effectiveness. Cost-benefit and cost-effectiveness analysis are analytical tools intended to serve this allegiance. The next chapter explains the notion of cost-effective medical care, defines CBA and CEA, and briefly examines the history of these analytical techniques.

NOTES

1. The gross national product is the monetary value of all goods and services produced in the economy.
2. This is not necessarily an index of the adequacy of care. In addition to possible variations in the quality of services received, the poor seem to have higher levels of morbidity and disability than the rich. Thus it is certainly plausible that the gap between need for care and receipt of effective services remains greatest for the poor. (U.S. Department of Health, Education, and Welfare, 1980).
3. The actual amount will depend on the taxpayer's marginal tax bracket.
4. The tax incentives may tip the balance between assuming one's own first-dollar risk and insuring against it. In the absence of the pro-insurance tax incentives, a risk-neutral individual would view the actuarial value of first-dollar coverage plus the administrative cost tacked onto the premium as too high a price for an expense for which the individual can budget. However, the present tax advantages of insurance may outweigh the administrative cost component of the premium. Keeler et al. (1976) have concluded that a comprehensive national health insurance program with deductibles would lead to almost no purchasing of first-dollar, supplementary insurance *if* the

tax incentives were eliminated. If the incentives were retained, however, the median individual might wish to purchase full supplementation.

5. These services were pathology tests, nuclear medicine procedures, anesthesiology, pharmacy items, laboratory tests (inpatient and outpatient), therapeutic radiology procedures, and blood bank units drawn.

6. The issues in caring for a growing elderly population are numerous and complex. Both the quality of and charges for nursing home care have been the basis of several recent investigations. Recognition that current financing mechanisms encourage institutionalization of large numbers of elderly who could live at home with limited assistance has led to attempts to redefine coverage of care for the elderly.

7. Note that this argument explains high prices and low quantities but not persistent increases in price; that is, unless supply becomes progressively more restricted over time, supply restriction helps to explain the level of prices but not continual *changes* in the level.

8. This introduction to the logic of health care cost inflation has been necessarily cursory and incomplete. Readers interested in a deeper treatment are referred to one of the recent textbooks on the economics of health care, including those of Eastaugh (1981), P. Feldstein (1979), Jacobs (1980), Newhouse (1978), Sorkin (1975), and Ward (1975). Additional data on the magnitude and nature of the health care cost problem are presented in U.S. Department of Health and Human Services (1981).

9. A detailed treatment of cost-containment efforts and their associated organizational entities would exceed the purpose and scope of this book. However, several of the organizations discussed below are considered further in Chapter 5, in which we examine the past and potential uses of cost-benefit and cost-effectiveness analysis.

10. The certificate-of-need process has been subjected to much criticism. Medical professionals question the ability of health planners to make socially desirable decisions on complex medical issues. In addition, the process is laden with political influence. Finally, several analysts have questioned whether the certificate-of-need process achieves its stated objectives. The best-known empirical study found that, from 1968 to 1972, certificate-of-need regulation succeeded in lowering the growth of bed supplies but that hospitals appear to have compensated by increasing plant assets per bed. As a result, no significant savings in hospital costs were realized (Salkever and Bice, 1979).

2

Introduction to Cost-Benefit and Cost-Effectiveness Analysis

IF COST-BENEFIT and cost-effectiveness analysis (CBA and CEA) are viewed as tools with which to search for cost-effective medical practices, an obvious point of departure for a study of these techniques is consideration of the meaning of cost-effective medical practice. We open this chapter, therefore, with an examination of this often misunderstood concept. Following that, we define the techniques of CBA and CEA. The remainder of the chapter provides historical background on the application of CBA and CEA, beginning with applications other than health care and then describing the limited role of CBA-CEA in the health care field. We close with some recent events indicating the intensity of interest in these techniques in both health professional and policy circles.

COST-EFFECTIVE MEDICAL CARE: THE CONCEPT

Awareness of the cost-of-care problem has made "cost-effective" an increasingly common adjective in discussions of health care. The term has come to have a legitimizing intent, conferring worthiness on the medical procedure or technology it modifies. The frequency with which the term is invoked has not been matched by a uniform understanding of its meaning. To some people, cost-effective means inexpensive; to others, it means technically effective. In either case, half the term is being neglected.

Cost-effectiveness relates to value for money. That is, a medical practice is considered to be cost-effective if it is "worth" the expenditure of the resources required to perform it. Assessing the value of a medical practice, and hence its cost-effectiveness, is a largely subjective undertaking. A given medical practice, standing alone, cannot be objectively labeled cost-effective because determination of the cost-effectiveness of a single medical practice requires a well-defined, generally quantifiable value system. For example, a procedure that saved a life and cost $100 would be labeled cost-effective by virtually everyone, yet implicit in this is the subjective judgment that a life is worth at least $100. The ambiguity, or subjectivity, becomes clearer by considering a different example: is a procedure that saves a life and costs $1 million cost-effective? Here one is unlikely to find unanimity in judgments of cost-effectiveness. What if the cost were $100 million? In short, the valuation of human life (discussed in Chapter 3) becomes a critical step in determining "inherent" cost-effectiveness, yet that step is necessarily subjective.

The concept of cost-effectiveness is more meaningful, and less subjective, when alternative uses of resources are being compared. That is, rather than considering the cost-effectiveness of medical practice X, standing alone, we examine the cost-effectiveness of X compared to Y and Z. Cost-effectiveness becomes a relative concept: practice X is cost-effective if it performs a specified task at less cost or use of resources than practices Y and Z; or, X is cost-effective if it produces more of the desired outputs than Y and Z when the same level of resources (cost) is invested in each. Note that, when the alternative practices are intended to achieve the same or highly similar types of outcome, the difficulty of valuing life, reduction in illness, alleviation of pain, and so on often can be avoided: the question is reduced to a relative determination of cost-effectiveness in producing a given (nonvalued) health outcome.

In general, cost-effectiveness rests on the basic economic concept of opportunity cost: that is, the true cost of an activity is the value of the alternative endeavors that might have been undertaken with the same resources. When two or more medical practices are compared, the opportunity cost of each is made explicit. If given resources could save ten lives using practice X and only five lives with practice Y, the opportunity cost of shifting the resources from X to Y is clear: five lives. When one refers to the cost-effectiveness of a single practice, opportunity cost becomes implicit. Thus, in the earlier example, it is unlikely that we could find better alternative uses for the $100 of medical care that saved a human life. By contrast, the $100 million procedure would appear to have a high opportunity cost: $100 million worth of resources should be able to do much more than save a single life. There are dozens of procedures that can save lives at a much lower cost; hence the resources represented by the $100 million could be redistributed to other uses that might save, say, 1,000 lives. Clearly, the single $100 million procedure would be less cost-effective than the alternatives.

To illustrate the difference between absolute and relative perspectives on cost-effectiveness, we refer to the often-discussed question of the cost-effectiveness of CT scanning (examined more fully in Chapter 4). While some authors have asserted that scanning is (or is not) inherently cost-effective, technically sound studies have assessed the cost-effectiveness of scanning by comparing its costs and diagnostic accuracy with those of alternative procedures. In the case of an intracranial mass lesion, CT scanning can be considered cost-effective when compared with angiography or pneumoencephalography. In terms of all of the medical costs associated with these procedures (including hospitalization), CT costs least and produces diagnoses of at least comparable quality; in addition, it avoids the pain and risk associated with an invasive procedure. By contrast, it makes little sense to say that scanning is (or is not) inherently cost-effective, since it is impossible to value the outcome of diagnosis objectively.

While we have emphasized that "cost-effective" should be a comparative adjective, applied after assessing a practice's costs and outcomes relative to those of alternative practices, we should also emphasize that, for the comparison to be meaningful, the outcomes must be directly comparable. For instance, if no other information is available, it does not make sense to say that procedure A, costing $1,000 and preventing one hundred days of disability, is cost-effective compared to procedure B, which costs $10,000 and prolongs one useful life for two years. When the benefits of the procedures are not commensurate, objective determination of cost-effectiveness is impossible.

At the risk of introducing confusion, we note two exceptions to the rule that the phrase "cost-effective" should be used in a comparative context. One is the truly unusual case of an inherently objective cost-effective procedure that saves money without imposing nonmonetary costs on anyone. For example, Centerwall and Criqui found that fortifying alcoholic beverages with thiamine in order to reduce Wernicke-Korsakoff syndrome (a thiamine-deficiency disorder) in alcoholics was inherently cost-effective because the hospitalization resources avoided by preventing the syndrome exceeded the costs of fortifying the beverages. If, however, thiamine fortification produced an undesirable taste or had other undesirable side effects, or if it prevented the drying-out of some alcoholics identified during episodes of the syndrome, the cost-effectiveness of thiamine fortification would be open to question (Centerwall and Criqui, 1978).

The second exception involves a relaxation of the strict definition of cost-effectiveness and an acceptance of common sense. For example, virtually everyone would concur that a $100 procedure to save a life is cost-effective. Furthermore, it seems obvious that such a procedure is more cost-effective than a $10,000 procedure that reduces a patient's bed disability by a single day. Even though this example requires us to compare medical apples and oranges, the quality and quantity of the fruit and the difference in costs are sufficiently great to produce unanimous, if subjective, judgments. In effect, the unanimity of these judgments substitutes for objective standards of comparison.

While we close with the notion that common sense can legitimize a technically inappropriate use of the phrase "cost-effective," we note the relative unimportance of this exception to the rule. Clear instances of cost-effective medical practices are not the ones that have created policy questions. Concern focuses precisely on those practices for which cost-effectiveness is at issue. The latter practices are the ones that seem to be appropriate candidates for CBA and CEA.

DEFINITIONS OF CBA AND CEA

Cost-benefit and cost-effectiveness analysis have come to refer to formal analytical techniques for comparing the negative and positive consequences of alternative uses of resources. Often enshrouded in technical jargon and mathematics, CBA and CEA are really nothing more than attempts to weigh logically the pros and cons of a decision. Each of us engages in such thinking every day, frequently subconsciously. The decision of how to spend a summer Sunday—going to the beach or working in the yard—is an implicit cost-benefit calculation. Business decisions on investments, marketing strategies, and so on have a distinct CBA-CEA character. "[U]ltimately, something like [CBA-CEA] must necessarily be employed in any rational decision" (Gramlich, 1981, p. 3).

While the logic of CBA-CEA is embedded in all rational decision-making, the terms themselves are most commonly applied to analysis of public sector resource allocation. In part, this reflects a popular view of CBA-CEA as a surrogate for the market's balancing of (private) costs and benefits. In the private sector, it is argued, the market serves as a rational resource-allocation mechanism. In the public sector, the absence of market forces creates the need to simulate an equivalent—hence CBA-CEA.

While the mechanics of public and private sector analysis are similar conceptually, there are notable differences between them. For example, the absence of a universally accepted bottom line in the public sector, something analogous to profit in the private sector, makes CBA-CEA in the public sector much more complex than evaluation techniques in the private sector. Furthermore, as we will discuss in Chapter 3, assessment of alternative allocations of public sector resources often requires analysts to examine more varied types of costs and benefits and to consider them from a variety of perspectives, perspectives reflecting the multiplicity of interest groups in the public sector. By contrast, the business manager serves a group of stockholders with shared objectives. Factors such as these hint at both the importance and the complexity of analyzing resource allocation in the public sector.

Both CBA and CEA require analysts to identify, measure, and compare all of the significant costs and desirable consequences of alternative means of addressing a given problem. A principal objective of CBA and CEA is to structure and analyze information in a manner that will inform, and thereby assist, policymakers. It is these individuals, not analysts, who will decide which, if any, of the competing programs will be proposed or implemented.[1] CBA and CEA are not formulas for making decisions. This reflects the subjective, often political, nature of the policies at issue and the conceptual and practical limitations of CBA-CEA. If judged according to the popular misconception that their purpose is to produce "correct" policy decisions, CBAs and CEAs will be found wanting. Viewed as information-generating techniques, as aids to decision-making, CBAs and CEAs can serve admirably as one of several inputs into the policy making process.

The principal technical distinction between CBA and CEA lies in the process of valuing the desirable consequences of programs. In CBA, all such consequences—benefits—are valued, like costs, in monetary terms. Conceptually, this permits an assessment of the inherent worth of a program (do the benefits exceed the costs?), as well as a comparison of competing alternatives (which of several programs generates the largest excess of benefits over costs?). Because all costs and benefits are measured in the same (monetary) unit, CBA can be employed to compare similar or widely divergent types of programs. Thus, in theory at least, CBA might be used to help decide whether certain public resources should be allocated to construction of a dam, construction of a hospital, or neither.

In CEA, some desirable program consequences are measured in nonmonetary units: in health care CEAs, common measures include years of life saved and days of morbidity or disability avoided. The reason for a nonmonetary measure of program effectiveness is either the impossibility or undesirability of valuing important outcomes in dollars and cents. Thus, the bottom line of a CEA is not, like that of a CBA, net monetary value; rather, it is expressed in units such as "dollars per year of life saved." CEA permits comparison of cost per unit of effectiveness among competing alternatives designed to serve the same basic purpose. Unlike CBA, it does not allow direct comparison of programs with different objectives (because the effectiveness or outcome measures differ), nor does it permit assessment of the inherent worth of a program (is a cost of $50,000 per year of life saved acceptable?).

Choice of CBA or CEA will depend on technical considerations and the predisposition of analysts and their clients. Neither technique is necessarily superior to the other. CBA is the theoretical ideal, since it permits direct comparison of the desirable and undesirable consequences of diverse programs, but, as we will discuss in the next chapter, problems of benefit valuation are myriad, particularly in social welfare areas such as health care. CEA avoids the difficult, arbitrary, and often distasteful job of assigning monetary values to such ostensibly nonmonetary "commodities" as years of human life. However, by rejecting the monetary measure, the CEA analyst loses a unifying metric with which to weight and compare different types of effectiveness. How are two programs to be compared when one averts several deaths but has limited effect on disability, while the other prevents considerable disability but averts only a couple of deaths?[2]

The distinctions between CBA and CEA are not quite as black and white as the above may suggest. In Chapter 4 we note an example of one generally well done CEA that its author has labeled a CBA. This apparent mislabeling cannot be dismissed simply as a mistake, however. Rather, it reflects what appears to be a trend in the health care CBA-CEA literature: unwilling to place dollar values on health outcomes, yet desirous of capturing all of a program's economic implications, several researchers are publishing analyses that merge elements of CBA with traditional

CEA. This evolving form of analysis still warrants the label CEA— the bottom line remains dollars per unit of health outcome—but indirect economic effects, ignored in traditional CEA, are being incorporated into the cost side of the equation. Indirect economic benefits are treated as negative costs; they are subtracted from the direct and indirect economic costs of a program. The example of thiamine fortification of alcoholic beverages was presented as a CBA, yet the principal purpose of the fortification—reduction of the number of cases of Wernicke-Korsakoff syndrome—was not valued monetarily. In effect, this was a CEA in which an indirect economic benefit of the reduction of the syndrome (the decrease in the costs of hospitalization of such patients) was compared with the cost of fortification. In this rare instance, the negative economic costs exceeded the direct program costs, leaving the analysts with a positive health outcome and a net saving of economic resources (Centerwall and Criqui, 1978).

We will return to this analytical development later. Suffice it here to note that the emerging concept of CEA does not appear to represent a conscious effort to combine the best elements of traditional CBA and CEA—at least the "new" CEA is not presented as such—yet it seems to be a promising development.

The purpose for which CBA and CEA are used has a time dimension. Both techniques can be used to plan for the future or evaluate past program performance. As planning tools, the techniques involve prospective analysis. That is, the analyst attempts to predict the costs and benefits (effectiveness) of alternative future programs. Analysis may draw on past or existing programs for data and ideas as to how to model the structure of the future programs, but the focus remains distinctly prospective. As evaluative tools, CBA and CEA involve assessment of the realized costs and benefits (effectiveness) of existing or past programs. Frequently, of course, a retrospective evaluation will have a prospective intent: should a program be continued into the future? If so, how should it be modified?

In this introductory glance at CBA-CEA it is useful to distinguish these techniques from others that are frequently confused with them. The two aspects of a CBA or CEA—assessment of a program's costs and desirable consequences—are important forms of analysis in their own right. Assessment of effectiveness is traditionally the focal point of evaluation in health care. A wide variety of evaluative approaches, including randomized clinical trials, epidemiological studies, and laboratory animal tests, forms the basis of assessments of the efficacy or effectiveness of numerous medical and public health practices (U.S. Congress, Office of Technology Assessment, 1978a). Similarly, though less commonly, the costs of certain programs or technologies are examined in a cost analysis that treats effectiveness only implicitly or tangentially. Risk-benefit analyses compare the desirable outcomes of a practice with the undesirable but noneconomic ones. Thus, the probability of a surgical procedure's alleviating pain or prolonging life might be compared with its operative mortality and postoperative morbidity. Technology Assessments, a new development in the health care evaluation field, strive to identify all of the consequences—health, economic, political, social, legal, and ethical—of emerging or prospective medical technologies. They rely on multidisciplinary teams to perform comprehensive analyses (Arnstein, 1977). Ideally, CBA-CEA would incorporate all of the concerns addressed by these other evaluative techniques, in essence becoming a Technology Assessment in which all effects are weighted by the same metric in order to permit comparability. In practice, CBA-CEAs tend to be less comprehensive than Technology Assessments, in that unquantifiable effects generally are left out of formal analysis (see Chapter 3); but CBA-CEAs succeed in making different effects comparable, whereas Technology Assessments merely enumerate effects.

The relative advantages and disadvantages of CBA and CEA, as well as the technical problems of each, are examined in detail in Chapter 3.

A Brief History of CBA-CEA

The commonsense principles of CBA-CEA have been promoted for centuries, and application of these principles to health care dates back at least 300 years. In the middle of the 17th century, Richard Petty, a prominent English physician, advocated greater social investment in medicine because, he had concluded, the value of saved human life far exceeded its cost (Fein, 1976). In the United States, a similar argument was made a century ago by Lemuel Shattuck in a famous report in which he applied cost-benefit logic to justify his proposal for sanitary reforms in Boston (Shattuck, 1850).

Nonetheless, formal application of CBA-CEA is a phenomenon primarily of the present century. In 1902, the River and Harbor Act directed the U.S. Army Corps of Engineers to assess the costs and benefits of river and harbor projects. In 1936, the federal Flood Control Act required that "the benefits [of projects] to whomsoever they may accrue [must be] in excess of the estimated costs," though the Act provided no guidance as to how benefits and costs were to be defined and measured. In the same decade, both the Tennessee Valley Authority and the Department of Agriculture implemented program budgeting systems that included rudimentary attempts at CBA-CEA. Official government criteria for appraisal of river development projects were first enunciated by the Bureau of the Budget in 1952 (Steiner, 1974).

Early in the Kennedy administration, the Defense Department, under Secretary Robert McNamara, adopted a program budgeting system that employed CBA-CEA to evaluate alternative defense projects. The perception that these endeavors assisted in rational defense planning, combined with a burgeoning federal budget, led President Johnson in 1965 to require the implementation of planning-programming-budgeting (PPB) systems throughout the federal bureaucracy. CBA-CEA represented both the spirit and the letter of the new initiative to rationalize government resource allocation (Schultze, 1968).

The PPB systems met with mixed and limited success because of lack of resources to implement them effectively, political and bureaucratic opposition, and unrealistic expectations of their role and potential (Gramlich, 1981; Marvin and Rouse, 1970). The formal system did not survive for long, though many Washington observers believe it left a legacy of continuing improvement in the use of rational analysis in government decision-making (Rivlin, 1971). During the Carter presidency, the philosophy and logic of CBA-CEA and PPB were reincarnated in the form of zero-based budgeting.

As formal evaluative techniques, CBA and CEA can assess decisions on public sector resource allocation in situations where conventional private sector techniques, such as capital budgeting and return-on-investment analysis, would not suffice. The inadequacy of these business evaluation techniques usually reflects the absence of a smoothly functioning market to allocate resources as desired, either because of technical problems or distributional considerations. Technical problems motivated early applications of CBA-CEA. For example, the provision of national defense does not occur in the private sector because national defense is what is known as a pure public good, one whose provision for one individual benefits all individuals. No one can be excluded from receiving the benefits of existing defense, and one person's consumption of benefits does not reduce their availability for other people. Consequently, it is impossible to "sell" national defense in a private marketplace. Consumers are aware that they will receive it for free if it is provided for anyone else, and if they were to buy it themselves, they would be providing it free to everyone else. (This is often referred to as the free-rider problem.) For national defense to exist, it must be supplied by the public sector.

Thus, it is no accident that the origins of CBA-CEA lie in the area of water resource management and that the Department of Defense was PPB's showcase in the 1960s. Dams, irrigation projects, and the like have significant characteristics of pure public goods,[3] yet market analogs permit the valuation of most of the projects' significant costs and benefits. For example, a dam may produce electricity, which has a direct market value, and at the same time provide flood control and irrigation; in this case, property values, insurance policies, and crop prices and yields are measures of benefits. In the case of defense, once an objective has been agreed upon, evaluation of alternative projects lends itself nicely to CEA, a technique used to compare programs oriented toward attainment of the same quantified, but not monetarily valued, outcome.

In the federal PPB era, CBA-CEA achieved less consistent success in social welfare areas, including education and health programs. In part, the limited success resulted from a lack of resources, particularly qualified analysts, to develop a high-quality analytical capability. It also reflected a failure to meet the unrealistically high expectations set for CBA-CEA. Specific technical problems in applying these analytical techniques included frequent disagreement on appropriate measures of outcome and on the valuing of redistributions—of money, educational resources, access to health care, and so on. The benefits of redistribution—the seeking of a more just and humane sharing of society's resources—are particularly difficult to quantify and value (Fein, 1977).

Nevertheless, there were many attempts to employ CBA-CEA in the social services areas. For example, analysts at HEW performed several CBA-CEAs oriented toward assisting in health program planning. In 1966, analysts prepared fairly rudimentary CBA and CEA comparisons of alternative categorical disease and accident programs, including cancer, syphilis, tuberculosis, arthritis, and motor vehicle injury prevention. The analyses were criticized on numerous grounds, but they were used, with caution, in developing policy recommendations (Grosse, 1970).

Prominent examples of health care CBA-CEAs were the 1967 studies of efforts to control kidney disease. One, undertaken by HEW, involved analysis of alternative mixes of research, prevention, and treatment of kidney disease (U.S. Department of Health, Education, and Welfare, 1967*b*). At the same time, the Bureau of the Budget appointed an advisory committee to study treatment alternatives for end-stage renal disease (U.S. Bureau of the Budget, 1967). The government was under considerable pressure to expand the nation's dialysis capacity, so the analyses were oriented toward a real and immediate health policy problem.

The studies concurred in finding transplantation preferable to dialysis in treating end-stage disease, and the HEW analysis emphasized the need for a multifactorial approach, including research, prevention, diagnosis, and early treatment. In the executive branch of the federal government, the studies dampened interest in mounting a national dialysis program. Such a program was viewed as extremely expensive and not a cost-effective means of dealing with the problems produced by kidney disease. The politics of the situation caused Congress to override the executive branch's approach, and, tied into a Social Security legislative package, the national dialysis program became a reality (Rettig, 1979).

From 1966 through 1968, HEW applied analysis to several other health policy issues. A major study of maternal and child health care programs proved both difficult to carry out and informative. Conclusions from it were embodied in the Social Security Amendments of 1967 (U.S. Department of Health, Education, and Welfare, 1966*c*; Grosse, 1970). Analyses related to providing health services for the poor and examining nursing personnel programs also occupied HEW analysts (U.S. Department of Health, Education, and Welfare, 1967*a*, 1968).

The middle to late 1960s were a high point for CBA-CEA in the federal health bureaucracy. Since that time, HEW (now the Department of Health and Human Services) has increased its in-house analytical capacities, as have many other departments and agencies at all levels of government, but explicit CBA-CEA seems to have become relatively less important. A notable exception is the work of the health program of OTA, which has produced the most comprehensive study of CBA-CEA in health care (U.S. Congress, Office of Technology Assessment, 1980*a*) and has examined the cost-effectiveness of several specific medical technologies. One such study, a CEA of pneumococcal vaccine (1979), played a central role in the evolution of legislation permitting Medicare to reimburse for pneumococcal vaccinations; the legislation was signed into law on December 28, 1980.

Aside from the work of OTA, the analyses of recent years that have attracted the most attention have come from outside the bureaucracy. Two prominent examples are the work of Weinstein and Stason on hypertension policy (1976b) and Eddy's assessment of optimal cancer screening programs (1980b). The latter is particularly noteworthy, for it is one of only a handful of CBA-CEAs undertaken with, and achieving, the specific intent of affecting nongovernmental policymaking. Supported by the national Blue Cross Association, Eddy developed computer models to examine the cost-effectiveness of alternative cancer screening strategies. As a result of the study, the national Blue Cross Association is developing a screening reimbursement package for distribution to member plans. Eddy's work has also caused the American Cancer Society to recommend less intensive screening than it did in the past. The Society will disseminate its new recommendations through an educational campaign aimed at both physicians and the general public.

The current level of interest in health care CBA-CEA is not matched by an ample supply of policy-related analyses. The examples discussed above are exceptions to the rule, not illustrations of it. Although thinking similar to CBA and CEA may play a large and growing role in public policymaking, there has been little formal analysis to date.

CURRENT INTEREST IN HEALTH CARE CBA-CEA

Interest in CBA-CEA has been growing rapidly in both health policy and professional circles. In general, the interest derives from concern about the mounting costs of health services, increased governmental spending, and the perception that the allocation of health care resources must be rationalized. Groups as disparate as providers and third-party payers have expressed a desire for cost-effectiveness information to aid them in promoting greater efficiency in the provision of health care services.

Several recent inquiries into the diffusion and use of medical technology have had evaluation of the cost-effectiveness of technology as an important implicit or explicit theme. In the latter category, the OTA recently completed a major two-year study on the implications of CEA applied to medical technology. Consisting of six documents, the overall study focused on the policy usefulness of CBA-CEA in rationalizing medical technology resource allocation (U.S. Congress, Office of Technology Assessment, 1980a). A similar theme occupied much of the proceedings of a conference sponsored by the National Center for Health Services Research (Wagner, 1979). Other activities with cost-effectiveness as an implicit theme include: A committee of the National Research Council devoted considerable attention to health care economics in its study of the diffusion of equipment-embodied technology (National Academy of Sciences, 1979); another National Center for Health Services Research conference focused exclusively on the issues of the cost of technology and what to do about it (Altman and Blendon, 1979); a Boston University conference entitled "Technology and the Quality of Health Care" found quality and cost issues inextricably linked (Egdahl and Gertman, 1978); a 1980 National Heart, Lung, and Blood Institute conference on the diffusion of technology, as well as several "consensus development exercises" at the National Institutes of Health (NIH), have addressed questions of cost-effectiveness.[4]

Thus the goal of identifying and encouraging cost-effective medical practices has risen high on the health policy agenda. For this reason, CBA-CEA represents an idea whose time has come. Further evidence of this is afforded by the fact that, in the 94th and 95th Congresses, over sixty-five pieces of proposed legislation related to health included words such as "cost-effectiveness" and "cost-effective medical care" (U.S. Congress, Office of Technology Assessment, 1980a). Both the Health Planning Amendments of 1979 and the Health Care Technology Act of 1978 called for the inclusion of cost-effectiveness in the deliberative processes of the agencies affected. However, despite the popularity of the idea, as the OTA study and this book suggest, it remains unclear whether, or how, the actual application of CBA-CEA will be an activity whose time has arrived. The need and desire for policy-relevant cost-effectiveness information are clear; the ability to produce and effectively use such information is not. This is not to disparage or discredit CBA-CEA. Rather, it is intended to suggest three major themes of this book: (1) Good CBA-CEA is not easy to do; (2) its usefulness to policy will depend on its intended purpose and will vary from setting to setting; and (3) its policy potential will depend on identifiable technical factors and the economic and political environment.

In health professional circles, as in the policy community, interest in cost-effective care and CBA-CEA is high. In Chapter 1 we offered action-oriented evidence of such interest. We close this chapter with a glimpse at another index of interest, one explored more fully in Chapter 4—the rapid growth in the health care CBA-CEA literature. Our review of that literature revealed that, prior to 1970, the total annual number of health care CBA-CEAs and related publications never exceeded fourteen. By the end of the 1970s, however, the number of annual contributions was approaching one hundred. The rate of growth was particularly rapid in medical publications. Prior to 1974, for example, the number of health care CBA-CEA contributions in medical journals exceeded the number in nonmedical journals in only one year. From 1974 on, however, the former exceeded the latter every single year, by an average of two-thirds. Finally, through 1974, the *New England Journal of Medicine* had published more than one relevant article in only one year (and in that year it published two). Since then, *Journal* readers have been exposed to an average of six CBA-CEA articles per year.[5]

In short, growth of interest in health care CBA-CEA—perhaps one is justified in calling it an explosion of interest—is a phenomenon of the 1970s, particularly the latter half of the decade. No longer merely esoterica for the academic economist, CBA and CEA have been thrust before health professionals and policymakers.

NOTES

1. By "policymakers" we refer to both individual professionals and persons in formal policymaking roles within organizations. The former may make their own private policy judgments as to how to practice their professions.
2. Note that, when decision-makers decide which of alternative programs to fund, they are implicitly assigning values to the ostensibly non-monetary commodities produced by the programs. In this policy-making context, one can question whether CEA is truly less arbitrary and capricious than CBA. At least the latter forces an explicit consideration of the valuation process.
3. Other sources of technical market failure are closely related to the pure public good problem. These include significant economies of scale—that is, decreasing average costs as the size of a project increases (for example, a dam)—and externalities—costs or benefits experienced by

other than the immediate decision-maker (for example, pollution of a downstream community's water supply by a firm dumping waste material upstream). We will not elaborate on these sources of market failure, but merely emphasize that they require nonmarket decision-making and hence are candidates for CBA-CEA. For further discussion, see Stokey and Zeckhauser (1978).

4. Proceedings of several of the NIH activities were not available at the time of this writing. One of the consensus development exercises, illustrative of this mode of professional interaction and inquiry, is discussed in Eden and Eden (1981).

5. See Chapter 4 for graphic portrayal of these growth phenomena and detailed discussion. The basis for and process of classifying literature as health care CBA-CEA are explained in Appendix A.

3

Principles:
The Methodology of CBA-CEA

IN THIS CHAPTER we present the "how to," the methodology, of CBA and CEA. The basic concept and purpose are simple and straightforward. In concept, CBA-CEA is a careful comparison of the negative and positive consequences of alternative means of addressing a given problem. Its purpose is to provide policy decision-makers with information and perspective to facilitate selecting wisely among the alternatives. Given its origins in economics, CBA-CEA is generally conceived of as an analytical tool intended to promote efficiency. We accept this concept of CBA-CEA, but in so doing we emphasize that efficiency means much more than financial profitability. In the context of social problem-solving, efficiency means the attainment of the greatest social good (however defined) permitted by the limits on resources.

In contrast to the conceptual simplicity of CBA-CEA, the actual design and performance of a specific analysis are fraught with difficulties, some surmountable through imagination and painstaking attention to detail, others inherent in the process of analysis and thus unavoidable. Nevertheless, whether one wishes to perform analysis or merely to understand it, one must possess an appreciation of its structural logic and problems. The purpose of this chapter is to provide such an appreciation.

The basic steps in CBA-CEA apply to all rational choices. The steps may strike the reader as obvious, but failure to address each of them systematically has been the downfall of many attempts at analysis. They are the following:

—Define the general problem of concern and the specific objective(s) to be sought in addressing the problem.

—Identify alternative (often programmatic) means of addressing the problem.

—Identify and, to the extent appropriate and feasible, measure and value all significant costs and benefits of each alternative.

—Compare the alternatives on the basis of criteria specified in advance; when possible, identify the dominant alternative.

—Present and interpret findings in a manner that will facilitate the reader's understanding of all important conclusions; this should include clear presentation of the limitations of the analysis.

Before delving into the individual components of analysis, we note two themes that will pervade our presentation and offer a concluding caveat about the methodology of CBA-CEA. The first theme is that, unless otherwise specified, we assume a societal perspective on costs and benefits, the traditional perspective of CBA-CEA. The analyst is charged with investigating, for a given activity, all of the costs and benefits accruing to all groups in the society. While this perspective appears to be appropriate for most public sector choices, one can imagine innumerable other choices in which the decision-makers' perspective will be narrower. For example, a firm considering building a new plant will focus its attention on the private profit implications. The firm's managers will not fully incorporate the social costs of plant-produced environmental pollution into their cost-benefit calculus, nor will they consider all of the social benefits of providing additional employment for the community. They will view the employment as a cost, totaling the wages, fringe benefits, and associated taxes they will have to pay.

Differences in evaluators' perspectives can and do play significant roles in assessment of health care activities. Analogous to the plant-construction case, private health insurers have a narrower perspective than does society on the value of a preventive health care practice. The insurer is concerned with comparing the current cost of the preventive measure with the costs of care averted in the future. Society may find inherent value in the avoidance of illness. Similarly, a hospital administrator will view acquisition of a new facility in light of its direct financial cost and its contribution to the hospital's revenue-generating capacity (and perhaps its image in the community), whereas a regional health planner, representing the society's broader interests, will be concerned with the facility's distributional implications, social costs, and so forth.

In short, legitimate differences in perspective reflect the interests and positions of decision-makers. Unless otherwise specified, our discussion assumes a broad social perspective on costs and benefits.

The second theme that pervades our presentation of methodology is the basic oneness of CBA and CEA. We acknowledge that there are several distinctive features of each technique, but the unity of basic concept and purpose, and indeed of much specific methodology, leads us to discuss the techniques as if they were a single technique. Where differences are important, we will elaborate.

Recent empirical developments in health care CBA-CEA have reduced the conceptual gap between the two techniques. A few years ago, CBA was often considered the complete form of analysis, with CEA an inferior technique employed when the problem at hand prohibited successful use of CBA. CBA represented an accounting, in a single metric (dollars), of all important costs and benefits; as such, it permitted one to determine a project's inherent value. By contrast, CEA was generally restricted to a comparison of the direct costs of a project with its effectiveness in achieving a specific, nonmonetary objective. Indirect costs and benefits (such as earnings lost because of illness or gained because of prevention of illness)[1] were usually ignored. The technique offered no hope of establishing the project's value since it compared apples (the dollars of cost) with oranges (nonmonetary effectiveness).

Two developments in the recent health care CBA-CEA literature have blurred these once-clear distinctions. There is a growing appreciation that CBA fails to incorporate important social values into its calculus. Specifically, while it considers the economic ramifications of illness or its prevention, it does not capture the nonpecuniary value of saving lives, avoiding pain, and so on.[2] As such, CBA is something less than the ultimate form of analysis. It yields the net economic value of a project but leaves it to decision-makers to value, subjectively and implicitly, the noneconomic aspects.

The second development in the literature is the increasing analytical sophistication and comprehensiveness of CEAs. Several competent analysts are including indirect costs and benefits in cost-effectiveness equations. Certain economic benefits are treated as negative costs—for example, averted hospitalization costs. In effect, the analytical trend is to include both economic costs and benefits—the two sides of the CBA equation—in a single net-cost calculation in CEA. Thus, the bottom line of a CEA becomes the net cost per unit of effectiveness. We will elaborate on this phenomenon later. For now, we hope that this glimpse at the development suggests why we perceive CBA and CEA as coming closer together.

We close this introduction to the methodology of CBA-CEA with a warning. Although the basic components of analysis presented below are (or should be) shared by all CBA-CEAs, the components may be addressed in a variety of ways. For example, prospective (planning) analyses differ from retrospective (evaluation) analyses; the latter involve observation of realized inputs and outputs, whereas the former require one to estimate the inputs and outputs of possible future programs. Similarly, consideration of emerging medical technologies involves a different kind of assessment of inputs and outputs than analysis of existing technologies. Perhaps most clearly, identification of types of costs and benefits and estimation of their values vary with the intended audience, or consumers, of an analysis: That is, analyses will differ depending on their purpose, technical considerations, and the perspectives and interests of their potential users.

These differences do not result solely from the immaturity of CBA-CEA. They often reflect the diverse technical and political purposes of analysis. For instance, in some political situations it may be difficult to rely on increased productivity as a measure of a program's worth: the Department of Health and Human Services could not base a decision on the funding of heart transplants primarily on the effect of transplants on recipients' future contribution to the economy. Other situations may make a productivity-based argument quite appealing—for example, if proponents of a drug-abuse treatment program could demonstrate that participants in the program not only kicked their habits but also began to make a contribution to the economy.

Thus, adherence to the methodological steps and format presented in this chapter does not assure a consistent analytical outcome. The handling of the steps makes it possible for different analysts to reach different conclusions. When the intent or perspective of the analyst is clearly biased, the analytical bias will be obvious. At other times, the bias will not be clear. Readers of analyses must never lose sight of the subjective and variable aspects of CBA-CEA. Indeed, they should search for such aspects whenever examining an analysis.

Now we turn to the specific components of analysis. We will attempt to clarify principles by explaining them conceptually and, frequently, by referring to cases in the literature.

DEFINING THE PROBLEM AND OBJECTIVE(S)

The necessity of identifying the problem toward which analysis is to be directed seems obvious, but experience with CBA-CEA suggests that this is not always true. The failure of analysts to consider carefully the varied dimensions of the problem has often produced analyses that have missed important, efficient means of attacking the problem. The case of end-stage renal disease is an excellent example. If one perceives the basic problem as the suffering and incapacity of current victims of kidney failure, analysis will focus on treatment alternatives. However, if one includes future victims of the disease in the analysis, additional alternatives become apparent: preventing the onset of future disease or reducing its severity. In the 1960s, the former perspective led one group of experts to study treatment alternatives (U.S. Bureau of the Budget, 1967; Klarman et al., 1968), while the latter produced a more comprehensive examination of prevention and treatment alternatives (LeSourd et al., 1968). To the extent that policymakers pay attention to analysis, their perspective on the nature of the problem and the alternatives available to address it can be significantly and unconsciously colored by the way in which the problem is defined by the analysts.

From the perspective of national health policy, the national health problem is all of the suffering associated with avoidable illness and accidents. Top-level health planning attempts to compare resource allocations across myriad health care activities; indeed, national health planning crosses the boundaries of the major federal departments. Virtually all departments engage in health-related activities, and some fundamental health activities fall wholly outside of the Department of Health and Human Services. Notable examples include worker safety, toxic substances control, transportation safety, and environmental control.

The logic of CBA-CEA is employed frequently at this level of resource allocation, but the ability to apply the techniques formally is restricted by the breadth and diversity of both the activities and the health objectives, as well as by the bureaucratic independence of both (that is, programs are housed in a variety of agencies and departments, each with its own budget). Traditionally, health care CBA-CEAs have started with a more specific health problem, such as premature mortality, avoidable disability, and unnecessary pain and suffering attributable to one or more identifiable causes. There is no right or wrong level of focus of attention. The higher level permits exploration of a wide range of alternatives and thus theoretically holds the promise of finding a socially optimal allocation of scarce resources. The lower level allows greater depth of analysis of the more restricted set of alternatives; as such, it has a greater chance of resulting in a technically sound and meaningful analysis. We can simply caution that analysts must contemplate the implications of their focus. Thus, attention directed toward alternative treatments of kidney disease was a meaningful focus in the context of the 1960s debate on national funding of kidney disease treatment, but it did not contribute to broadening legislators' perspectives to encompass the prevention of kidney disease. Recent consideration of revising public dialysis funding to include center and home dialysis called logically for analysis of the costs and benefits of alternative methods of dialysis; nevertheless, we would not want to lose sight of the apparently greater cost-effectiveness of transplantation (Klarman et al., 1968; Stange and Sumner, 1978; Roberts et al., 1980). Analyses of all delimited problems can and should assist policymakers by emphasizing what is excluded from consideration. Indeed, in the case of the study of the full range of approaches to kidney disease, including research, prevention, and early treatment, analysts should put their work in context by noting the relative importance (impact on health and social cost) of kidney disease and other illnesses.

While the starting point of health care CBA-CEAs is best formulated as a health problem, in recent years the starting point often has been a specific medical technology—a piece of equipment, a facility, or a procedure. Instead of considering alternative means of ameliorating a social problem, analysts examine the ability of a given technology to accomplish a social objective efficiently. Technology as the starting point permits very detailed, potentially more rigorous analysis, but it sacrifices the ability to compare alternative approaches to basic health problems. In essence, it risks missing the forest for the trees. An analysis of alternative forms of kidney dialysis is a case in point. Probably the most difficult of all types of technologies to analyze are diagnostic techniques, such as CT scanning, since their ultimate impacts on health often remain a matter of conjecture. Analysis of diagnostic technologies frequently must resort to intermediate outcomes that are hoped to contribute to health (for example, the number or quality, or both, of diagnoses).

Identification of the health problem or technology obviously defines many of the limits of ensuing analysis, but a closely related second step has at least comparable influence on all that follows. This is the setting of one or more concrete objectives against which programmatic alternatives are to be evaluated. The fundamental health problem may not be readily susceptible to measurement or formal specification; for example, the suffering and incapacity of victims of kidney disease has many dimensions, several clearly not quantifiable. Thus specific objectives must be selected in order to evaluate the effectiveness of alternative means of alleviating the suffering and incapacity. In the case of kidney disease, the common objective specified in most analyses has been the extension of life expectancy. Both direct and indirect attempts have been made to reflect the quality of the additional years.

Selection of an appropriate, measurable objective is not always easy. When HEW investigated alternative investments in illness prevention, the analysts recognized that the objective of saving lives was not a wholly suitable basis for comparing alternative programs. Alleviation of the pain and disability associated with arthritis would represent a major milestone in the history of health care, and a cost-effective one according to the analysts' cost-benefit calculations; but arrayed against other disease programs on the basis of dollars per life saved, the arthritis program understandably looked undesirable (Grosse, 1972b).

Another example clearly indicates the importance of careful attention to the link between general health problem and specific objective. The mortality and morbidity attributable to myocardial infarction certainly constitute an important health problem. However, approaches to reducing the problem may vary radically, depending on which of two ostensibly reasonable objectives an analyst selects: reducing the mortality rate of victims or reducing the incidence of myocardial infarctions. The former objective suggests a variety of emergency treatment alternatives, including improved mobile emergency medical service units, better equipped and accessible hospital emergency rooms, a 911 emergency telephone system, and a community cardiopulmonary resuscitation

(CPR) education program. The latter objective suggests prevention efforts, including patient education and community media programs promoting healthful behavior. Neither specification of the objective, however, has room for the alternative programs recommended by the other. In other words, a prevention program will have relatively little impact on reducing postinfarction mortality, while treatment efforts will not reduce the incidence of myocardial infarctions.

The incompatibility of these objectives does not imply that one is not valid or is inferior to the other. Rather, the two are independent and complementary. Each addresses the basic health problem—mortality and morbidity due to myocardial infarctions—but from a different point in the history of the disease. When analysts encounter this dilemma, they must decide whether to suboptimize (focus on one of the subproblems represented by the different objectives) or to search for a measurable objective that incorporates all relevant concerns. In the case of myocardial infarctions, a useful objective might be to reduce the number of years of life lost because of them. Both prevention and treatment alternatives are consistent with this objective.

The ideal objective, or outcome measure, is often elusive. In the case just mentioned, morbidity is considered only inadvertently, if at all. Postinfarction years of life, in which activities are restricted, are weighted equally with years saved due to prevented myocardial infarctions. When confronted with such inadequacies in an objective, some analysts will attempt to fine tune it (weighting years of life saved by a quality-of-life index, for example); others will employ multiple objectives; still others will simply acknowledge the limitations of their objectives. We discuss the various approaches later in this chapter.

The selection of a measurable objective sets the tone for the remainder of the analysis. Given the multiple dimensions of most health problems, it is particularly important that the objective(s) specified directly address the most important dimension(s). Further, it is desirable that the objective(s) be representative of nonspecified health impacts. For example, seeking a reduction in deaths caused by traffic accidents may imply a proportionate decrease in serious disability.

One common set of dimensions of health problems raises a special challenge for the analyst: the nonmeasurable goals and outcomes of many health programs. Certainly the reduction of pain and suffering is a central goal of much health care, yet success in this regard often must be evaluated subjectively or limited to a nonquantitative ranking of accomplishment. This puts the health care analyst in something of a quandary: it is commonly assumed that outcomes must be measurable in order to carry out a successful CBA-CEA, yet many important health care problems do not lend themselves readily to quantification. What should the analyst do? Ignore such problems? Evaluate them only according to their measurable dimensions? There are no easy answers to such questions. To ignore the problems altogether or to concentrate on their measurable dimensions—common practices in health care CBA-CEA—could be to relegate analytically messy health problems to the bottom of the resource allocation priority list, or, at best, to focus policymakers' attention solely on the quantifiable dimensions of problems. Yet trying to quantify the unquantifiable may be a waste of scarce analytical resources.

An example should help to clarify the nature of this quandary. Should the government help develop and fund care in hospices? The goal of hospice care is to allow the dying to die in comfort and with dignity, two objectively unquantifiable outcomes. If government analysts restricted their attention to an economic comparison of high quality hospice care and the more traditional means of dealing with death, with number of deaths as the objective measure of outcome, the analysts might find the traditional system more cost-effective (that is, cheaper) and recommend against hospice care. But, of course, such an assessment would miss the point of the hospice care movement.

Occasionally analysis can produce a meaningful result relying on a secondary, but measurable, objective. When the alternative that dominates quantitatively in terms of the secondary objective also dominates qualitatively in terms of the primary (but unmeasurable) objective, that alternative clearly will be preferred. For example, suppose there is agreement that, for a significant proportion of the population, the quality of the death experience in hospice care is at least as satisfactory as, and probably more satisfactory than, that in the traditional system. If cost analysis revealed that hospice care was less expensive than traditional care, clearly funding of hospice care for those who desired it would represent a socially cost-effective decision.

IDENTIFYING ALTERNATIVES

Health problems can be addressed through a variety of qualitatively different approaches. When analysts speak of "alternatives" in the context of problem-solving, most often they have in mind explicit programs with budgets, organization, inputs, and outputs. Nevertheless, it is important to recognize that such flesh-and-blood programs represent only one type of approach to a health problem. Other types include legal requirements (such as prohibiting the sale of alcohol to minors), economic incentives (imposing a large excise tax on cigarettes), and persuasion (exhorting the public to wear seat belts). Such nonprogrammatic alternatives do not always lend themselves neatly to CBA-CEA because their costs are often quite difficult to assess. For example, a principal cost of prohibiting consumption of a given substance is the loss of the freedom to choose, but how is this to be valued? What is the social cost of increasing an excise tax on a deleterious product? Regardless of such measurement problems, analysts always should investigate the possibilities of nonprogrammatic alternatives, simply because they may be quite cost-effective.

As we discussed in the preceding section, defining a health problem and specific objective(s) delimits the alternative means of attacking the problem. If the problem is the consequences of kidney disease, all alternatives examined must address specifically those consequences. If the objective is to increase the life span of victims of kidney failure, prevention alternatives are precluded from consideration. If the objective is narrowed further, to finding cost-effective means of dialysis, kidney transplantation is eliminated from the set of relevant alternatives.

Circumscribing alternatives does not invariably define the alternatives an analyst will study. Most often, it simply identifies feasible alternatives from which the analyst will select a subset for the analysis. When the health problem and objectives are broad—for example, reducing mortality and morbidity caused by myocardial infarctions—the set of feasible alternatives is so large as to prohibit meaningful analysis of all of them, given the time and resources most analysts will have at their disposal. In such situations, it is incumbent upon analysts to select alternatives wisely, since alternatives excluded from the analysis may consequently drop out of contention for policy consideration. The following are useful rules of thumb:

— Select all alternatives believed to be potentially quite cost-effective.

— Select a variety of types of alternatives. For example, in investigating means of combating the ravages of kidney disease, analysts could include examples of research, prevention, early treatment, and treatment of end-stage disease. It would be less enlightening to focus solely on end-stage treatment alternatives. Similarly, in the case of reducing the toll of myocardial infarction, analysts should consider prevention alternatives (such as health education programs) and nontraditional treatment alternatives (such as community-based CPR education), as well as examples of traditional treatment modalities (such as emergency services). The exception to this rule occurs when analysts have good reason to believe that alternatives of one class dominate those of other classes.

— As representatives of classes of alternatives, select only those that are not clearly (or probably) dominated by others within their classes. For example, the evidence on kidney disease treatment techniques indicates that transplantation, when possible, is more cost-effective in prolonging useful life than any method of dialysis and that inpatient dialysis is the least cost-effective mode of dialysis. It would be illogical, therefore, to select inpatient dialysis as the only representative of end-stage treatment in a comparison of prevention, early treatment, and end-stage treatment of kidney disease.

— Select a sufficient number of alternatives to permit a broad understanding of the options available, but do not select so many that analytical depth must be significantly sacrificed. In other words, be sure that the analysis team can handle the alternatives selected in a manner that will prove technically meaningful.

— Finally, be aware of subtleties that may affect the comparability of alternatives. For example, a program to treat victims of myocardial infarction will benefit an older population more than would a prevention effort oriented toward altering deleterious life-styles early in life. If one is interested in benefiting only one of these age groups, one of the alternatives will be inappropriate. However, if all years of life are viewed as comparable, the difference in target groups may not matter for purposes of the analysis.

Selection of alternatives can be influenced by the alternatives' political and legal feasibility. A pragmatic analysis oriented toward short-term results may exclude all alternatives considered to be politically infeasible or at variance with the existing legal or bureaucratic structure. We referred above to the programmatic independence of many government agencies. Such independence suggests, for example, that a health planner might conclude that greater law enforcement or safer highway construction was the most cost-effective means of reducing highway fatalities; yet, if the planner wished to influence policy directly, he or she might feel compelled to concentrate on means of achieving a more responsive emergency medical care system, an effort in which the planning agency could exert its influence. The alternative to such a pragmatic, short-term perspective is a longer-term perspective, one that takes into consideration the potential for political change, for example. This perspective recommends that otherwise attractive alternatives not be dismissed on the grounds of short-term feasibility. Thus, the health planner interested in highway safety might examine a broad range of programmatic alternatives, including those under the purview of such agencies as the state police and highway department. The hope would be that relevant findings could be conveyed to these agencies and eventually translated into meaningful policy actions. We believe that an important role of analysis is to broaden perspective. As such, we feel that analysts, who undoubtedly must be attuned to the practical needs of their clients, should take advantage of their analytical hunting licenses and explore a full range of possibilities.

DESCRIBING PRODUCTION RELATIONSHIPS

Defining the health problem, objective(s), and alternatives establishes the conceptual framework of a CBA-CEA. The next step in analysis—describing production relationships—creates the technical framework for the quantitative assessment and comparison of costs and benefits of the alternatives. A description of the production relationship of a given alternative entails identifying the resources required by the alternative (for example, specific types of labor, equipment, supplies), explaining how they are combined, and predicting the outcome(s). Once this production relationship, or function, has been characterized, the analyst will have a specific basis for estimating costs and benefits.

Specifying production functions is one of the most technically challenging aspects of analysis. Production processes are frequently black boxes: we can see what goes into them (inputs) and what comes out (outputs) without knowing how inputs are transformed into outputs. Therefore, we cannot evaluate the efficiency of the process. Were the inputs combined in the right proportions? Were some of them unnecessary? In the case of a newly proposed program, the problem appears still more difficult because we may not even know which inputs are required to produce the desired output.

There are several methods for characterizing production relationships. Each involves developing a model that specifies how inputs are combined and how much output a given input configuration produces. A model is a representation of the production process, a characterization of its essential elements. A model can be as simple as a flow chart denoting inputs and their quantities, the points at which they are combined, and the resultant output, or it can be a sophisticated, multi-equation computer simulation.

Complexity in modeling production processes is not a virtue; sometimes, however, it is a necessity. As a rule of thumb, analysts should strive for the most straightforward characterization consistent with the demands of the problem. Often analysts can draw directly on past or existing experiences to model one or more of the alternatives they are investigating. For example, if a city is contemplating alternative means of reducing cardiovascular mortality, its analysts can turn to the experiences of other cities to gain understanding of a communitywide CPR program, to learn about upgrading emergency vehicles and the skills of their staff, or to explore hypertension detection and treatment programs.

In such cases, abstracting from the operational programs permits analysts to model hypothetical programs for their own communities. However, analysts must be careful not to assume that production processes transfer perfectly from one setting to another. In borrowing from the experiences of others, analysts must always pay attention to differences between existing programs and the potential new program. Examples of differences that should be taken into account include:

— Scale factors: The ratio of inputs to output will not necessarily remain constant as the size of the program changes. A program intended to serve a city of 100,000 may not require twice the inputs needed to serve a city of 50,000. Economies of scale—loosely, greater efficiency associated with greater size—may mean that fewer than twice as many inputs are needed. Conversely, coordination problems or the like may translate into input requirements more than twice those of the smaller city—diseconomies of scale. Analysts must attempt to anticipate such scale effects—they should be expected whenever program sizes differ significantly.

— Technical change: If relevant technology is changing, analysts have to adapt their models to account for it. For example, a hospital planner studying acquisition and installation of a new CT scanner in 1981 surely would not want to reproduce a CT facility dating from 1976. Technological change must be accounted for, and analysts should attempt to anticipate relevant changes in the near future.

— Market characteristics: Even if the existing program is not technically outdated, local market characteristics may recommend a different configuration of inputs. For example, if a community is experiencing a serious nursing shortage and must pay correspondingly high salaries to nurses, analysts should examine the possibility of substituting other personnel or even equipment in a hypertension clinic. An input mix that is efficient in one community may not be in another. As another example, consider the implications of heating costs for designing programs and structures in Minnesota modeled on programs in Arizona.

— Client, or patient, population characteristics: Different types of program populations will respond differently; such variations must be taken into account in modeling all aspects of program production relationships. For example, compare a hypertension program in a white-collar work setting and one offered in a black ghetto clinic. With hypertension more prevalent among blacks than whites, the latter program should identify a higher proportion of hypertensive persons among the population screened. However, differences in attitudes, beliefs, support systems, and so on might cause rates of compliance with instructions to seek care or take medicine daily to be greater in the white-collar work setting. All such differences will affect the productivity, and possibly the structure, of an optimal program.

— Inefficiency in the existing program: Just because a program exists, analysts should not assume that it is structured or functioning efficiently. Analysts should attempt to get inside the black box of the existing program to determine if it could be operated more efficiently. If the existing program employs physicians at tasks that could be handled equally effectively by nurses or technicians, and hence at considerably lower cost, the analyst should model the potential program with nonphysician personnel performing the relevant tasks.

— Unique inputs in the existing program: Existing programs may benefit from resources that cannot be made available for a new program. The former may have a monopoly on the requisite expertise or a facility that cannot be duplicated economically. A prominent illustration is the case of heart transplantation, a procedure now performed with moderate success by the team at Stanford, but one that other medical teams have not been able to match. Analysts must ascertain whether or not existing programs, examined for modeling purposes, depend fundamentally on inputs that will become unavailable in the new setting.

Techniques frequently applied in modeling production relationships go by such forbidding names as Monte Carlo and Markov Chain models, queuing models, decision analysis, and linear programming. We do not intend to familiarize the reader with these techniques—that task requires a book in itself[3]—but we do wish to emphasize that a variety of mathematical approaches exists. Effective use of these techniques is an integral component of the science of analysis; selection of appropriate techniques is an element of the art of analysis. The frequent need for, or benefit from, using mathematical modeling techniques underscores the advantage of analysts' having relevant technical training. Whether or not they are so trained themselves, they should appreciate the potential for enriching CBA-CEAs by using technical consultants in assessing production processes.

Several technical aspects of assessing production relationships span the variety of modeling techniques. Here we discuss two issues frequently encountered in health care CBA-CEA.

One is the need to analyze production from the perspective of marginal inputs and outputs; that is, for each additional unit of an input or complement of inputs, how much additional output will be gained? The tendency is to examine a single total program and then rely on average rather than marginal assessment of inputs needed to produce a unit of output. This tendency has two weaknesses: first, by failing to observe what occurs at the margin, the analyst generally cannot determine optimal program size. A given total output might appear quite attractive compared with the total inputs required to produce it, but the program might appear still more attractive if one had the information that, on the margin, a reduction of output of, say, 1 percent would decrease input needs by 25 percent.[4] Second, the health policy question is often whether an existing program or activity should be expanded. In such cases, the only relevant analysis is a comparison of the prospective additions to both inputs and output. Consideration of the total or average inputs and output for the enlarged program has little relevance, since the question is whether expansion should occur given the base program. The basic principle—assessment of inputs and outputs, costs and benefits, at the margin—lies at the heart of all economic analysis.

The second technical issue relates to marginal analysis, but it is not as easily resolved. This is the problem of joint production, a process in which a single production effort produces multiple outputs. Although each output may be valuable, only one is of interest. For example, a blood sample can be drawn to test for a given disease, but when the blood is put into an automated, multichannel chemistry analyzer, the sample will receive up to thirty-eight tests, for multiple diseases. Hence it would not be appropriate to attribute all of the technology's cost to the single diagnosis of interest; neither is it obvious how to separate out the diagnosis-specific inputs. The principle is that described in the preceeding paragraph: identify the marginal inputs needed for the diagnosis. But it is not clear how this principle should be implemented in the case of joint products. While there is a conceptual difficulty here, the practical problem involves accounting, and there are standard, albeit often arbitrary, accounting procedures available. At the very least, the analyst has a clear responsibility to explore and enumerate the other joint products.

Conceptually, the basic features of production relationships do not vary across substantive fields. Practically, however, the health and other social service fields confront analysts with certain specific problems regarding the modeling of production relationships. First and foremost among these is the relative intangibility of the intended output—in this case, health. As we noted above and discuss below, analysts invariably must settle for some incomplete index of health, such as life expectancy or days of morbidity. Second, and often most perplexing, is the difficulty of associating specific health care activities with objective health outcomes. Illustrative of this problem are attempts to relate diagnostic procedures to their ultimate health effects. What effect do electrocardiograms (EKGs) have on health? How about CT scans?[5]

In such instances, a common, if imperfect, resolution is to assume the health relevance of the intermediate outcome—in this case, the diagnosis—and then structure the production relationship to run from inputs to intermediate outcome. This, of course, is relatively straightforward. The assumption of health relevance follows in the tradition of health care evaluation, in which the structure or process of care has constituted the focal point for the attention of would-be evaluators (Donabedian, 1969). Early efforts to evaluate health care concentrated on assessing the amount and quality of program inputs—structure. Having more doctors and nurses was regarded as better than having fewer, board-certified specialists represented higher quality than general practitioners, and new facilities were superior to old ones. More recently, process measures—assessment of the manner in which health care is practiced compared to a specified norm—have come to dominate health care evaluation. Peer review and medical audit are examples, both the work of PSROs. Process evaluation seems to be a more valid measure of the quality of health care than is structure evaluation; nevertheless, each assumes the value of the output of the process. In recent years, strides have been made toward evaluating the outcomes of care, but, for a set of medical activities, including many diagnostic techniques, successful outcome assessment seems distant.

Regardless of the method chosen, description of production relationships for each alternative in a CBA-CEA establishes the framework for the remainder of the analysis. Identification of inputs and outputs and specification of the linkage between them provides the basis for estmating costs and benefits (or effectiveness).

COSTS, BENEFITS, AND EFFECTIVENESS

At the heart of every CBA and CEA is the identification, measurement, and valuation of the costs and benefits (or effectiveness) associated with the production process. The identification and measurement procedures for both techniques are essentially the same; it is during the valuation process and in the final accounting that they differ. As the reader will recall, the principal difference is that CBA requires all costs and benefits to be valued in monetary terms, whereas CEA requires only costs to be so valued.

There are other, less obvious differences, however. One of the inherent difficulties of describing the elements of both CBA and CEA simultaneously, as we do in this chapter, is that, despite the fundamental conceptual similarities of the two methodologies, details sometimes differ for technical reasons. The classification of costs and benefits is one such example. It is convenient to look upon costs as those resources that one must give up in order to gain some benefit or desired effect. Conversely, benefits are desired outcomes derived from the expenditure of resources. These definitions hold for the costs of buying or implementing the activity being assessed and for the health benefits attributable to the activity. But what of the medical cost savings that may result? Are they benefits, or are they negative costs (that is, are they to be subtracted from the activity's cost)? The answer is either. In CBA, costs are commonly considered to be only those costs directly associated with the activity being assessed (which includes the expenditure of indirect costs such as time and lost productivity). All desirable changes in resources resulting from those costs, including medical cost savings, are treated as benefits. In CEA, on the other hand, all net changes in medical and health costs, measured in dollars, are compared with all net changes in health benefits, measured in some nonmonetary unit(s). This requires that medical cost savings be treated as negative costs rather than as benefits. In this chapter, for the convenience of exposition, we will consider medical cost reduction under the discussion of benefits. Later in the chapter, we will investigate the potential importance of these different ways of handling such outcomes.

In the following two sections, we examine costs and benefits (effectiveness) in terms of their identification, measurement, and, where appropriate, valuation. Separating cost and benefit analysis into these three steps permits us to consider intangible or non-quantifiable costs and benefits, which can be identified but not measured, as well as the more traditional measurable costs and benefits of CBA-CEA.

COSTS

Identification

It is often suggested that costs are easier to determine than benefits. The manner in which many analysts assess costs supports this perception. A common practice is to take an accounting approach to estimating costs, simply identifying and adding up dollar expenditures. As we shall see, this practice is far from the theoretically desirable approach to assessing costs.

A principal concept of economics is opportunity cost, the basis for estimating costs in a CBA-CEA. The opportunity cost of a resource is its value in another use. That is, if we did not use resource A in project X, what would its value be in project Y? Thus the true cost of a resource is not necessarily its market price tag. Rather, it is what we must give up elsewhere if we choose to use the resource here.

An illustration should help to clarify the difference between a market price tag and a resource's opportunity cost. To a hospital accountant, volunteers' time is free; it is not found on the hospital's wage bill, and the accountant would ignore it. But is not volunteer labor a true cost of running the hospital? Volunteers definitely contribute to the output of the hospital. If their labor had been donated elsewhere, it would clearly have had value. In essence, the opportunity of using the labor productively in other activities has been foregone. In a social CBA-CEA, the volunteers' time should be included in an assessment of costs. Although determining an appropriate dollar value may be difficult, the social value of volunteer time should not be ignored.

To identify the costs of a given activity, analysts must enumerate all resources expended to produce the desired benefit (effectiveness). Some of these, perhaps most, will be obvious, including program labor, supplies, capital equipment, and so on. These are direct costs, resources purchased directly to run the activity. Indirect costs—resources consumed indirectly in the production process—may be less obvious. An example of the latter is the value of patients' time, the value of patients' using their time in other productive activities. Another indirect cost is the fear induced in prospective patients or, for example, the pain resulting from an inoculation. Again, from the program manager's perspective, these costs may be irrelevant. From a social point of view, however, they command attention. Indicative of the importance of indirect costs such as pain is the fact that they are often sufficient to convince people not to seek a service that they perceive to be of some value, even when it is provided free of charge. An example is the large number of people who choose not to receive publicly provided immunizations. These indirect costs of health care illustrate the kind of cost that can be identified but that is extremely difficult to measure or value.

It is crucial that analysts begin cost analyses by identifying the actual inputs used and, where possible, their quantities. In essence, this should be reflected in a well-specified production function. There is a temptation, yielded to frequently, to skip this step and use available data on the costs or charges for relevant services. In the discussion of valuation, we shall see how misleading this can be in evaluating health care program costs.

Several resource identification problems arise in many cost analyses. Some of these are generic in CBA-CEA; others are more specific to the health care setting. Among the generic problems are the following:

— How does one treat resources devoted to research and development (R&D) activities? Where the R&D is an integral component of the immediate program in question (for example, when analyzing the costs and benefits of a new technology in a medical research center), its resources should be included with the program's operating inputs. When the R&D has preceded the program being evaluated (that is, its existence is independent of the immediate policy decision) its resources should be excluded from consideration.

— How should analysts deal with overhead? There is no easy answer to this question. If the production process at issue is truly marginal to the overall enterprise, one might be tempted to ignore overhead, to look only at the marginal resource needs associated with the program. However, if the existence of some of the overhead depends on the program in question, clearly it must be identified and included. The general principle of seeking the marginal inputs still holds, but often analysts may have to attribute to the program a share of overhead proportional to the program's share of the total enterprise.

— How does one determine resource usage when the production process produces two or more joint products? Analytically this problem is quite similar to the preceding one, and one must attempt to follow the marginal resource consumption principle, recognizing the possible need for averaging. In both this instance and the proceeding one, consultation with accountants may prove helpful.

A fourth resource identification problem, although not unique to health care, occurs so frequently in the health care context that it is worthy of special attention. This is the case of an expensive resource being used to perform a function a less expensive resource could perform at least as well. Examples are physicians giving immunizations (instead of nurses), registered nurses making hospital beds (instead of aides), and dentists cleaning teeth (instead of hygienists). In each of these cases, use of the more expensive resource is clearly socially inefficient, yet law or custom may preclude realization of the more efficient resource allocation. Therefore, how should the analyst identify inputs? Where the less expensive inputs truly cannot be employed, whether for legal or other reasons, we would recommend counting the physician's (or nurse's or dentist's) time as the relevant input, for this is indeed the input on which a future program will have to rely. If, however, the more efficient resource allocation is a possibility, the analyst should identify the efficient input mix. Often there is a fine line between whether or not a given input can be used. If analysts feel uncomfortable drawing that line, they can identify costs under two different conditions: one using the customary input, the other using the more efficient input.

Measurement

The process of quantifying—measuring—the inputs of a given programmatic alternative is generally straightforward. It should result from the specification of the production process and identification of inputs. Commonly, measurement takes the form of simply counting the number of hours or days required of each of the types of labor, the physical quantities of the various supplies, the amount of use of capital goods and facilities, and so on. In order to compare alternative programs, analysts should seek to determine the most efficient input mix for each. Thus, the measurement process should assume efficiency and count the minimum resource needs rather than the quantities consumed in existing, inefficient operations. Of course, resource needs will vary according to several factors, such as the scale of the program. These should be imbedded in the specification of the production process, but they warrant repeated attention at the stage of estimating specific resource needs.

As the preceding discussion suggests, some costs are relatively intangible or unquantifiable. To date, techniques for reliable and valid measurement of quantities of pain or fear must be deemed no more than a remote prospect for the future; this is why it is important that such costs receive emphasis in the identification stage of cost analysis. The tendency in cost analyses is to relegate such unquantifiable costs (and, for that matter, benefits) to a footnote. That is, hard-to-measure costs are identified qualitatively and then dropped out of the analysis. We acknowledge the difficulty, even impossibility, of quantifying such costs, but, rather than dismiss them, the analyst should keep them simmering on a back burner, to be poured back into the analytical stew at the conclusion of the analysis. As we will discuss later, indirect values for such costs often can be ascertained once all readily measured variables have been taken into account.

Even the tangible, quantifiable inputs can be a source of frustration for analysts. Particularly when analysis has a prospective intent, the need to estimate quantities often arises. While an ultimate goal of analysis is precision, analysts should recognize the value of even rough estimates in permitting completion of an otherwise unapproachable analysis. We do not advocate indiscriminate guessing, but we do perceive a role for educated guesses supported by sensitivity analysis, an important CBA-CEA tool that permits determination of the importance of precision in measuring variables. Sensitivity analysis is discussed in detail later in this chapter.

Valuation

The conversion of quantities of inputs into dollars of cost is the final step in basic cost analysis. Many analysts take a rather cavalier approach to the conversion, relying directly and uncritically on market prices for this purpose. In a theoretical world of perfect competition, market prices do reflect the true opportunity costs of resources. In many parts of our nontheoretical and imperfectly competitive world, market prices constitute adequate measures of true opportunity costs, with no obviously preferable measures coming to mind. If analysts do not find the need for adjustments after they have contemplated problems with market prices, the market prices can be used to reflect opportunity costs and convert quantities of inputs into dollars.

Uncritical use of market prices, however, can lead to large gaps between cost estimates and true costs. Illustrative of this problem is the use of hospital charge data to reflect the costs of hospital care. A common practice, this form of pricing ignores the known idiosyncrasies of hospital accounting, in which hospitals charge well above true marginal costs for certain services and use the profits therefrom to subsidize other services for which charges do not cover marginal costs. If the deviations from marginal costs were small, one might reconcile acceptance of imperfect hospital data as a readily available source of information providing a qualitatively valid picture. However, studies of the discrepancies between charges and true costs show dramatic differences. For example, hospital pharmacy charges can range from 10 to 1,000 percent of the true costs of drugs, depending on the frequency of their use, level of cost, purpose, and so on.

When we dealt with the question of whether volunteer labor should be treated as a regular input for purposes of a CBA-CEA, we concluded that it should be, when concern is with the true social opportunity costs of the project in question. The problem in the valuation phase of cost analysis is that the market obviously does not provide direct price data to guide the analyst in valuing volunteer labor. In such cases, the analyst must impute a price, a value approximating the true opportunity cost of the volunteers' time. Often this is neither as difficult nor as capricious as it might sound. If the volunteers' efforts have close market analogues—paid employees who perform similar tasks—one can use the paid employees' wage rate as the price of the volunteers' time. The most common illustration of this approach to imputing the value of unpriced labor is the use of domestics' wage rates to value the time of persons engaged in unpaid housework in their own homes. Obviously, this is not the only conceivable, nor even necessarily the most logical, means of determining the cost of unpriced labor, but it does have conceptual appeal. Furthermore, the precision with which this imputation captures true social value may not be of great importance. As we shall see in the discussion of sensitivity analysis, substantial deviations from true value often will not affect the qualitative findings of an analysis.

A final issue in valuing costs relates to the treatment of the standard use of inefficient inputs. As we noted above, law or custom often restrains less well trained health care personnel from providing in the health care field services they are quite capable of providing with the highest of quality. Social efficiency might call for use of the less well trained individuals, hence their wage rates would constitute an appropriate means of valuing the opportunity cost of the relevant input. However, if it is clear to the analyst that the more expensive professionals will have to perform the tasks in question, it seems prudent in cost analysis to use the value of their time, which is indeed the opportunity cost of their engaging in these activities. Such programs will appear more expensive or less efficient than necessary, but they will constitute the appropriate basis for comparing these activities with alternative uses of resources. In general, the cost chosen will reflect the purpose of the analysis. If the analysis is oriented toward resolving a practical, short-term resource allocation issue, use of the higher cost will represent the necessary reality. If, however, the analysis is targeted toward a policy level at which established practices can be challenged, use of the lower cost estimate can serve to inform the health care community, a legislative body, or the public how attractive a program might be. In any case, it is always safe, and often enlightening, to test the effects of both cost estimates.

We close the discussion of valuation by reiterating a caveat that analysts must keep in mind constantly: certain costs cannot be valued in a meaningful fashion—for example, pain and suffering—but analysts' inability to take them to and through the valuation stage is no excuse for ignoring them in the final cost-benefit calculus. Even when it is not possible to indirectly or implicitly value such costs, it is incumbent on analysts to bring the immeasurable to the fore when measured costs and benefits are being compared.

BENEFITS AND EFFECTIVENESS[6]

Identification

The benefits of health care programs are numerous, diverse, often obscure, and often hard to measure. Trying to identify benefits is a rewarding component of the analytical process, especially for the nonmedical professional interested in health care. For example, a CEA of alternative diagnostic techniques forces analysts to come to grips with the potential indirect benefits of diagnosis—that is, benefits other than a direct improvement in prognosis or even in patient management. An analysis of noncurative therapeutic techniques confronts analysts with the intangible benefits associated with the caring function, the alleviation of pain, and so on.

There is no single "right" way to categorize benefits, but the following classification scheme may assist analysts in contemplating the full range of types of benefits that may be associated with given health care activity.

Personal Health Benefits

The primary function of health care is to enhance the health and well-being of individuals. Thus, principal benefits considered in health care CBA-CEAs are improvements in health. Notable among these are increased life expentancy, decreased morbidity, and reduced disability. Most often, of course, analyses address specific health problems, hence benefit assessments focus on a subset of one or more of these outcomes. Other elements of enhanced well-being, such as reduced pain or suffering or lowered anxiety, constitute common and important benefits of health care that are not often found in CBA-CEAs, usually because of the difficulty of measuring them or because of the misspecification of the objectives of the health care program.

Health Care Resource Benefits

Many health care activities have an impact on the consumption of health care resources beyond the activities themselves. Treatment of high blood pressure can decrease the number of later medical crises and the consumption of associated medical resources. Indeed, this is a basic intent of such treatment. While the principal purpose is realization of the personal health benefit, the health care resource savings constitute both a predictable benefit sought by planners and a potential source of interest to health insurers. These potential savings are often cited as benefits of disease prevention and health promotion activities.

It must be realized that not all effects on health care resources will be positive. For example, screening programs often find disease in asymptomatic individuals. The resource consumption required to care for such persons must be considered a cost.

In both cases—medical resource savings and resource consumption attributable to the program—the shift in health care resources must be taken into account in identifying costs and benefits.

Other Economic Benefits

Many of the desirable outcomes of health care programs cannot be identified as either health or health care benefits. A major benefit of numerous health-enhancing activities is an increase in work productivity. Illness restricts both the time individuals can work and their productivity on the job. Thus decreases in morbidity and disability can translate into improvements in work output. Similarly, reductions in or avoidance of various disabilities can reduce accident rates, with an attendant savings in property damage.

Such effects are clear benefits of the programs in question, making an economic contribution to both the individual and society. Often that contribution can be as significant as, or more significant than, the contribution to better health. However, in that such benefits are indirect—removed from the immediate health effects and from the health care arena—they are less obvious. Analysts must take special care to identify all of the major benefits in this category.

Other Social Benefits

Health care activities can confer benefits related to broad social objectives. For example, Medicare and Medicaid were intended to foster more equitable access to society's health care resources. Thus, in addition to any improvements in health that might be attributed to these programs, one must count the increased access to services of the poor and elderly as a social benefit in and of itself. Similarly, legislation in the late 1960s providing for public funding of kidney dialysis reassured the nation of its collective compassion. This, too, ranks as a benefit above and beyond the greater longevity experienced by dialyzed patients. All such positive social effects should be identified in an accounting of benefits.

Intermediate Outcomes

Whenever possible, the benefits of health care programs should be identified in terms of final outcomes, the kinds of outcomes discussed in the four preceding classes of benefits. Unfortunately, as we have noted above, final outcomes cannot always be ascertained. In many diagnostic procedures, the clearly identifiable outcome—the diagnosis—does not invariably define the final health outcome. The link between this intermediate outcome and its effects on health is often a matter only for conjecture. In such cases, analysts may have to restrict their attention on the benefits side to the quantity, quality, or both, of the intermediate outcome. Thus one can discuss the relative cost-effectiveness of CT scanning, angiograpy, and pneumoencephalography as means of diagnosing intracranial tumors, but assessing the ultimate impact on the health of the patient remains a matter of educated guesswork. In such cases, analysts may have to accept the intermediate outcome as the focal point in assessing effectiveness, but they should explore other outcomes as well. In the case of diagnosis, some benefits are easy to overlook: diagnoses can resolve nagging uncertainty for both patient and physician; they can define, or for that matter avoid, therapeutic interventions; and they can contribute to the growth of medical knowledge. Of course, whenever it is possible to link soundly a diagnostic procedure to a final outcome, it should be done. Several analysts have used probabilistic approaches to specifying pathways linking diagnosis to treatment and outcomes (Eddy, 1980b; Knox, 1976; Luce, 1981; McNeil et al., 1975a). Refinements in such work should close the gap between diagnosis and its outcomes.

Diagnostic procedures are not the only health care activities in which analysts commonly rely on intermediate outcomes on the benefit side of CBA-CEA. Short-term studies of activities to promote health often assess outcome in terms of behavior changes—an intermediate outcome with the link to health status assumed. Examples are efforts to decrease cholesterol intake or reduce weight. In any such case, analysts should explicitly state their assumptions about impacts on health.

Measurement

The measurement of many types of benefits is straightforward. Tangible personal health benefits can be measured in terms of years of life saved, months of disability avoided, or days of morbidity averted. Theoretically, health care resource benefits should be measured in physicial units reflecting the resources saved, such as hours of physician time, days of hospital bed occupancy, and so on. In practice, health care resource benefits commonly are measured directly in dollars and cents, thereby blending the benefit measurement and valuation tasks. Other economic benefits are counted in terms of obvious units; in the case of productivity losses averted, days of work loss avoided serves as a useful measure. In the case of intermediate outcomes, measurement again relies on obvious units, such as the number of accurate tests, in the case of diagnostic techniques, or pounds lost, in the case of a weight-control program.

A major roadblock to benefit assessment is the measurement of intangible benefits. Examples are important personal health benefits, such as alleviation of pain and suffering, and social benefits, such as achieving a more egalitarian distribution of health care services. These illustrate important outcomes of health care programs that should not be ignored but often are because their measurement is controversial. Frequently, analysts must accept the fact that some benefits cannot be quantified and find ways to proceed with the quantitative analysis without losing sight of these benefits. Later in this chapter we explore means of accomplishing this.

Often the quantities of benefits deriving from health care activities can be estimated only with a great deal of uncertainty about the estimates' validity or reliability. Lack of precision is a hazard associated with many, if not most, social policy analyses. While it must always remain a conscious concern, we have techniques that permit determination of the importance of the imprecision. Collectively known as sensitivity analysis, these techniques are examined below in the discussion of dealing with uncertainty. Here we suggest simply that analysts should not be intimidated by the need to estimate the magnitude of benefits (or costs). They should strive for reasonable, logical estimation procedures.

As a final issue in the measurement of benefits, we note that many health care activities have multiple important outcomes and therefore the measurement of an activity's benefits may require several quantified outcomes. Thus an illness-avoidance immunization program should be evaluated in terms of the number of deaths it prevents, the amount of morbidity and disability it averts, the quantity of future health care resources it saves, and so on. The process of valuing benefits in monetary terms, the next step in CBA and the next topic in our presentation, allows analysts to combine such divergent outcomes into a common benefit metric. In CEA, in which effectiveness is measured in nonmonetary units, this is not always possible; one may be left with an effectiveness package of two dozen apples and three dozen oranges. Toward the end of this chapter we address the question of how one deals with multiple, noncommensurate effectiveness measures. Here we simply acknowledge that this can and will happen and that, unless analysts can settle on a single effectiveness measure as representative of the entire package of benefits, they will have to deal with the problem in presenting and interpreting their findings.

Valuation

In CEA, analysts do not attempt to value program effectiveness in monetary units. Consequently the task of effectiveness assessment ceases when the measurement phase is completed.[7] In CBA, by contrast, translating outcome quantities into dollar values constitutes a central feature of analysis. In this section we discuss the procedures for valuing benefits, some well accepted and straightforward, others quite controversial.

For those benefits directly associated with market prices, benefit valuation is easy, assuming that one accepts the market prices as reflecting opportunity costs. Health care resource savings represent a common use of market prices to establish the economic value of benefits. In the case of certain indirect economic benefits attributable to health care programs, market values are also generally accepted as good indices of benefits' values; the use of wage rates to value hours of work-loss averted is a prominent example.

In instances where market prices are not associated directly with realized benefits, imputed prices can serve to value the benefits. For example, hospital volunteers may not be paid for their work, yet it is clearly productive activity. The market for similar labor, both inside and outside of the hospital, provides a value for unpaid volunteer time. Thus, if a health program reduces illness among hospital volunteers, this benefit can be valued by multiplying the work hours saved by the appropriate market wage rate.

Certain basic health program benefits, such as the avoidance of premature mortality or unnecessary morbidity, do not lend themselves to a single, obvious method of monetary valuation. Nevertheless, they are central to health care activities and valuation of them is essential if one is to undertake a CBA. If placing a value on such benefits is regarded as impossible or undesirable, CBA can be rejected and CEA adopted. However, the desire to value these outcomes for purposes of CBA has created a substantial theoretical and empirical literature on the dilemma. It is safe to say that this dilemma, inappropriately labeled the "value of life" problem, constitutes one of the most controversial issues in health care CBA.

We now examine the basic techniques for valuing health benefits.

Human Capital

The oldest and most common means of valuing personal health benefits is the human capital approach. As its name suggests, this approach views the value of personal health benefits as the economic productivity they permit to take place. That is, by avoiding a fatal or debilitating illness, a program allows individuals to remain productively employed in the labor market. The value of their economic contribution, measured as earnings, constitutes the value of avoiding work loss. In essence, the human being is viewed as a capital investment, the sole purpose of which is economically productive output. This indirect benefit is added to health care resource savings to determine total benefits.

The technical steps in the human capital approach are

straightforward, though not devoid of assumptions and occasional rough estimates. First, analysts aggregate years of work loss that would occur without a health program, loss caused by premature mortality and avoidable morbidity and disability. Work loss is categorized by age, sex, and occupation. Appropriate wage rates, reflecting the value of productivity, are applied to the hours of work loss in each group and added up. For those groups lacking a market wage, values are imputed from related market data—for example, the wage rates for housecleaners are applied to hours spent by individuals working in their own homes.

Almost all CBAs use this gross measure of productivity savings. Years ago, a debate raged briefly in which some analysts argued in favor of using net productivity savings—gross productivity minus the affected individuals' own consumption. Use of net productivity would mean that the human capital approach would attribute no value to the years saved for individuals who consumed goods and services equal in value to their productivity. The gross measure won out on the argument that the individuals' own consumption provided them with utility (loosely, satisfaction) and that, as members of society, their utility should count in an assessment of social welfare. A literal view of the notion of human capital might suggest that essential, or subsistence, costs of living should be deducted from gross productivity. These costs would be much less than those represented in typical consumption patterns in industrialized countries. To date, this variant has never been applied in the health care CBA-CEA literature.

The human capital approach has raised the ire of numerous observers. Critics note that the approach values years saved for working-age white males more than those saved for the elderly, the very young, women, and blacks and other minorities. This reflects the typical employment and wage patterns of these groups in today's marketplace. Thus, the critics argue, the human capital approach thereby attributes more value to the life of a white male than to that of other people. Aside from this being distasteful, the human capital approach means that programs benefiting the health of working-age white males will look better on cost-benefit grounds than programs having equal or even superior health effects on other population groups.

A second major problem with the human capital approach is that it does not measure the value of life; rather, it measures the market value of livelihood. To be sure, the productive potential in an individual represents something of value to society, but it is not the full measure of either the individual's self-valuation of life or of society's valuation of the individual's life. This limitation of the human capital approach is particularly important in that it strikes at the very characteristic of CBA which proponents cite as making the technique so appealing: all benefits are measured in a common metric (dollars), thereby allowing assessment of inherent program worth and direct comparison of programs having different objectives. Yet here we observe that the human capital approach, and hence the vast majority of CBAs that have relied on it, omits a major benefit—the value of life above and beyond economic productivity. Many analysts share the misconception that the approach attributes a value to life itself.

Willingness to Pay

In order to address this weakness of the human capital approach, some analysts have been struggling to develop a method to value life itself. Called the willingness-to-pay approach, the notion is to measure the value that individuals place on reducing risks of death and illness. Conceptually the approach has much appeal: within the determined values rest individuals' valuation of the physical and emotional costs of illness, for themselves and others. That is, one can value a reduction in risk for its benefit to someone, even if that someone is not oneself. Practically, the difficulty of translating concept into reliable numbers is enormous. Analysts have tried several techniques, most commonly asking people to value small reductions in the risk of death or debility and then imputing the value of life from such numbers. Unfortunately, imputed values of life can vary dramatically depending on the wording of substantively identical questions.[8] Another technique of the willingness-to-pay approach is to attempt to assess the risk premium paid to workers engaged in high-risk occupations—for example, comparing the wages of construction workers building bridges with those of other construction workers performing similar tasks in less risky circumstances. This technique, which conceptually allows an objective measurement of how people value risk, has several problems, including the myopia of the risk-takers, the fact that they may be less averse to taking risks than other people, and the fact that the technique does not apply to important segments of the population, including young children and the elderly. Thus, there is no satisfactory means to date of generating consistent and useful numbers for willingness-to-pay valuation of life. Furthermore, even if valid and consistent numbers could be developed, willingness to pay shares with the human capital approach the problem of rating the life of a wealthy individual higher than that of a poor person, since the former would be able, and hence willing, to pay more to reduce risk.

Other Approaches
There are still other methods of estimating the value of life. One is to use court awards in civil cases as estimates because they combine productive value lost and emotional costs. Unfortunately, court awards vary substantially from one case to the next, with the variations unrelated to probable productivity and emotional cost differences. Still another method suggested to value life is to impute values from life insurance holdings. But life insurance measures individuals' perceptions of risks and assessments of their value to others, not themselves; insurance does not decrease their own risks.

Whatever its limitations—and they are significant—the human capital approach continues to predominate in health care CBA. However, this approach—and hence most CBAs—cannot be construed as incorporating the value of life in the cost-benefit calculus. In effect, CBA is not necessarily more complete or comprehensive than CEA, since the former fully excludes the nonmarket value of life, while the latter includes it, implicitly yet quantitatively, in measures such as deaths averted or years of life saved. The possibility of combining the merits of both CBA and CEA has led in recent years to several analyses that retain a nonmonetary effectiveness measure as the bottom line but that include monetary economic benefits on the cost side of the equation as negative costs. While we are not aware of many examples, it would certainly be possible to estimate all economic benefits, including the value of productivity losses averted, and include them in a CEA as negative costs. In such a case, the nonmonetary effectiveness measure could be judged against a more comprehensive assessment of economic impacts.

Notwithstanding the elusiveness of a value of life measure, the search for one is likely to persist. Herbert Klarman (1974*a*, p. 335) characterized the importance of this search as follows:

> As Mishan observes, a rough measure of a precise concept is superior to a precise measure of an erroneous concept. It is agreed that the notion of the value of human life, apart from livelihood, is sound. And a numerical estimate of this value would be useful in comparing how worthwhile alternative programs are. Comparisons of programs would gain in relevance and aptness if all benefits were counted,

including saving of human life or gains in life expectancy. This potential gain is much more likely to be realized if all benefits are entered into the model, rather than having some appear only in footnotes.

Cost-effectiveness analysis seems to attempt to avoid this valuation controversy by simply counting health benefits (such as years of life saved) and not transforming the numbers into money. However, once money is allocated (or not allocated) to save lives, the implicit minimum (or maximum) value of life can be imputed, an important point that is often overlooked. For example, if a program is estimated to cost $25,000 per year of life saved and the program is implemented, the policymakers are stating implicitly that they believe a year of life to be worth at least $25,000 (assuming, of course, that they believe the analysis). By contrast, if a program costing $50,000 per year of life saved is rejected, the decision-makers are announcing, again implicitly, that they do not believe the years are worth that much. Thus the conceptual difference between CBA and CEA appears to be less than their definitions might suggest: in CBA, analysts explicitly place values on life; in CEA, analysts provide decision-makers with data that assist them in valuing life implicitly.

A common misconception about the two techniques' approaches to valuing personal health benefits is that CEA avoids value judgments, while CBA requires them. In fact, the value judgments in CEA are often subtle, implicit, and, as in the preceding discussion, diverted from analyst to decision-maker. Selection of CEA effectiveness measures frequently entails value judgments so subtle that the analyst may be oblivious to them. For example, "lives saved" fails to differentiate between young and old people or to consider the quality of life. "Years of life saved" seems to represent an improvement in the former dimension—it does distinguish between young and old—but it, too, fails to consider the quality of life. Further, it does not distinguish between a substantial extension of life in a few people versus a brief extension of life in many: is six months of life saved for each of twenty people better than, the same as, or worse than ten years saved for one person? The answer is not obvious to us, yet the issue is seldom considered in CEAs.

Health Status Indexes

Quality of life is a central issue. It has been recognized in the literature for years. Over a decade ago, CEA analysts weighted a year of life with a transplanted kidney higher than a year on dialysis (Klarman et al., 1968). In recent years, much attention has been devoted to developing a health status index to adjust years of life saved to reflect their quality. Such weighting represents a clear attempt at relative valuation, with the metric being something like quality-adjusted years of life (Bush et al., 1973; Weinstein and Stason, 1977b) instead of dollars. In general, health status indexes attempt to combine multiple indicators, such as death and types of disabilities, into a single index. Often a scale is used, with, for example, a range from zero, representing death, to ten representing perfect health.

Development of a widely accepted health status index has been hindered by several methodological problems. Health status indexes suffer from problems of reliability (that is, do repeated measurements provide the same information?), validity (is the relative weighting system correct?), and definitional consistency (what constitutes health?). There has been considerable progress in addressing these problems (Bergner et al., 1976a, 1976b; Brook et al., 1979; Kaplan et al., 1976, 1978), yet with notable exceptions (U.S. Congress, Office of Technology Assessment, 1979; Stason and Weinstein, 1977), the health care research community has exhibited considerable reluctance to accept the validity of health status indexes. In part, this undoubtedly reflects the relative immaturity of the research effort, the fact that, whereas there are several researchers working on development of health status indexes, their approaches differ significantly from one another. In part, the lack of acceptance of health status indexes also seems to reflect a lack of understanding of the techniques. Many CBA-CEA analysts are aware of the literature on health status indexes and of its potential relevance to their own work, but few have examined for themselves the validity of the indexes.

Health status indexes represent only one more attempt to measure health benefits. In general, the valuation of benefits in CBA-CEAs, be it through monetary or nonmonetary measures, represents a crucial, often controversial feature of CBA-CEA. It is incumbent on analysts to comprehend fully the implications—the strengths and limitations—of the valuations they make, including both explicit and implicit ones. Sensitivity analysis can help to evaluate the importance of some valuation procedures, but nothing can replace analysts' conscious attention to the meaning of their approaches.

VALUING COSTS AND BENEFITS OVER TIME: DISCOUNTING

CONCEPT AND PROCEDURE

The costs and benefits of health care programs rarely occur entirely in the present. More often, costs are incurred over several years and benefits are realized for an even longer period. If one is to compare costs and benefits, one must be able to add up, separately, the costs and benefits occurring throughout the effective life of the program.[9] If a dollar of cost or benefit ten years from now were the same as a dollar today, the summation process would be trivial. But current and future dollars are not the same, even once one has controlled for inflation. As we shall show in this section, current dollars are worth more than future dollars; thus future dollars must be discounted to make them commensurate with current dollars. The rationale and process of discounting, a necessary step in almost all CBA-CEAs, are often not well understood.

We can demonstrate in two ways why future dollars are valued less than current dollars. One is the concept of time preference, which is that people prefer current consumption to future consumption, all other things being equal. To illustrate this, answer the following question: If we offered to give you $100 right now or to give you $100 next year, which would you prefer?[10] If you are like the vast majority of people, you answered "Now". Having the money now gives you the option of spending it or saving it, or doing some of both. Deferring receipt of the money until next year eliminates the possibility of spending or investing it now. In essence, waiting a year to get the money reduces your options without offering any compensating advantages. By preferring the money today, you are providing evidence that you do not value identically a dollar today and a dollar in the future; rather, you value the dollar today more highly.

There is a logic other than simple time preference that helps to explain your preferring current dollars. If you have the money now, one of your options is to invest it in some productive activity that will yield more dollars in the future. Thus, if you find an investment yielding, say, 3 percent,[11] you could invest the $100 in this project and end up with $103 at the end of the year. In essence, then, $100 a year from now is worth less than $100 today because if you had the money today, you could convert it into *more* than $100 in a year.

The process of discounting involves deflating some future number of dollars by the rate at which investments have been growing. It is the reverse of the process whereby one calculates the future value of a current investment. For the latter, a $100 investment today grows to $103 next year because the principal ($100) is multiplied by the rate of growth (3 percent) and this interest, or rate of return, is added to the original principal. That is, $100 × (1 + .03) = $103. More generally, for an amount of principal invested now (P_0) at an interest rate of r, the value of the investment next year (P_1) will be

$$P_0 \times (1 + r) = P_1.$$

The following year, the value of the investment (P_2) will be

$$P_1 \times (1 + r) = P_2$$

or

$$P_0 \times (1 + r)^2 = P_2.$$

At the end of n years, the investment will be worth

$$P_0 \times (1 + r)^n = P_n. \tag{1}$$

The present value of $103 a year from now is $100. This we determine by reversing the process we have just worked through. We divide the future amount, $103, by 1 plus the interest rate to calculate the present value: $103 ÷ (1 + .03) = $100. More generally, to determine the present discounted value (P_0) of P_n dollars n years from now,

$$P_0 = \frac{P_n}{(1 + r)^n}$$

All that we have done is to divide both sides of equation (1) by $(1 + r)^n$, thus isolating the present value (P_0) on the left side of the equation. The discount rate is r; n years from now, the discount factor will be $(1 + r)^n$.

The application of discounting to the costs and benefits of health care programs is straightforward. If a program has costs of C_0 immediately, C_1 in year 1, C_2 in year 2, and so on through year n, the present discounted value of the entire stream of costs, C_{pdv}, is found as follows:

$$C_{pdv} = C_0 + \frac{C_1}{(1 + r)} + \frac{C_2}{(1 + r)^2} + \ldots + \frac{C_n}{(1 + r)^n} , \qquad (2)$$

where each of the components of the right side of the equation is the present discounted value of one year's costs. Another way to write equation (2) is

$$C_{pdv} = \Sigma_{j=0}^{n} \frac{C_j}{(1 + r)^j} , \qquad (3)$$

where Σ indicates addition and j indicates the year from the immediate time through year n.

The present discounted value of the stream of benefits (B_{pdv}) is identical, except that B should be substituted for the C in equations (2) and (3):

$$B_{pdv} = B_0 + \frac{B_1}{(1 + r)} + \frac{B_2}{(1 + r)^2} + \ldots + \frac{B_n}{(1 + r)^n} , \qquad (4)$$

and

$$B_{pdv} = \Sigma_{j=0}^{n} \frac{B_j}{(1 + r)^j} . \qquad (5)$$

Table 3.1 illustrates the discounting process and its effects. Its footnote presents equations (2) and (4) as applied to the specific problem. The last column in the table gives the results of these calculations. Note that undiscounted benefits exceed undiscounted costs, but that the effect of discounting is to make discounted costs greater than discounted benefits. This is a reflection of the fact that benefits in the example are deferred several years, so the discounting process reduces their dollar value more than that of costs, which occur soon after initiation of the program.[12]

DEALING WITH INFLATION

If the numbers used as examples above have an air of unreality, that is most likely a reflection of our being conditioned to expect inflation. While certain kinds of inflation can pose tricky problems in calculating present discounted values—for example, differences in the rates of inflation of medical care and food prices—general

Table 3.1:   Hypothetical Example of Discounting Costs and
Benefits*

	Year				Sum ($)	
						Undis- Discounted
0	1	2	5	10	counted	at 3%†
Benefits ($) 0	0	0	70,000	25,000	95,000	78,985
Costs ($) 50,000	10,000	10,000	20,000	0	90,000	86,387

*Assume that no costs or benefits are realized in any year other than those
presented.

$$\dagger \quad B_{pdv} = \frac{\$70,000}{(1.03)^5} + \frac{\$25,000}{(1.03)^{10}} = \$78,985$$

$$C_{pdv} = \$50,000 + \frac{\$10,000}{1.03} + \frac{\$10,000}{(1.03)^2} + \frac{\$20,000}{(1.03)^5} = \$86,387$$

inflation is not a source of technical difficulty. In general, the best
procedure is to deflate dollar figures to the price level of a single
year before one begins the discounting process.[13] By bringing
dollar values into constant dollars, such as today's prices, the
messiness of inflation can be avoided. Besides, while we expect
inflation, we tend to think in terms of current values. For example,
if we anticipated 10 percent inflation over the next year, we would
think of $1.10 next year as meaning one of today's dollars.

SELECTING THE DISCOUNT RATE

There is widespread agreement among economists and policymakers about the need for discounting. There is less consensus,
however, about the rate that should be used. The rate is more than
an academic concern, since the choice of discount rate can have a
substantial impact on the relative assessment of alternative programs. This is illustrated in table 3.2, in which no discounting or
discounting by 2 percent makes program Y look better than program X, whereas discounting at 4 percent makes X preferable to Y.
The higher discount rate has a more significant impact on the
program that has significantly deferred benefits.

The discount rate for public sector activities is a social opportunity cost. In effect, it should represent the rate of return on
society's best alternative uses of its resources. Thus, if a project not
undertaken could have produced a 3 percent real rate of return, the
opportunity lost must be at least matched by whatever programs
are implemented.

Table 3.2: Example of the Effect of Discount Rate on Program Ranking

	Year			*Sum ($) at Discount Rate*		
	0	*5*	*20*	*0%*	*2%*	*4%*
	Program X					
Benefits ($)	0	125,000	0	125,000	113,216	102,741
Costs ($)	100,000	0	0	100,000	100,000	100,000
Net Benefit ($)				25,000	13,216	2,741
	Program Y					
Benefits ($)	0	0	200,000	200,000	134,594	91,278
Costs ($)	100,000	0	0	100,000	100,000	100,000
Net Benefit ($)				100,000	34,594	-8,722

Translating this into a concrete number is more difficult than espousing the theory. Many analysts advocate that the social discount rate should be the opportunity cost of private sector capital, subject to some adjustments (for example, reflecting the social cost of pollution produced by the private sector). These analysts argue that public sector resources are withdrawn from the private sector, primarily through taxation, and hence public sector activities ought to yield a return at least comparable to that which the private sector must forego because of taxation.

An alternative view argues that the discount rate for social programs should be lower than the private-sector opportunity cost measure since society's interests include consideration of future generations. That is, the social rate of time preference is lower than our individual rates of time preference. Recalling the example presented in table 3.2, one can see that this discount rate would favor programs with long-term benefits, as compared with the higher opportunity cost discount rate.

Regardless of which of these two positions one favors, a specific number for the social discount rate remains undetermined. Academic and government analysts have used a wide range of discount rates, with the tendency having been toward higher rates as inflation has increased, despite the fact that the discount rate should be independent of the rate of inflation (because the discount rate should reflect the real rate of return). In general, the best strategy seems to be to seek a reasonable number (for example, 3 percent) and then test the sensitivity of findings to both higher and lower rates (see the discussion of sensitivity analysis below).[14]

VALUING NONMONETARY EFFECTIVENESS OVER TIME

The logic of discounting monetary costs and benefits is fairly easy to understand. But what does one do in the case of a stream of nonmonetary outcomes in a CEA—for example, years of life saved? Health care CBA-CEA analysts have engaged in considerable debate on this issue. The notion of discounting lives strikes many observers as distasteful, if not downright illogical. However, Weinstein and Stason (1976b) have presented a compelling argument as to why effectiveness measures, like dollar benefits, must be discounted. To illustrate the argument, suppose that a program costing $10,000 could save, immediately, ten years of life, or $1,000 per year of life saved. Assume a linear relationship between costs and effectiveness; that is, for every additional $1,000 (or fraction thereof) an additional one year of life (or fraction thereof) could be saved. If, instead of mounting the program, policymakers invested the money at 3 percent, at the end of a year they would have $10,300 which would permit them to save 10.3 years of life. However, if they held their investment for another year, the kitty would grow to $10,609, permitting them to save 10.609 years. And so on, year after year. In effect, if a year of life today is valued no higher than a year of life in the future, there is an incentive to defer lifesaving efforts forever; they would never appear desirable compared with the alternative of waiting one more year. In short, effectiveness, like monetary benefits, is valued more highly in the present, and discounting is appropriate.

Addressing Problems of Uncertainty

By now it must be abundantly clear that CBA-CEA is pervaded by assumptions and uncertainties. Understanding of production relationships is often imprecise, and unpredictable behavior can alter that which analysts think is known. Measurement and valuation of costs and benefits require numerous imputations and rough estimates. No one knows *the* appropriate discount rate. In effect, myriad assumptions and uncertainties accumulate and can leave one with a sense of despair. How does one deal with all this uncertainty? Should we reject CBA-CEA as not useful?

The answer is not to discard CBA-CEA, but to place the results obtained from it in perspective, to examine closely the assumptions upon which the analysis rests, and to test the sensitivity of the results to reasonable changes in these assumptions. Only then can one be confident of the credibility of the analysis and its ability to provide additional information regarding the health problem being evaluated.

There are several techniques for dealing with uncertainty in a CBA-CEA. Before discussing these, we need to distinguish two types of uncertainty: the presence of random events or a basic lack of knowledge. Random events occur according to a known probability distribution. We know, for example, that flipping a coin will result in heads roughly half of the time and tails the other half. Thus we know the probability distribution of heads and tails, but the result of a single flip of the coin remains uncertain. By contrast, when uncertainty reflects a lack of knowledge, we do not know the probabilities with which various outcomes will occur; we may not even know which types of outcomes can occur. Thus, administering a new chemotherapeutic agent to a terminal cancer patient may have any of several therapeutic and toxic effects; the latter might include side effects never previously experienced in cancer chemotherapy.

Uncertainty reflecting a basic lack of knowledge can be addressed in several ways. When time or other resources, or both, are available, analysts often can buy additional information. In the case of the cancer drug, additional tests on laboratory animals might yield information that could decrease (but not eliminate) uncertainty about the likely effectiveness and side effects of the drug. When direct testing is impossible, opinions can be solicited from experts in the field, either formally or informally. Two examples of formal solicitation methods are the Delphi technique and Consensus Development Exercises. The Delphi technique involves eliciting confidential written opinions from each member of a panel of experts and then circulating each member's responses to the other panel members. This process is repeated, often several times, always preserving the anonymity of the panel members. The procedure permits each expert to think through his or her own opinions in light of those of the other panelists, with the hope that revised opinions will approach a consensus, if not a unanimous conclusion. The principle of maintaining anonymity is intended to avoid direct interpersonal influences. By contrast, Consensus Development Exercises, as practiced by NIH, bring together a diverse group of experts to listen to and evaluate the scientific evidence on a given subject. Following presentation of the evidence, the group is isolated, much like a jury, to collectively weigh the evidence and reach a consensus as to the current state of knowledge. Sensitivity analysis (discussed below) can help to determine the importance of any remaining uncertainty.

Although its effect on the usefulness of CBA-CEA can be equally significant, uncertainty due to random events often seems less frustrating analytically, since analysts have a small arsenal of techniques to deal with it. A common approach is to use decision analysis, diagramming possible courses of action on a decision tree, with branches in the diagram associated with known or imputed probabilities and payoffs (the positive or negative values of the outcomes) associated with each pathway. Thus analysts can trace plausible paths to determine the probability and expected value of each final outcome. In addition to decision analysis, a variety of computer simulation techniques allows analysts to model real phenomena and estimate their consequences over hypothetical periods of time. By manipulating all such models until outcomes mirror empirical findings, analysts may be able to acquire valuable insight into real processes.[15]

The potential usefulness of modeling techniques is great, but analysts and policymakers always must retain an awareness of the influence of underlying assumptions. Technical sophistication can mask tenuous assumptions, particularly for those individuals to whom the analytical approaches appear alien and complex.

SENSITIVITY ANALYSIS

The myriad uncertainties in CBA-CEAs have caused many analyses to be scrapped prior to completion. Often, awareness of the considerable need for assumptions has deterred potential analysts from even beginning CBA-CEAs. Further, the apparent tenuousness of assumptions has led many readers of analysis to ignore otherwise good studies. Rather than viewing uncertainty as a source of despair, analysts and readers should accept it as a fact of analytical life and approach the determination of its importance as an interesting challenge.

Sensitivity analysis is a conceptually simple but powerful tool with which to address that challenge. Actually a series of techniques, sensitivity analyses test whether variations in assumptions affect the qualitative conclusions of a CBA-CEA. Thus, if an analyst assumes a discount rate of 2 percent and concludes that the program in question is desirable, he or she can try discount rates of 0 and 4 percent to determine whether the program's basic desirability is a function of, or is sensitive to, the discount rate.

Referring back to table 3.2, we can illustrate two different outcomes of such a sensitivity analysis. Each of programs X and Y appears desirable at a discount rate of 2 percent; discounted benefits exceed discounted costs. Program X continues to look desirable even at the higher discount rate of 4 percent. Thus, assuming that 4 percent represents an upper bound on reasonable discount rates, the finding of positive net benefit is not sensitive to the discount rate used. By contrast, program Y's net benefit becomes negative when the 4 percent rate is tested. In this case, the finding of positive net benefit *is* sensitive to the discount rate selected. This sensitivity analysis suggests that program X is a desirable program, despite the fact that there was uncertainty about the "correctness" of the discount rate assumed. With regard to program Y, however, we found that the choice of a discount rate did matter; we might be reluctant, therefore, to draw any conclusions about the program on the basis of our analysis.

These examples illustrate that sensitivity analysis can shed light on the importance of certain assumptions. In the case of program X, it tells us that an analysis is meaningful despite the presence of uncertainty. In the case of program Y, we have learned that the uncertainty does matter and therefore that the CBA is ambiguous in terms of providing policy guidance.

Sensitivity analysis can also be applied to several programs simultaneously. For example, a group of analysts might be interested in examining which of five lifesaving programs was most cost-effective, yet they lack confidence in their selection of a discount rate. By testing alternative high and low rates, they can ascertain whether the rank order of the programs is affected by the discount rate. If not, they can identify one program as preferred to the others. If the rank ordering changes as the discount rate is varied, they will appreciate the limitations of the analysis in assisting decision-making.

Selecting high, low, and best estimates of uncertain variables is only one method of sensitivity testing. Two others can assist analysts in determining the importance of uncertainty. In worst-case analysis, analysts assign to uncertain variables values that will bias the analysis against what otherwise appears to be the more desirable program. For example, suppose that a CEA concludes, under the best set of assumptions, that program V will reduce morbidity by 1,000 days for an expenditure of $10,000 in resources. Under the same assumptions, program W requires $15,000 in resources to achieve the same reduction in morbidity. However, suppose that the analysts were uncertain about the amount of labor needed to run each program; in each case they had estimated a need for $2,000 worth of labor. To apply worst-case analysis, they might try cutting that estimate in half for program W and doubling it for program V, thus doubly biasing the analysis against program V. After the new costs are taken into account, however, we still find program V superior to program W. Under the assumptions biased against program V, it costs $12,000, while program W costs $14,000. The CEA is not sensitive to the uncertain estimate of labor cost. Of course, if the relative desirability of the programs had been reversed, we would have been concerned that the analysis *was* sensitive to the estimation of labor cost.

Break-even analysis offers an attractive means of examining sensitivity, particularly in cases in which analysts are reluctant to assign, or incapable of assigning, any value to a variable. Suppose that, in comparing two alternative transportation systems, S and T, analysts can value all costs and benefits in monetary terms except the fact that system T will save ten lives compared to system S (and the analysts are reluctant to place a dollar value on life). Suppose further that their CBA found that system S offered net benefits of $1 million, while system T offered net benefits of $950,000 plus the ten lives. Break-even analysis calls for the analysts to determine the dollar value that would have to be placed on the lives saved to make the systems appear equally attractive. In this case, the ten lives would have to be valued at $50,000, or $5,000 per life, to make the systems break even. Since virtually anyone would agree that a life is worth at least $5,000, the break-even analysis suggests that system T is preferable to system S. One can imagine examples in which the opposite conclusion would emerge. For instance, repeat the same example except substitute ten days of slight disability for ten lives. Our guess is that most people would be unwilling to spend $5,000 to avoid a day of limited disability and hence would prefer system S. The result of a break-even analysis can be ambiguous. Suppose that instead of the ten lives, the nonmonetary benefit had been one healthy year of life for a parent with three children. Would system T dominate system S or vice versa? Our guess is that it would be difficult to achieve consensus on this question. The analysis, in this instance, is sensitive to the perceived implicit value of the year of life.

To summarize, sensitivity analysis can produce four important results:

— It can demonstrate the substantial dependence of a conclusion on a particular assumption; this suggests that the overall analysis cannot be viewed as definitive.
— It can demonstrate that an assumption does not significantly affect a study's conclusion, and hence that the tenuousness of the assumption is not a source of concern.
— It can establish a minimum or maximum value that a variable must have for a program to appear worthwhile.
— It can identify issues (uncertainties) deserving of research attention.

EQUITY

Throughout this chapter we have emphasized the technical steps and problems in CBA-CEA. It is imperative, however, that we not lose sight of the nonefficiency content of the subject matter. Problems studied with CBA-CEA often relate primarily or secondarily to social distribution goals, yet CBA-CEA is often not well suited to analyzing this dimension of health issues. In the context of CBA-CEA, how can equity—concern with the distribution of health care resources—be incorporated into policy analysis?

Several major national health care initiatives have had equity as their principal objective. Medicare and Medicaid were passed with the intention of increasing the access to care of the elderly and the poor, thus redistributing the nation's health care resources toward these groups. Evaluations of these programs that focused on their impact on the health status of the elderly and poor might find the programs not entirely successful. But by the criterion of increasing access to care, independent of implications for health, the programs are clear successes.

Many health care activities have implicit distributional implications. Research on sickle-cell disease, for example, redistributes resources toward blacks, while occupational safety efforts channel resources primarily toward blue-collar workers. The redistributional impact of some activities is so subtle, or secondary, that it often goes unnoticed: cardiovascular research benefits a group at risk, but the group is not clearly and readily identifiable.

A first issue, therefore, is how the distributional benefits (or, occasionally, costs) of health programs can be taken into consideration in CBA-CEA. When a particular distributional goal is the principal objective of a program, one can measure attainment of that goal by a CEA that assesses the costs of alternative programmatic approaches. For example, the effectiveness of a program intended to provide health care services for the poor might be measured in any number of ways: the proportion of the relevant (target) group seeing a physician each year; the number of physician visits per target group member, compared with the number for people who are not poor; and so on. Alternative means of achieving the desired effectiveness measure might include a financial entitlement program (like Medicaid), a system of publicly funded neighborhood health centers, and so on.

When the distributional objective is implicit or secondary, it becomes much more difficult to take it into account in a formal CBA-CEA. Surely the effectiveness of a sickle-cell research program will be evaluated primarily in terms of progress against the disease and, ultimately, the number of lives saved. But a sickle-cell research program has a clear, if unquantifiable, equity benefit associated with it: it redistributes resources to attack a problem that afflicts members of a disadvantaged minority population. How can one incorporate this benefit into a CBA-CEA?

Although there are theoretical means for examining distributional benefits,[16] in practice most unquantifiable costs and benefits tend to get suppressed or relegated to footnotes in formal analysis (Fein, 1977; U.S. Congress, Office of Technology Assessment, 1980a). Occasionally one of the sensitivity analysis techniques discussed above may be helpful. For example, in comparing sickle-cell research to a research effort that is not obviously associated with a social redistribution, one could employ break-even analysis to determine the minimum value one would have to attribute to the distributional benefit in order to make the two research programs equally attractive. Break-even analysis cannot resolve the question of how equity should be quantified and valued, but it can provide an empirical framework for policy assessment of alternative programs.

Frequently our bag of analytical tricks will not contain any meaningful quantitative approaches to considering equity, which is why the basic structure of an analysis is so important. When a distributional goal is identified as a significant objective at the outset of an analysis, it will be difficult for analysts and readers to ignore it at the end. Similarly, if analysts explicitly address each stage of the analysis of costs and benefits—identification, measurement, and valuation—they are more likely to emphasize those costs and benefits, such as distributional consequences, which can be identified (and possibly measured) but not valued. Hence the identification stage will accord such consequences a prominence commensurate with their importance. That importance can and should be reemphasized in the conclusion of an analysis.

In this brief glimpse at equity, we have noted difficulties in incorporating recognized equity impacts into analysis. Now we turn momentarily to the inadvertent introduction of equity problems into an otherwise neutral analysis. As we noted in the discussion of benefits and effectiveness, measurement and valuation techniques can introduce unintended values into analysis. The most blatant example is the use of the human capital approach, which, through use of age- and sex-specific wage rates, places a higher value on avoidance of morbidity and mortality among working-age white males than among any other group. While use of prevailing wage rates may present an accurate picture of market conditions, encoding that distribution in a health-oriented analysis is an understandable source of controversy.

Other distributional issues that get embedded inadvertently in CBA-CEAs often reflect selection of effectiveness measures without due contemplation of their meaning. Earlier we noted how failure to distinguish the quality of life saved or even its length can lead analysts to favor resource allocations that society as a whole might find undesirable. In this instance, the subjective and often unarticulated algorithm in citizens' minds may be superior to that which the analysts have committed to paper.

The issues involved in dealing with equity are complex and troublesome. Our failure to devote more attention to them here is a reflection of the state of the art, not our assessment of their importance.

PRESENTATION AND INTERPRETATION OF FINDINGS

Throughout this chapter we have catalogued the technical problems that plague most CBA-CEAs: uncertainty about the values of many key variables; difficulty in identification and measurement; lack of consensus on the valuation process; and so on. All such problems can lead to misinterpretation of the results of analysis, both by readers and the analysts themselves. The latter are in jeopardy of misinterpreting their own analyses because they may lose sight of, and eventually ignore, the assumptions and uncertainties that arise in the course of analysis. Unless they have tested these with sensitivity analysis, they cannot make a judgment on the usefulness of their findings.

The solution to analysts' erring in interpreting their findings is general familiarity with the pitfalls of analysis and careful attention to specific problems in their own studies. Readers of CBA-CEAs have fewer defenses against misinterpretation. Often they are exposed only to summaries of analyses—abstracts, news briefs, and the like. Even if they have entire analyses at their disposal, many readers, including public officials and health care professionals, do not have the technical expertise to discover and comprehend all of the nuances in an analysis. This places a special burden on analysts to present and interpret findings clearly, carefully, and fully.

The presentation of the findings should identify the important variables and discuss the confidence the reader can place in the values that were used. In this discussion, a review of the findings and the significance of the sensitivity analysis is critical. Analysts should also be sure to emphasize relevant considerations that have not been addressed by the formal analysis, including equity or distributional issues and the existence of other important but nonquantified variables. The perspective of the analysis (for example, social or institution-specific) should be made clear and its significance noted.

In addition to such expository concerns, analysts must be aware of certain technical considerations when selecting means of presenting findings. A popular misconception is that the benefit-cost ratio serves as an adequate and appropriate index of a program's desirability relative to competing alternatives. While the ratio will suffice under certain specific conditions, the measure of program desirability in CBA should be net benefit (discounted benefits minus discounted costs), not the benefit-cost ratio. The net benefit measurement will always identify the preferred ranking of programs; the benefit-cost ratio sometimes will be misleading.

To see why net benefit should be used, consider the following example.[17] Program X costs $2,000 and yields gross benefits of $4,000. Program Y costs $2 million and yields $3 million. Using the benefit-cost ratio as a criterion, one would prefer program X to program Y, since the ratio for the former is 2 to 1 ($4,000 ÷ $2,000), while that of the latter is 1.5 to 1 ($3 million ÷ $2 million). Note that the ratio gives the reader no indication of the size of the expected net benefit. Program X produces a net benefit of only $2,000 ($4,000 −$2,000), compared with program Y's net benefit of $1 million ($3 million−$2 million). Assuming that we had the resources to mount either program, and assuming the program X could not be replicated, clearly we would prefer program Y, the program identified by the net benefit criterion.

The benefit-cost ratio is also sensitive to whether an effect of a health program is considered as a benefit or a negative cost. The net benefit measure is not sensitive to this. Earlier we noted that medical cost savings, resulting from an investment in disease prevention or health promotion, can be treated either as negative costs (the savings are subtracted from the other costs) or as regular benefits. This distinction is technically important only when a benefit-cost ratio is employed; when costs and benefits are combined and a net figure is used, it makes no difference whether a particular item is considered a benefit or a negative cost. To illustrate, suppose that a program costs $1,000 to implement and operate, saves $500 in future medical costs, and results in a direct health benefit valued at $1,500. If the future medical cost savings are treated as regular benefits, the benefit-cost ratio will equal 2 to 1 [($1,500 + $500) ÷ $1,000]. If the cost savings are treated as negative costs instead, the ratio rises to 3 to 1 [$1,500 ÷ ($1,000 − $500)]. Nothing has changed in terms of the program's costs and benefits, but the two different calculations produce significantly different ratios. By contrast, the net benefit criterion produces the same net benefit regardless of the treatment of the cost savings: ($1,500 + $500) − $1,000 = $1,500 − ($1,000 − $500) = $1,000.

In CEA, the lack of a common metric for costs and effectiveness makes it impossible to speak of net effectiveness. As a result, almost all CEAs have relied on a cost-effectiveness ratio as an index of relative program desirability. However, this ratio should not be used uncritically; indeed, like the benefit-cost ratio, it can mislead. Under a limited set of circumstances it provides a reliable index of relative desirability. Without those circumstances, analysts are well advised to characterize program alternatives in terms of their costs and effectiveness, without converting them into ratios. The strength of such analysis is simply in conveying the consequences of alternative programs to decision-makers.

Table 3.3 can assist in demonstrating the circumstances under which a cost-effectiveness ratio is meaningful and those under which it is not. According to the simple cost-effectiveness ratio

Table 3.3:   Cost-Effectiveness Ratio and
Ranking of Program Desirability

Program	Cost ($)	Effectiveness (Number of Lives Saved)	Cost Effectiveness Ratio ($ per Life Saved)
S	100,000	10	10,000
T	100,000	12	8,333
U	200,000	12	16,667
V	200,000	15	13,333

criterion, program T is the best program (it costs least per life saved) and program U is the worst (it costs most per life saved). But is program T really best? Comparing it with program V we find that the latter could save three more lives than the former for $100,000 more. The marginal cost per life saved, $33,333, is relatively quite high, but who is to say that those lives are not worth the money? In other words, focusing solely on the average cost per life saved—the ratio—misses the possibility that a program both costing and producing more would be deemed socially desirable. Valuing the extra lives is a social or political function, not an analytical one. Indeed, the decision to perform CEA instead of CBA implies an analytical rejection of valuing life.

Table 3.3 also shows circumstances under which the cost-effectiveness ratio does provide useful information for ranking alternatives. Program T clearly dominates program S, since the former saves more lives for the same cost.[18] For the same reason, program V is clearly superior to program U. We can also conclude that program T is better than program U, since each saves the same number of lives, yet T costs half as much as U. Thus, overall, the analysis represented in table 3.3 helps to narrow the set of alternatives. Programs S and U are eliminated from consideration, leaving Programs T and V in contention. The relative desirability of these two programs cannot be established by objective empirical policy analysis.[19] In general, the cost-effectiveness ratio serves as an accurate gauge of relative program desirability only when costs *or* measures of effectiveness are the same across programs. Then one seeks the least costly program to achieve a given level of effectiveness, or the most effective program given a level of costs.

Figures such as those presented in table 3.3 conceal potentially important information on the marginal costs and effectiveness (or benefits) of alternative programs. Whenever such information can be made available, it can offer substantial assistance to users of CBA-CEA. For example, as specified in table 3.3, program T clearly dominates program S. Yet suppose one had available the more detailed information on these two programs presented in table 3.4. These figures indicate that the first half of program S is highly

Table 3.4: Marginal Analysis in CEA

Cost Level ($)	Effectiveness (Lives Saved)	Cost Effectiveness Ratio ($ Per Life Saved)
Program S		
50,000	8	6,250
100,000	10	10,000
Program T		
50,000	6	8,333
100,000	12	8,333

productive, even more than the first half of program T. The entire program T is better because its second half is productive, while the second half of program S results in saving only two lives. If policymakers had the option to select portions of programs, their optimal use of $100,000 to save lives would entail implementing half of each of programs S and T. Investing $50,000 in each of these programs would save fourteen lives, more than either program could achieve at a cost level of $100,000.

The phenomenon of concern here involves programs' returns to scale: as some programs expand, their output increases more rapidly than their costs (increasing returns to scale); for others, costs rise more rapidly than output (decreasing returns to scale); for some, both costs and effectiveness increase at the same rate (constant returns to scale). Most commonly, returns to scale vary as programs expand. A typical pattern might be increasing returns first, followed by a period of constant returns and then decreasing returns. Information on returns to scale can permit decision-makers to refine their appreciation of the potential of alternative programs and, with refined appreciation, to strive for still greater efficiency than single aggregate numbers permit.

In the discussion of benefits and effectiveness, we noted that analysts may find it difficult, if not impossible, to reduce diverse outcomes to a single measure of effectiveness, be it dollars in CBA or an index of health status in CEA. In such cases, it may prove desirable to work with multiple effectiveness measures (for example, years of life saved, days of morbidity avoided, and days of disability averted). The bottom line of such a study can be presented as an array of outcomes associated with a total cost. Table 3.5 illustrates this approach. As in table 3.3, when alternative

Table 3.5: Arraying Multiple Effectiveness Measures in a CEA

		Saved		
Program	Costs ($)	Years of Life	Days of Morbidity	Days of Disability
W	100,000	5	25	30
X	100,000	5	20	25
Y	100,000	4	400	35
Z	200,000	7	60	80

programs' costs and effectiveness differ, with one program having more of each, objective ranking is impossible. This is the case in comparing program Z with either program W or X. When costs are the same, as for programs W, X, and Y, objective rankings are possible only when one program dominates another in at least one measure of effectiveness and is not worse in any other; thus program W is clearly superior to program X, since the former saves more days of morbidity and disability and the same number of years of life. By contrast, value judgments are required to rank program W against program Y, since the former saves 1 more year of life than the latter but at the cost of 375 days of morbidity and 5 days of disability. Which is worth more? Objective analysis cannot provide an answer. Note, however, that subjective rankings occasionally may be so consistent as to establish one program as clearly preferable to another. For example, if program W saved 400 days of morbidity (instead of the 25 recorded), we conjecture that almost all people would rank it ahead of program Y, since now the trade-off would be 1 more year of life in program W compared with 5 days of disability saved in program Y. In short, few people would rank these outcomes as comparable; almost all would agree that 1 year of healthy life is worth more than 5 days without disability.

Whether outcomes are merged into a single index or kept

distinct, presenting costs and positive consequences provides potentially useful information. Occasionally it may produce a definitive identification of an optimal approach to a problem. Most often, it will add information and perspective to a search for a good approach. Even when program effectiveness is presented as an array of outcomes, the data make trade-offs explicit, in itself a useful analytical outcome.

We close this consideration of how findings should be presented by reiterating our emphasis at the outset: regardless of the formal mechanism selected (for example, a table of discounted costs, benefits, and net benefit), analysts should use the concluding discussion to emphasize the context of the findings. Critical assumptions and uncertainties should be identified and their importance, as measured by sensitivity analysis or other means, should be noted. If analysts can accept CBA-CEA as an information-generating technique rather than as a decision-making one, they will be more comfortable with qualifying the empirical results of their studies. Properly presented and carefully interpreted, such results can lend valuable insight into the nature of resource allocation problems.

From Analysis to Implementation

In the main, CBA-CEA is intended to be a practical tool, dedicated to assisting decision-makers in evaluating resource allocation issues. Yet this purpose stands in striking contrast to experience in CBA-CEA in general and particularly in health care. Relatively few CBA-CEAs have contributed to the policy analysis process, and only a handful of these have played central roles in policy decisions. In this concluding section of our chapter on CBA-CEA methodology, we take a glance at why this is so and how analysis can be adapted to the exigencies of decision-making. In essence, we attempt to build a bridge between the principles of analysis and the potential of analysis in the world of decision-making.[20]

The inherent technical limitations of analysis, discussed throughout this chapter, restrict its direct applicability in many situations. Beyond this, as we have emphasized, the credibility of a CBA-CEA reflects the analysts' success in dealing candidly and effectively with the assumptions and uncertainties that pervade analysis. Beyond the technical features of analysis, the link between analysis and decision-making is affected by a variety of personal factors. Are the decision-makers familiar with and sympathetic to analysis? Have the analysts striven to address the concerns and needs of the decision-makers throughout the analytical process? And so on (Quade, 1975).

All such factors can influence the use of analysis, but one reason that CBA-CEA has had relatively little policy impact relates to the perspective from which analysts view costs and benefits in CBA-CEA. At the outset, we argued that a CBA-CEA should consider all costs and benefits, regardless of to whom they may accrue. In general, CBA-CEAs are performed from a societal viewpoint; that is, they should reflect the aggregate interests of the society rather than the special interests of identifiable groups within that society. While this social perspective represents the theoretically correct perspective for questions of social resource allocation, it fails to recognize that the interests of flesh-and-blood decision-makers are not always (indeed, rarely) perfectly congruent with those of society. Government bureaucrats have the interests of their agencies, as well as their own career goals, at heart. Hospital administrators often have to deal with powerful competing group interests and undoubtedly find it difficult to represent freely and completely the community's concerns. Physicians have to worry about their institutions' needs, their colleagues' concerns, and the business aspects of their profession and hence cannot always fully represent their patients' best interests. And the patients' best interests are frequently in conflict with the public's. By viewing costs and benefits from "society's" perspective, analysts fail to focus on the subsets of costs and benefits that are important to given decision-makers. As such, their analyses acquire an aura of irrelevance, or at least limited relevance.

To address this problem, Luft (1976) proposed a positive variant on the generally normative CBA-CEA. His notion was to assess costs and benefits from the perspectives of the various interested parties and then to weight them by the influence each group had on the decision-making process. Luft suggested that such an analysis would have considerable predictive value. Unlike conventional CBA-CEA, it might not say what society ought to do with regard to resource allocation, but it *could* predict what would happen given the configuration of interests and power.

This approach to analysis can be used to redesign program alternatives so that the distribution of costs and benefits conforms to the power structure. While this does not seem desirable in itself, it represents a mechanism whereby a socially attractive but politically infeasible program can be restructured to become feasible. The trade-off becomes social desirability versus feasibility; if one can gain a lot of the latter without sacrificing much of the former, some compromise might be quite useful.

Luft presented two examples to illustrate his concept of relating analysis to policy implementation; otherwise the literature is devoid of conscious examples of this interesting approach to CBA-CEA. Nevertheless, it, or something like it,[21] has the potential for moving CBA-CEA in a direction more relevant to policy. The principle in Luft's positive analysis certainly emphasizes the logical gap between analysis and decision-making.

Analysts can also try other adjustments to make CBA-CEAs more relevant to decision-makers. For example, in the case of a major construction project, such as building a university hospital, analysts might use break-even analysis to determine how much of a cost overrun could be tolerated before the project became economically infeasible. Construction projects are notorious for cost overruns, and a decision-maker would be only prudent to avoid uncritical reliance on an analysis that presented only the best estimate of costs. In short, the analyst should make the analysis meaningful to the decision-makers, should give them the kind of information they would seek on their own, and should try to anticipate their questions and answer them before they are asked.

NOTES

1. Concepts such as direct and indirect costs and benefits are discussed in the section on costs and benefits.
2. This limitation of CBA refers to the predominant method of valuing health benefits, the human capital approach. An alternative approach, willingness-to-pay, addresses this deficiency conceptually, but severe practical problems have restricted its application to date. Both of these benefit valuation techniques are discussed in the section entitled Benefits and Effectiveness.
3. One such book is that of Stokey and Zeckhauser (1978). This is one of the few books that provide a solid introduction to most of these techniques without requiring much mathematical sophistication of the reader. The book opens with helpful discussion of the nature and purposes of models.
4. The issue of the relationship between marginal input and output is termed "returns to scale." We discuss it later.
5. It can be argued that diagnostic procedures ought not to be evaluated on health-outcome criteria for reasons other than the difficulty of such evaluation. For example, diagnosis produces learning among physi-

cians, which one day might contribute to significant therapeutic breakthroughs. Also, diagnosis removes uncertainty for both patient and physician (see McNeil, 1979).

6. In this section and throughout the remainder of the book we will use the word "benefits" generically to refer to the positive outcomes of health care programs. Thus "benefits" can refer to the economically measured benefits of a CBA or to the program effectiveness of a CEA. When we mean only the former (the CBA context), we will state that explicitly.

7. As the preceding paragraph hinted, analysts may attempt to combine different effectiveness measures through some arbitrary weighting scheme. In a sense this is valuation, though of a nonmonetary sort. Here we focus exclusively on monetary valuation.

8. For example, survey respondents will provide different answers to a typed question referring to risk reduction of .001 than to one described as one in a thousand.

9. By referring to effective life, we include a period following formal program closure during which derivative benefits continue to be realized.

10. Throughout the discussion in this section we are controlling for inflation. Thus, in the present instance, the option is for $100 in today's purchasing power, taken today or next year. If inflation ran 10 percent over the next year, the number of inflated dollars that would be required to produce the equivalent purchasing power would be $110. So that inflation will not confuse the basic issue, think in terms of a single year's value of the dollar.

11. In the 1980s we are conditioned to expect yields on investments of 10 to 20 percent. Most of these percentage points, however, reflect inflation rather than true productivity. In periods of no inflation, or once one has controlled for inflation, real rates of return tend to be quite small, from 1 to 4 percent.

12. Discounting tables are available in most standard accounting or finance textbooks. These tables facilitate discounting calculations.

13. Inflation indexes can be found in several federal government publications, including the annual report of the Council of Economic Advisors.

14. Another strategy is indirect: rather than discount by a social discount rate, one can calculate a program's internal rate of return and see how the rate corresponds to a plausible range of social discount rates. The internal rate of return (IRR) is the rate of return on investment in a program. It is calculated by finding that discount rate (the IRR) which precisely equates discounted costs and discounted benefits. The IRR is found by solving the following equation for i:

$$\Sigma_{j=0}^n \frac{B_j}{(1 + i)^j} = \Sigma_{j=0}^n \frac{C_j}{(1 + i)^j} .$$

If benefits occur later than costs (a common experience in health programs), the IRR represents the highest interest rate by which costs and benefits can be discounted and net benefit remain nonnegative. Thus if the IRR is large, one can rest confident that the program is desirable.

15. Again, we refer the reader to Stokey and Zeckhauser (1978) for an excellent, nontechnical introduction to several popular modeling techniques.

16. The notion of a social welfare function could handle equity conceptually but is of little practical use in empirical policy analysis. See, for example, Steiner (1974).

17. Throughout this discussion we will assume that all costs and benefits have been properly discounted to their present value.

18. Throughout this discussion we are assuming that the lives saved by the different programs are equally valuable.

19. In this example, we are assuming that programs cannot be repeated. If program S could be doubled—that is, its costs and effectiveness each increasing 100 percent—it would dominate both programs U and V, since it would save more lives (twenty) for the same $200,000. Whenever programs can be expanded or contracted such that the cost-effectiveness ratios are preserved, then those ratios will constitute meaningful guides to relative program desirability. But such is rarely the case, so marginal analysis becomes relevant. Here we treat the programs as all or nothing.

20. Exceptions to the rule of limited policy impact were noted in the preceding chapter and will be considered in Chapter 4. The why of CBA-CEA's limited role in health care decision-making is discussed in detail in Chapter 5. Here we are concerned with formal techniques for adapting CBA-CEA methodology to social decision-making in general.

21. Another possibility is a system in which competing and "biased" CBA-CEAs are brought before a policy tribunal in an advocacy proceeding. In essence, the various parties at interest perform, and attempt to sell, their own CBA-CEAs on an issue of policy concern.

4

Practice:
A Review of the Literature

THE PRECEDING CHAPTER established the technical criteria with which the quality of contributions to the health care CBA-CEA literature can be evaluated. Such evaluation is a basic purpose of this chapter. Before turning to the quality of the literature, however, we feel it would be useful to acquaint the reader with the size, composition of, and trends in that literature. Although familiarity with this more "empirical" dimension may be inherently interesting, we present it principally because we believe that an appreciation of the composition of the literature and of the magnitude and nature of its growth will lend insight into characteristics of the quality of the literature, both positive and negative. To preview later discussion, we believe that the rapid growth of interest in CBA-CEA among the health care community has led to many technically deficient analyses which are being performed by practitioners and analysts who often do not possess an appreciation of the complexity of the techniques. At the same time, the growth in interest has spurred some new work in health care CBA-CEA methodology.

GROWTH AND CHARACTER OF THE LITERATURE[1]

DIFFUSION

Growth in the health care CBA-CEA literature has been explosive, with the numbers of contributions increasing exponentially throughout the 1970s. The annual magnitude and rate of growth of this literature are indicated in figure 4.1. The solid line plots the annual sum of references clearly identifiable as CBAs and CEAs,

Figure 4.1:   Growth of Health Care CBA-CEA Literature

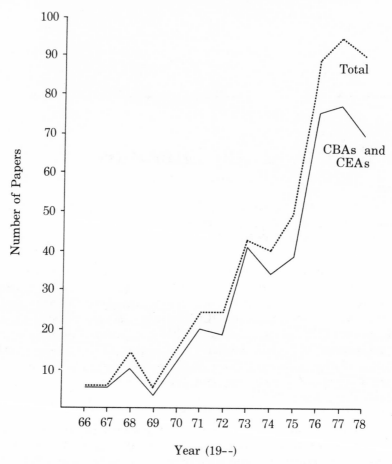

Year (19--)

while the dotted line traces the total of all references related to CBA-CEA (that is, including general methodology papers and clearly related references not readily identifiable specifically as CBAs or CEAs). As the data vividly demonstrate, significant interest in health care CBA-CEA is a phenomenon of the 1970s. Before then the annual number of health care CBA-CEAs and related publications never exceeded fourteen; after 1970, there were never fewer than twenty-five; and since 1976, the total has always exceeded eighty-eight.[2]

The general proliferation of professional health care journals might be expected to result in increased numbers of articles on many subjects without representing a genuine increase in relative interest in this subject. To provide perspective, one can compare the increase in CBA-CEA literature with that of the total increase in number of citations in *Index Medicus*. Over the entire period studied (through 1977, since 1978 was not fully indexed when we acquired our data), *Index Medicus* citations increased from 157,000 to 260,000 articles, a growth of two-thirds. By comparison, the CBA-CEA literature grew by a factor of fourteen to eighteen. Even recently, growth in the latter has considerably outpaced that of the overall medical literature. For example, from 1975 to 1977, the number of contributions to the CBA-CEA literature nearly doubled, while *Index Medicus* citations increased less than 10 percent.

Will health care CBA-CEA literature continue to grow? The number of contributions dropped in 1978, and preliminary analysis of 1979 data suggests that the number did not rebound significantly in that year. However, several recent influences might be expected to promote growth. Publicity associated with a variety of governmental efforts should increase awareness and interest (Altman and Blendon, 1979; U.S. Congress, Office of Technology Assessment, 1980a; Wagner, 1979). Of great potential importance are numerous efforts within the medical community, many discussed in Chapter 1, that should spark interest and promote analysis. Continued public concern about the high and growing costs of care should itself generate numerous attempts to assess the cost-effectiveness of medical procedures and technologies.

The federal government's direct interest in supporting health care CBA-CEA appears to have shifted considerably with the transition from the Carter administration to the Reagan administration. When Congress established the National Center for Health Care Technology in 1978, its mandate to assess the safety, efficacy, and cost-effectiveness of medical technologies was interpreted as fostering analytical activities such as CBA-CEA. The Reagan administration's elimination of the Center, combined with severe cutbacks in other health services research funding, implies substantial reduction in both the direct financial support for analysis and the indirect leadership role the government had been developing in the area of health care CBA-CEA. Other things being equal, this should dampen future growth in the performance of analysis.

PUBLICATION VEHICLES

Figure 4.2 plots the annual number of articles in medical and nonmedical journals. Its purpose is to examine the proportion of the literature that has been intended primarily for a physician audience and to determine how this proportion has changed over time. The graph shows a shift from rough parity before 1973 to a clear majority of medical journal articles after 1973. In other words, the rate of growth of medical journal literature has exceeded that of nonmedical journal literature, particularly in recent years. This shift is statistically significant at $P = .05$.

In categorizing references by publication vehicle, we kept track of a subset of medical articles, namely those published in the *New England Journal of Medicine*. We isolated these articles because of

Figure 4.2: Diffusion of CBA-CEAs by Type of Journal

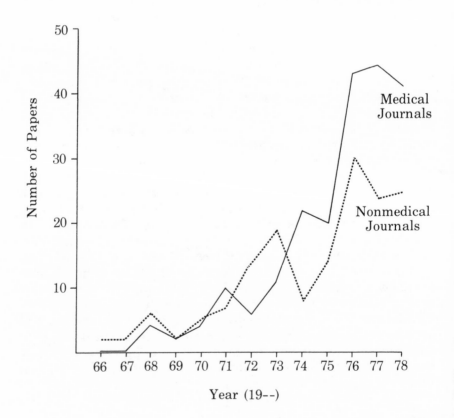

the journal's general position of leadership in the medical literature and because several of the best, most influential health care CBA-CEAs have been published there. It is interesting to observe that, prior to 1975, the number of contributions related to CBA-CEA in the journal exceeded one only once (in 1968, when two contributions were identified). It published seven relevant articles in 1975 and four or more each year since.

For the reasons discussed in Chapter 1, we anticipate continued growth in physician interest in issues of cost containment and cost-effectiveness. As a result, we expect the growth in medical journals' share of the literature to persist, although possibly at a slower rate because of increasing interest in CBA-CEA among nonphysician health professionals. At present, most nonphysician health professional groups seem to be lagging behind physicians both in terms of cost consciousness and involvement with CBA-CEA. Consequently, there seems to be potential for relatively more rapid growth in CBA-CEA contributions written by and directed toward nurses, health educators, and so on. If this occurs, the medical journal share of the literature might diminish. Nevertheless, the health care journals' share of the literature will almost certainly continue to increase.[3]

MIX OF CBAS AND CEAS

Whereas in the earlier years (1966–73) the annual number of CBAs generally exceeded the number of CEAs, since the mid-1970s the reverse has been true. The difference in the mix in the two periods is statistically significant (see table 4.1). This provides support for Weinstein's conclusion that CEA "has been gaining in acceptance relative to benefit-cost." The reason, however, is not obvious. Weinstein attributes the shift to "the conceptual limitations of the [human capital] approach and the empirical barriers to the willingness-to-pay approach" to valuing benefits in CBAs (Weinstein, 1979, p. 58). Other explanations relate to the apparent simplicity of CEA relative to CBA: analysts use CEA because it is easier for the economic layperson—such as the physician—to understand. The recent relative growth of CEA in medical journals appears to include more contributions by physicians, who may find CEA easier and more acceptable to perform than CBA.[4] We anticipate that the trend toward CEA will persist, although the distinction between CBA and CEA seems likely to diminish. As we observed in the preceding chapter and will discuss again later,

Table 4.1:   Trends In Health Care CBA-CEA, 1966–73 and 1974–78

Publication Classification	Years	
	1966–73	*1974–78*
Average annual number of publications	17.0	73.2
Publications in medical journals as percent of total journal publications	40.2	62.7
CEAs as percent of combined CEAs and CBAs	42.1	53.2
Percentage of articles on:		
Prevention	44.7	22.0
Diagnosis	18.8	30.9
Treatment	36.5	47.2
Percentage of articles with orientation toward:		
Individual	8.3	15.8
Organization	21.3	10.8
Society	70.4	73.4

All differences significant at $P = .05$.

increasingly sophisticated CEAs will incorporate elements of CBA that were traditionally ignored in CEAs.

MEDICAL FUNCTION

Of three broad categories of medical functions, prevention and diagnosis each account for slightly more than a quarter of classifiable studies in the bibliography, while treatment accounts for just under half.[5] However, comparing earlier and more recent years, we find a significant shift in the relative mix away from prevention and toward diagnosis and treatment. Between 1974 and 1978, the number of both diagnosis- and treatment-oriented papers has exceeded earlier totals by a factor of four or five. By contrast, the number of prevention-oriented contributions is only 50 percent greater between 1974 and 1978 than it was earlier (see table 4.1).

This shift seems consistent with the relative growth in the medical journal share of the literature (assuming that physicians are relatively more interested in diagnosis and treatment, compared with prevention, than are nonphysician health professionals). Also, early health care CBA-CEAs concentrated relatively more on the "public good" aspect of health care[6] (particularly communicable disease control) than on individual patient care. Several excellent communicable disease prevention studies can be found in recent medical literature (Schoenbaum et al., 1976*a*, 1976*b*), but this is one of the few substantive areas in which the number of pre-1974 papers exceeds the number from 1974 through 1978.

The permanence of the shift away from prevention is problematic. The widespread perception that technology is a major villain in medical cost inflation, combined with the general medical orientation toward diagnosis and treatment, has contributed to growing interest in the CBA-CEA literature in diagnostic and treatment technology and in individual physician decision-making concerning the use of such technology. These interests should be sustained in the near future. However, increasing public acceptance of the idea of health promotion should encourage renewed interest in prevention-oriented CBA-CEA. This might reverse the relative decline through the 1970s in prevention's share of attention in the literature.

In addition to examining the mix of contributions oriented toward prevention, diagnosis, and treatment, we investigated the mix of types of treatment. Half of all papers on treatment were concerned with curative treatments; the remaining half were divided roughly equally between rehabilitation and maintenance. Perhaps reflecting the inherent subjectivity and difficulty of quantifying "relief from pain," "comfort," and so on, the literature included not a single contribution that we could identify as dealing with palliation. The relative mix of treatment functions does not appear to have changed significantly in recent years.

PHYSICAL NATURE OF SUBJECTS OF STUDY

In attempting to categorize subjects by their physical nature, we found ourselves incapable of definitively assessing the vast majority as technique, drug, procedure, equipment, personnel, or system. Most seemed to represent a mix of two or more categories; consequently we included them in the "miscellaneous" category.[7] Even some which we did manage to categorize left us feeling uncomfortable. For example, a study of the cost-effectiveness of CT scanning appears on the surface to belong under "equipment" (where we did categorize it), yet that same study will emphasize the important role—and cost—of the technicians needed to operate the scanner.

Our principal impression is that the literature covers a broad spectrum of types of programs and technologies, with procedures being the best represented category. In recent years, there appears to have been distinct growth in the attention devoted to equipment-embodied technologies, though that growth has been heavily concentrated on one such technology: CT scanning.

DECISION ORIENTATION

The original intent of CBA-CEA was to assist in social decision-making, to identify and value program costs and benefits from a societal perspective, but the CBA-CEA label seems to be applied with increasing frequency to narrower analyses. Often the perspective is that of an organization, such as a hospital or a government agency. Frequently, it is that of an individual, most often a medical practitioner.

Our data suggest that the social perspective has dominated the literature over the entire period studied, accounting for roughly 70 percent of all publications in both the early and more recent years. However, articles oriented toward individual decision-making have increased rapidly in recent years. Comparing the pre-1974 period with the years 1974 through 1978, one observes a near doubling of the share of papers oriented toward the individual perspective, balanced by fewer papers with an organizational orientation. While the two categories together account for fewer than 30 percent of the contributions to the literature, the shift is statistically significant (see table 4.1). It represents a trend we expect to continue while the medical profession's interest in cost concerns continues to expand.

SUBSTANTIVE TOPICS AND AREAS OF INTEREST[8]

Health care CBA-CEA literature covers a vast array of health problems and all of the major medical functions. Yet despite the diversity, a few subjects and concerns account for a large share of the literature. In this section, we identify topics that have been the object of multiple studies, as well as a few topics that have received little or no attention. In many instances, we discuss plausible explanations for the relative amount of attention devoted to the various topics. In general, there are certain factors that stimulate or restrict interest in performing a CBA-CEA. The importance of the health problem is often reflected in the amount of literature addressing it. The availability of viable alternative means of preventing, diagnosing, or treating the problem is another factor affecting the frequency with which the problem is addressed in the CBA-CEA literature. Cost alone may be of sufficient importance to encourage analysis of whether a procedure can be justified on the grounds of anticipated benefits.

A few factors serve to restrict analysis. For example, although a topic may be a prime candidate for CBA-CEA in terms of its importance or cost, ethical or political considerations may serve to limit the number of relevant analyses undertaken (witness the case of abortion). Finally, an obvious hindrance to analysis is difficulty in quantifying important outcomes, as is the case in our finding not a single instance of analysis of treatment for purposes of palliation.

POPULAR SUBJECT AREAS

The disease class that has captured the most attention in the literature is also the nation's number one killer: cardiovascular disease. Nearly three dozen papers in the bibliography concern this disease, while an additional nineteen citations relate to hypertension screening and treatment. Other major diseases have also received considerable attention. Cancer screening programs have been the subject of over thirty papers, including a dozen on breast cancer screening. Twenty-one papers have addressed mental illness problems and programs, with a similar number of citations relating to dental care. Together, drug abuse and alcoholism account for two dozen references. Renal disease has received an amount of attention (roughly twenty papers) disproportionate to its incidence but reflective of the political and economic importance associated with public funding of dialysis. The federal government's mid-1960s interest in disease control programs, and in kidney disease in particular, made this the only disease to have more than one citation prior to 1969.

Two general classes of health problems have captured considerable attention. Communicable diseases have been the subject of some thirty papers. Since communicable disease and its treatment have distinct social characteristics, this is a logical subject for CBA-CEA; it is not surprising, therefore, to find that a large proportion of all the communicable disease papers were published prior to 1974. By contrast, the second class of problems—the prevention of birth defects—has been studied much more in recent years, with only two of nineteen papers published before 1974. Several diseases have received isolation attention, but at least one—phenylketonuria (PKU)—has been the subject of three studies. Except for PKU and rheumatic fever, there were no multiple studies of any single disease.

Several diseases emerge in the guise of surgeries intended to treat them. Each of the following surgeries is the focal point of at least one reference in the bibliography: radical cystectomy, tonsillectomy, cholecystectomy, herniorrhaphy, appendectomy, synovectomy, joint replacement, and hysterectomy. In addition, there is a substantial number of papers related to surgery and CBA-CEA, but they are not identified with a specific surgery. Many of the surgery papers were contributions to a book on the subject (Bunker et al., 1977).

We classified nearly twenty papers as relating to each of screening and prevention, in addition to the papers referring to specific subjects noted above. Some of these papers dealt with particular activities (for example, multiphasic screening), while others discussed CBA-CEA issues more generally. A few represented attempts to cover several separate activities.

In recent years, a great deal of policy discussion and regulatory activity have concentrated on the adoption and diffusion of expensive, sophisticated capital equipment. Thus, it was with considerable interest that we explored whether such equipment had been the focal point of numerous CBA-CEAs. With one exception, the answer is a striking no. The exception, the CT scanner, was the most talked-about medical technology of the 1970s, and both the quantity and nature of the general interest are reflected in the CBA-CEA literature on CT. Nearly two dozen citations concern this technology, all but two of them published after 1976.

Will other equipment-embodied technologies emerge as the subject of much attention in the literature? As controversy over specific technologies grows, particularly controversy over their cost implications, additional CBA-CEA papers can be anticipated. Electronic fetal monitoring is an example of such a technology, and it has already been the subject of a few papers. The emphasis of several federal agencies on technology, combined with general interest and concern, should increase the proportion of CBA-CEA literature focusing on equipment-embodied technologies.

A variety of health-related services accounted for a significant proportion of articles. Some of these services have relatively tangible outcomes and hence are good candidates for CBA-CEA; for example, we found over half a dozen studies of pharmaceutical services. The literature review also yielded several articles on family planning and on maternal and child health programs. We classified over twenty articles in a broad category labeled "hospital services and systems."

Other services address social needs that are extremely difficult to quantify. In general, one would not expect such services to receive a great deal of attention in a literature that places a premium on quantification and measurement. Exceptions would be likely to reflect an unusual policy or social importance. We noted that there are twenty-one articles related to CBA-CEA in the mental health area. Similarly, we found eleven papers on geriatric services and five on institutional versus home care, with patient type not indicated. Given current problems and anticipated growth in the elderly population, continued interest in this subject matter would not be surprising. Another area of considerable current interest, occupational health and rehabilitation, includes both tractable and difficult-to-measure outcomes. We identified a dozen literature contributions on relevant topics.

Program services are not the only area in which social importance recommends analysis while quantification problems limit it. Manpower programs are another instance in which technical innovations—often, in this case, substitution of one type of personnel for another—produce outcomes that are difficult to quantify. Nevertheless, analysts have made sixteen contributions on this subject.

UNPOPULAR SUBJECT AREAS

In terms of importance, there are a few diseases that are conspicuously absent from the CBA-CEA literature. Cancer therapy and diabetes are prominent examples. A topic on which we found not a single CBA-CEA article before 1981, cancer therapy is a sensitive subject, one that evokes so much fear that the public (and hence analysts) may not be receptive to questioning on whether costly therapy should be attempted. Nevertheless, the parameters of the cost-effectiveness of cancer treatment would seem to warrant attention, as a more recent study suggested. Studying bone-marrow transplants, Schweitzer and Scalzi (1981) found that conventional therapy for adult acute leukemia costs more than $30,000 for the patient's last year of life and yet is highly ineffective. There must be numerous other examples of cancer therapies with extremely high costs and very little, if any, effectiveness, yet our social and political response to cancer seems to preclude consideration of alternatives to such therapies.

In the case of diabetes, we found only one directly relevant article (Tunbridge and Wetherill, 1970). The dearth of CBA-CEA literature on diabetes may reflect the relative absence of treatment alternatives or questions about the effectiveness of variations on insulin therapy. With the evolution of technologies that could infuse insulin automatically, it would not be surprising in a few years to see this understudied topic become a focal point of some CBA-CEAs.

We noted above that CT scanning serves as the one major exception to the rule that CBA-CEAs specific to sophisticated capital equipment are less common than policy interest might lead one to suspect. Continuing interest in this subject should prompt more analysis.

Related to the paucity of equipment-specific studies, relatively few diagnostic procedures, other than screening procedures, have been the subject of CBA-CEA attention. A few procedures have received isolated discussion, but only radiology has received frequent attention. We found some sixteen papers relating to diagnosis other than CT and screening, a relatively small number when one considers the variety and importance of diagnostic procedures. Weinstein (1979) has identified the evaluation of diagnostic procedures as deserving of CBA-CEA efforts. His finding is supported by the growing body of literature that indicts the increasing use of diagnostic tests as a major source of medical cost inflation (Scitovsky and McCall, 1976). The evidence suggests that common tests which are individually inexpensive are, in the aggregate, at least as significant in total cost increases as the more sophisticated and individually expensive technologies (Fineberg, 1979; Redisch, 1974), yet the former have received very little CBA-CEA attention. We suspect that the low unit cost of such tests has obscured their collective importance. Problems of measuring and valuing the outcomes of diagnostic procedures inhibit ready application of CBA-CEA.

A few health care services with measurable costs and effectiveness have received much less attention than their social importance would seem to warrant. For example, reproduction and contraception issues have been the subject of much public debate for many years. When one abstracts them from their moral context, several such issues should lend themselves to reasonably objective CBA-CEA. Yet moral overtones may dominate the potential for objective consideration of appropriate topics for analysis. An obvious example, abortion, has been the subject of only two papers (Catford and Fowkes, 1979; Mandel, 1975).

Two other areas seem underrepresented in the literature. For the last several decades, drugs have epitomized the scientific growth of medicine and dramatically altered the practice and outcomes of health care. Drugs have been the subject of hundreds of biochemical and medical studies and, within the social sciences, numerous analyses of medical technical change. Yet, aside from implicit and tangential interest in them (as a component of hypertension management, for example), drugs have not often concerned CBA-CEA analysts. An explanation may be that drugs are usually paid for directly by millions of individuals, so their cost-effectiveness has not been perceived as a major public sector concern.

The literature reveals very little evidence of attempts to compare specific medical and nonmedical means of dealing with health problems. Although our bibliographic search focused on medical approaches, we might have expected to find a few studies that cross the medical-nonmedical border. Yet with the exception of the early HEW efforts, the principal mechanism for crossing that border is the reader's location and comparison of separate, independent studies. For both conceptual and empirical reasons, this is not a highly rewarding analytical strategy. Conceivably, heightened awareness of prevention alternatives will motivate formal efforts to grapple with medical-nonmedical comparisons in the future.

PUBLICATIONS CONVEYING PRINCIPLES AND PRACTICE

The vast majority of studies referred to in the preceding section have never been considered in other reviews, primarily because those reviews concentrated on the twenty, thirty, or forty analyses that experts would classify as technically sound, high-quality studies—the tip of the CBA-CEA iceberg. Many earlier reviews acquainted the health care community with both the principles and practice of analysis, or at least practice that conformed well to the principles. Any student of CBA-CEA would find his or her appreciation of these techniques and their applications significantly enriched by consulting these reviews.

We have documented the dearth of health care CBA-CEAs found in the literature prior to the 1970s. Not surprisingly, efforts to convey the principles of analysis to the health care community are few and recent. Methodology and review publications addressed specifically to an audience of medical professionals are still fewer in number and of very recent vintage.

Of publications written solely to present or evaluate health care CBA-CEA, the first we found appeared in the mid-1960s. In 1966,

Crystal and Brewster (1966) wrote an introduction to CBA-CEA in the health field. The following year, Klarman (1967) published the first of two prominent reviews he has written, this one appearing in the *American Journal of Public Health.*

From 1967 until 1972, no significant health care review or methodology contributions appeared in print, with the exception of a chapter by Grosse (1970) in a book oriented toward students of economics and policy analysis. This chapter is particularly noteworthy for its review of CBA-CEA applications done at HEW during the author's tenure there. Grosse conveyed much of the same material in an article published two years later (1972b); again, the audience was not health care professionals. In that same year, however, a book that became one of the health care community's most widely read and frequently cited contributions, Cochrane's *Effectiveness and Efficiency: Random Reflections on Health Services* (1972), was published. In our estimation, this short book profoundly influenced the thinking of health care professionals concerning issues of resource scarcity and the link between efficiency and equity. It is at least possible that Cochrane's book played a significant role in the rapid growth in health care CBA-CEA that began the following year.

In 1974, Klarman published two articles on CBA methodology and its application. One is the most often cited review and discussion of health care CBA-CEA (1974a); the other was the first such article to appear in a medical journal (1974b). The following year, Dunlop published a review in *Social Science and Medicine* (1975). The year 1975 also witnessed publication of a controversial issue of the *New England Journal of Medicine.* The issue was devoted to a discussion of CBA-CEA and related methodology (McNeil et al., 1975b) and several illustrations of its application (McNeil and Adelstein, 1975; McNeil et al., 1975a; Neuhauser and Lewicki, 1975; Pauker and Kassirer, 1975). To many observers, this issue stands as a landmark in the evaluation of medical practice.

Two years later, the *New England Journal of Medicine* offered readers a discussion of CEA methodology (Weinstein and Stason, 1977b), a sophisticated application of it (Stason and Weinstein, 1977), and a thoughtful treatment of the limitations of formal analysis (Fein, 1977). Many health services researchers judge this package, combined with Weinstein and Stason's book on hypertension policy (1976b), to be a milestone in health care CBA-CEA. In December 1977, the Arthur D. Little Company completed the "Introduction to Cost-Benefit Analysis Applied to New Health

Technologies" (Harris, 1977), which was intended to assist health planners and others and which was prepared under a contract with the Bureau of Health Planning and Resources Development in the Health Resources Administration, HEW.

In December 1978, at the Urban Institute Conference on Medical Technology, Weinstein (1979) assessed the literature and reviewed "a nonrandom sample" of health care CBA-CEAs. The most noteworthy feature of the paper is the author's discussion of remaining methodological issues. While several of these have been of concern since the inception of formal CBA-CEA, others represent subtle, sophisticated problems, the existence of which is testimony to progress on more basic issues. Indeed, the paper serves as a vivid reminder both of the frustrating, seemingly intractable problems of CBA-CEA and of their gradual yielding to sustained conceptual and empirical struggle.

The past few years have witnessed several attempts to convey the principles of CBA-CEA to various elements of the health care community. In the fall of 1979, Dittman and Smith published an article in *Health Care Management Review* that presented a conceptual framework for consideration of costs and benefits (1979). Like the Arthur D. Little "Introduction," this work was supported by the Bureau of Health Planning and Resources Development and was addressed to health planners. Around the same time, Shepard and Thompson contributed a discussion of CEA principles to *Public Health Reports* (1979). More recently, Hellinger (1980) reviewed past applications and future prospects for CBA in health care, and Warner and Hutton (1980) examined the growth and composition of the health care CBA-CEA literature.

A theme of national health policy that emerged in the late 1970s—health promotion and disease prevention—constitutes the substantive focus of three recent reviews of CBA-CEA understanding. One, by Scheffler and Paringer, first appeared in the Surgeon General's report on prevention and health promotion and was later published in *Medical Care* (1980). Another, by Warner, was published in *Social Science and Medicine* (1979b). Rogers et al. contributed the third, to *Preventive Medicine* (1981).

Within the federal government, OTA recently completed a two-year study of *The Implications of Cost-Effectiveness Analysis of Medical Technology* (1980a), one component of which discussed the methodology of CBA-CEA and reviewed the health care CBA-CEA literature. The OTA report devoted considerable attention to the numerous CBA-CEA contributions that have escaped attention in the review literature, but that because of their numbers and publication vehicles, have constituted the principal exposure of many practicing health professionals to the language, concepts, and application of CBA-CEA. As the title suggests, the OTA report examined the implications of using CBA-CEA to establish or implement health care policy in the areas of reimbursement, planning, quality control, and premarketing approval of drugs and devices. The OTA study includes three volumes of case studies reviewing understanding of the costs and effectiveness of several important medical procedures (U.S. Congress, Office of Technology Assessment, 1981; Saxe, 1981; Wagner, 1981*b*).

QUALITY OF THE LITERATURE

The rapid growth in the health care CBA-CEA literature indicates considerable interest in, and even enthusiasm for, applying CBA-CEA to health care problems. Perhaps more important, it suggests increasing cost-consciousness within the medical community.

Unfortunately, growth in the size of the literature does not imply commensurate maturation in the technical quality of published analyses. Indeed, two opposite trends are detectable in the literature of the 1970s. On the positive side, a number of well-trained analysts, including several physicians, have been grappling seriously with difficult CBA-CEA problems in the context of specific health care applications. As a consequence, methodological progress is detectable on several fronts. Examples include the definition and quantification of multiattribute effectiveness measures (Bergner et al., 1976*b*; Brook et al., 1979; Kaplan et al., 1978), incorporation of indirect economic costs and benefits into increasingly comprehensive CEAs (Cretin, 1977), and substantive dealing with the unique problems of evaluating diagnostic technologies (McNeil, 1979; Wagner, 1981*a*). Multidisciplinary collaboration (including, for example, economists, sociologists, engineers, and physicians) has resulted in analyses that combine technique and substance in a particularly harmonious and sophisticated manner (Schoenbaum et al., 1976*b*; Weinstein and Stason, 1976*b*). All in all, these analyses have conceptually and substantively enriched the literature and have further defined the nature and sophistication of remaining methodological issues (Weinstein, 1979).

On the negative side, some of the rapid growth of the literature has come about because new practitioners of CBA-CEA include many individuals with interest, but little training, in analysis and only a rudimentary appreciation of its subtleties. Their enthusiasm is admirable, but it has not been matched by adequate skill in application. As a result, our impression is that the literature has included a higher proportion of technically low-quality analyses in recent years than in the early years of the period we studied. Numerous published studies reveal serious technical flaws or conceptual weaknesses in structure or interpretation. As CBA-CEA diffuses to nonphysician health care professionals, this tendency can be expected to persist.

An assessment of the quality of the literature depends on the yardstick by which it is measured. Here that yardstick is the technical characteristics of high-quality analysis identified in the preceding chapter. We wish to emphasize that technical virtuosity is not synonymous with usefulness. Usefulness refers to positive contributions to the thinking or behavior of health care providers and policymakers. We hope that influential studies are technically sound. Nevertheless, we must recognize the possibility that a technically elegant study might contribute little to the practice of medicine, while a "quick-and-dirty" analysis might stimulate useful cost-consciousness in those responsible for delivering health services—it might even have a direct impact on health policy. Consideration of the uses and usefulness of CBA-CEA is deferred until the next chapter. Here we focus exclusively on the technical merits of the published literature.

Two contextual aspects of the evaluation presented in the remainder of this chapter warrant emphasis at the outset. First, many of the limitations of health care CBA-CEA are inherent in almost all CBA-CEA. For example, the inability of health care CBA-CEAs to incorporate distributional considerations (Fein, 1977) is shared by CBA-CEAs on education, defense, energy, transportation, and so on. We will attempt to identify generic problems and distinguish them from those that are specific to health care CBA-CEA. We will also strive to distinguish between problems that can be resolved and those that are inherent in the process of analysis. Nevertheless, the reader should bear in mind that, although some criticisms are specific to health care literature, most are inherent in the process of analysis.

Second, reviews of literature often restrict their attention to the most prominent articles and books, as is the case in the earlier reviews of health care CBA-CEAs. There is a logic to this approach:

These publications reflect, and indeed create, the state of the art. Because they are widely read, their influence on professional thinking and on future contributions to the literature is disproportionate to their numbers. Nevertheless, as we noted above, such publications constitute only the most visible portion of the literature. The ten, twenty, or thirty articles repeatedly cited in health care CBA-CEA reviews represent considerably fewer than one-tenth of the publications that can be readily identified as part of this literature. The remaining nine-tenths of the literature provides the principal exposure of many practicing health professionals to the language, concepts, and application of CBA-CEA.

In order to capture the essence of what CBA-CEA means to health professionals, we believe it important to critique the entire literature. The basis of our review is an assessment of general tendencies in the literature as a whole, including the 90 percent of the iceberg that has escaped attention in previous reviews; but our emphasis on common problems and deficiencies is frequently counterbalanced by identification of successful attempts to address the deficiencies. We refer to these successful attempts specifically in order to identify for the reader the most prominent contributions to the literature. Thus, while we have adopted a generally critical stance toward the literature, we acknowledge the many examples of technical proficiency in the practice of health care CBA-CEA. For a review that concentrates on this high-quality end of the spectrum, we recommend the paper by Weinstein (1979).

Finally, rather than bury readers in the details of specific studies, we emphasize the general tendencies in health care CBA-CEA with regard to each of the components of analysis discussed in the preceding chapter. Thus the organization of the remainder of the present chapter parallels that of Chapter 3. References to specific studies, made throughout our discussion, are intended to illustrate phenomena of interest. Most of these studies are abstracted in Appendix D, but readers may wish to refer to the original publications for clarification or amplification.

DEFINING THE PROBLEM AND OBJECTIVE(S)

Most of the contributions to the early health care CBA-CEA literature focused on problems and specific objectives that had a distinct health (or disease) starting point (Dunlop, 1975). At the extreme, HEW analysts used CBA and CEA to examine resource allocation across a wide variety of disease- and accident-control programs (Grosse, 1970, 1972b). Narrower definitions of the problem implied fewer and less disparate alternatives, but the health relevance of the objective was generally clear. Thus Weisbrod's (1971) examination of the costs and benefits of medical research was restricted to the case of polio, but the analysis centered on the health consequences of polio research and consequent prevention of the disease.

In recent years, there have continued to be numerous attempts to use CBA-CEA to analyze programs having clear health relevance (for example, Cretin, 1977; Schoenbaum et al., 1976b; Weinstein and Stason, 1977b), but two factors seem to be increasing the proportion of studies whose health relevance is implicit, tangential, or simply unclear. First, and most distressing to us, is a tendency to assume that certain programmatic outcomes are desirable, without questioning their ultimate health implications. For example, Dawson et al. (1976) assumed that finding cases of certain childhood illnesses was socially desirable in itself, without exploring the health implications of medical follow-up. As a result, they interpreted the finding that case-finding was inexpensive as meaning that it was cost-effective. In addition to assuming a positive impact on health, they failed to examine the costs of follow-up.

The second factor is a technical one, directly reflecting the cost-containment emphasis of current health policy. Rather than focusing on promoting health, many studies today emphasize concern with efficiency in the provision of existing services, including particularly a group of intermediate medical services whose ultimate health impact is neither known nor questioned. Illustrative of this phenomenon is the CBA-CEA literature on CT scanning, which, as we observed in Chapter 3, is the only expensive, equipment-embodied technology to have been the subject of considerable CBA-CEA attention. The scanner exemplifies the difficulties involved in evaluating diagnostic procedures (McNeil, 1979; Wagner, 1981a), an area that has been identified as deserving much greater CBA-CEA effort (Weinstein, 1979). Despite their studying the same piece of equipment, the authors of the numerous CBA-CEAs diverge significantly in their perceptions of the objectives of scanning and, hence, in their evaluations of its cost-effectiveness. At one extreme, the diagnostic effectiveness of scanning is assumed, with no attempt to link diagnosis to either patient management or outcome; cost-effectiveness is measured as the cost savings of using CT, as opposed to alternative techniques, to perform a given volume of diagnoses (Gempel et al., 1977). At the other extreme, effectiveness is defined in terms of effects on disease management and patient outcome (Baker and Way, 1978). The latter seems the socially most desirable conception of effectiveness, but the problems in its determination are substantial, and it misses additional benefits such as those associated with decreasing patients' uncertainty, directing short-term patient management, and contributing to greater medical understanding (Abrams and McNeil, 1978; Banta and McNeil, 1978*b*). Needless to say, the differing objectives result in widely varying assessments of the social desirability of scanning.

Determination of objectives for purposes of analysis is frequently regarded as a trivial exercise, but the literature provides examples which illustrate that failure to appreciate the limits of a selected objective can mislead both analyst and reader. For example, when HEW analysts decided to compare the cost-effectiveness of alternative disease-control programs, they selected lives saved as the measure of effectiveness. The analysts discovered the limitations of this common measure by observing that an arthritis control program could never be justified on the basis of lives saved, yet the program ranked as one of the better investments when the benefits associated with disability avoided were taken into account in a CBA framework (Grosse, 1972*b*). Relatively few health care CEAs make explicit reference to the nature of the biases their effectiveness measures introduce. One suspects that many analysts do not even realize that such biases exist.

Distinctive efforts to capture in quantified objectives the subtle, often intangible goals of health services have been made in recent years. Perhaps most notable is the attempt to adjust for quality the number of years of life saved, an analytical tack discussed below under Benefits and Effectiveness.

IDENTIFYING ALTERNATIVES

By beginning with clearly articulated problems, early health care CBA-CEAs were able to explore a wide range of alternative interventions. For example, the interest of LeSourd et al. (1968) in identifying efficient means of grappling with kidney disease led them to compare the costs and benefits of a variety of programs, ranging from prevention of disease to treatment of renal failure. Similarly, Acton (1973) employed both CBA and CEA in examining several alternative prehospitalization programs for reducing deaths due to myocardial infarction. Even in studies of more limited problems—for example, the treatment of existing diseases—comparison of alternatives characterized much of the early analysis. Thus, the focus of Klarman et al. (1968) on kidney disease treatment precluded consideration of prevention alternatives, but the authors examined all of the major therapeutic alternatives.

In recent years, there appears to be a narrowing of problem definition in health care CBA-CEA. Accompanying this has been a reduction in the number and scope of alternatives examined in CBA-CEAs. The extreme—an analysis of a single program or procedure, with the only alternative being its absence—has become reasonably common in the literature (Schweitzer and Scalzi, 1981). Another development is exemplified by Eddy's (1980*b*) analysis of optimal cancer screening and the assessment by Schoenbaum et al. (1976*b*) of the desirability of mounting a national swine flu immunization program. Analyses such as these represent an intermediate position between single-program analysis and comparison of numerous qualitatively diverse alternatives: Analysts are striving to design or determine the optimal (most cost-effective) structure of a program by analyzing the effects of changes in several parameters and assumptions (such as compliance rates, diagnostic accuracy, and therapeutic effectiveness). In essence, such analysts are examining an infinite number of programs of a single type. While confining analysis to a single program type implies limitations, the approach holds the promise of making significant contributions to policy understanding and program development.

Narrowed problem definitions and the resultant reduction in the number and breadth of alternatives examined in analyses are subtly altering the character and purpose of CBA-CEA in the field of personal health services. The original purpose of CBA-CEA, to assist in broad societal resource allocation, seems to be yielding to more concern with efficiency in the small. Today, analyses more often focus on individual technologies or diagnostic or treatment modalities. And, closely reflecting the increasing concern about the costs of health services, CBA-CEA authors appear to be according relatively more attention now to cost containment than to optimal benefit expansion. We would characterize the latter as the predominant theme of the early years of health care CBA-CEA.

DESCRIBING PRODUCTION RELATIONSHIPS

As we observed in the preceding chapter, the process of specifying production relationships is the most technically demanding phase of analysis. As such, it serves as one of the principal features distinguishing high-quality analyses from the more typical contributions. We discuss characteristics and examples of the former below. Here we note characteristics of the much larger pool of typical studies.

The most common approach to describing future production relationships for a prospective (planning) analysis is to assume that existing relationships and conditions will apply to a similar program in the future. That is, analysts identify the inputs and outputs of existing programs similar in nature and purpose to the alternatives they are studying and use these to characterize their alternatives' production relationships. This process can lead to significant miscalculations if the analysts fail to account for a myriad of factors, identified in Chapter 3, which recommend modification (scale effects, technical change, market conditions, and so on). For example, in one study, the per-case costs of existing small, urban programs for case-finding and follow-up treatment of several health problems were multiplied by the number of untreated cases throughout the country to estimate the total costs of nationwide efforts to address these problems. Similarly, success rates from the existing programs were assumed to apply for the millions of untreated cases around the country. Regarding both costs and effectiveness, the study ignored the differences between the small, well-run urban programs and the variety of programs, in diverse settings, that would be necessary to mount a nationwide effort. Many important production issues were ignored, such as differences in compliance between eager volunteers and the rest of the population at risk, ease of case-finding in industrial work sites and elsewhere, and variations in resource availability, and hence costs, from one location to another. Implicitly, constant returns to scale were assumed for a scale increase of at least 100,000 times. Analytical errors such as these are found throughout the literature, though usually on a less dramatic scale.

The literature also reveals numerous examples of more intractable production-specification problems. Evaluations of CT scanning are plagued by the analysts' inability to predict technical changes in scanning and improvements in the efficiency with which a given generation of scanner is used. The severity of many similar problems of ex post facto evaluation for prospective planning increases the more novel the technology or program in question. A familiar, established, and successful program is more likely to represent a good model for planning purposes than is a new, conceivably experimental program. Yet a major role of forward-looking CBA-CEA ought to be to assess the potential costs and benefits of a program. As we noted in the previous chapter, the earlier analysis is done in the life (real or conceptual) of an innovation, the easier it is to have a desired influence on the diffusion process—to expedite or retard it or direct it toward a particular set of potential adopters—but the harder it is to assess costs and benefits with confidence. This problem is generic to CBA-CEA. In the health care literature, it is particularly obvious in the ex post facto analyses intended to influence future planning. The CT case illustrates this point well. Given an appropriate policy lever, early analyses might have influenced the diffusion process.[9] But the analyses based on early use of CTs evaluated experience and assumed that it would persist into the future, ignoring all of the problems noted above. Thus, some of the negative assessments of CT do not allow for more rationalized use of improved, and conceivably less expensive, equipment in future years (Baker and Way, 1978).

CT also serves as an excellent example of the great difficulties of undertaking analysis early enough to influence planning and decision-making. These difficulties span the spectrum of applications of CBA-CEA, but they are particularly severe in an area like medical care, in which technological change occurs rapidly and frequently. It would have been exceedingly difficult to perform an intelligent analysis of CT scanning prior to its diffusion. All of the studies in the literature relied on that early experience for data, and most of the early studies failed to anticipate changes which occurred only a couple of years following publication of the studies. Furthermore, anticipated changes in radiological technology may make CT scanning technically obsolete within a few years, yet the nature and amount of relevant information have not, to date, been adequate to incorporate this factor into an analysis intended to assist planning. Not a single study in the CBA-CEA literature on CT has addressed this issue.

The handling of joint production issues represents another generic CBA-CEA difficulty. Illustrative is the case of evaluating the cost-effectiveness of Pap smears, an activity that frequently takes place during a complete gynecological examination. Cervical cancer is only one of several diseases for which the patient is screened during the visit. How much of the cost of the visit should be assigned to the Pap smear? Luce (1981) developed a method of assigning costs on the basis of the purpose of the visit, recognizing where possible the marginal resource consumption attributable to the Pap tests. However, Luce's study is the exception to the rule in the literature: most analyses suggest limited understanding of the important differences between marginal and total resource consumption and their relationship to outcomes of interest.

Formal modeling is difficult, a fact that undoubtedly accounts for the lack of imaginative, useful characterization of production relationships in much of the literature. At the least, formal modeling requires talent in disciplined conceptualization; frequently, it also necessitates application of specific mathematical or formal modeling skills. The latter, in particular, are not abundant. Medical education generally includes no consideration of such skills, and few analysts with appropriate training from other disciplinary backgrounds have devoted their attention to health care CBA-CEA issues. There are, of course, notable exceptions. Specific CBA-CEAs in the literature have illustrated skillful conceptualization, use of mathematics, and formal modeling techniques (for example, Averill et al., 1977; Cretin, 1977; Deane and Ulene, 1977; Eddy, 1980b; U.S. Congress, Office of Technology Assessment, 1979; Schweitzer, 1974). As presented, many of these studies are beyond the comprehension of readers lacking the requisite technical background. Only a minority of the authors of technically sophisticated studies seriously try to explain for the unsophisticated reader both the methods and limitations of the techniques they use. Good examples of analyses in which authors demonstrate concern for effective communication are Cretin's analysis of treatment and prevention of myocardial infarction (1977) and Weinstein and Stason's package of a primer on CEA (1977b) and an assessment of optimal resource allocation for hypertension management (Stason and Weinstein, 1977). Other primers have also accompanied technically sophisticated studies (McNeil et al., 1975b), and review articles have communicated basic principles of modeling (for example, Klarman, 1974a). As interest in CBA-CEA grows in the health care community, both analytical and critical sophistication should increase.

High-quality analysis of production relationships does not require sophisticated modeling efforts. A few studies have exhibited both elegant conceptualization and structural simplicity. For example, in their analysis of the national swine flu immunization program, Schoenbaum et al. (1976b) considered the effects of varying acceptance rates, the probability of an epidemic, and so on in a manner that was technically sound and readily understandable. Particularly in the medical literature, the comprehensibility of studies such as this one probably serves to educate and build interest.

In closing our examination of the assessment of production relationships, we should emphasize that many evaluation issues have not been resolved conceptually. The handling of joint production inputs is one example. Another relates to the question of whether analysts should be concerned with theoretically optimal production processes and true opportunity costs or with those that reflect typical practice, often with built-in inefficiencies. The cardiologist's over-read of an automated EKG adds to the charges for this diagnostic procedure and to the true resources used, but how should such time be valued? If reliable and valid automation is achievable, but cardiologists persist in a pro forma over-reading, should over-reading be included at all in assessing the true production of an EKG? An exploration of the different possibilities demonstrated that assessment of this technology is quite sensitive to the empirical handling of such questions (Arthur D. Little, Inc., 1976).

COSTS

Although authors demonstrate much more interest in and concern about assessment of benefits, the literature reveals numerous examples of poor or inaccurate measurement and valuation of costs. Such deficiencies are frequently more insidious than those associated with benefit assessment, because authors commonly do not discuss cost analysis problems, thus failing to alert readers to them. Often the analysts themselves seem unaware of the deficiencies of their approach, data sources, and so on. Yet the outcome of many CBA-CEAs hinges on cost-accounting techniques (Luce, 1981).

Costs are a reflection of resources consumed. Thus many of the difficulties that have plagued cost assessment are perfectly analogous to those just discussed in the examination of analysts' handling of production relationships. Rather than repeat that discussion here, we simply note a few common problems: Often analysts have measured realized costs in an analysis intended for prospective planning, without allowing for learning, technical, and economic changes that seem likely to occur; they have failed to distinguish the cost implications of running programs under optimal versus average conditions; and they have not always accounted for the differential valuation of costs occurring at different times (the discounting problem, discussed below).

Certain problems particularly hinder sound cost analysis. Chief among these in the health care literature is the use of inaccurate or inadequate proxies for true costs, an insidious problem because of its pervasiveness and the failure of many investigators even to be aware of it. A major source of inaccuracy is the use of market prices as measures of costs. Published charges (for example, from hospital billings or insurance charges) are often used as the index of cost in health care CBA-CEAs. Occasionally analysts recognize that charges may not accurately mirror costs (Charles et al., 1978), but most often the problem is not even acknowledged. Use of hospital charges is particularly objectionable because of the large body of evidence that charges often are not based on costs. Thus, charges for certain laboratory tests exceed their costs and subsidize other hospital functions; frequently used, inexpensive drugs are often marked way up to subsidize less commonly prescribed, expensive drugs; prior to social insurance for the poor, private room charges exceeded costs in order to subsidize ward costs, which were not fully covered by charges; charges for the less resource-intensive later days of hospital care subsidize the high-cost earlier days; and so on. The vast majority of health care CBA-CEAs employ charges uncritically, frequently introducing potentially large errors into the estimation of the true costs of the programs in question. Of course, we must recognize that charges will be the costs of interest from some perspectives, for example that of the payer of a charge. Thus charges may be a good measure of cost in an analysis developed for a health insurance company. However, from a societal point of view, the correct cost is the real resource cost or opportunity cost; and the societal perspective is both the traditional point of departure in CBA-CEA and the perspective we have adopted in discussing methodological issues. At the minimum, analysts ought to explore the relationships between charges and actual market costs.

Inadequate cost assessment in the literature often results from failure to take into account costs that are real but hidden. For example, very few health care CBA-CEAs account explicitly for the costs of patients' time traveling to medical facilities and waiting for and receiving services. CBAs occasionally capture some of this by valuing lost productivity, but most commonly lost productivity measurement relates only to days of morbidity, disability, or mortality avoided, and not to hours involved in seeking and receiving care. Furthermore, lost productivity is not the only time cost associated with health care services.[10] This problem is exacerbated, however, by the fact that many employees are covered (through sick leave, for example) for time off from work for medical visits. Thus, neither the physician nor the patient perceives the time as lost, and analysts sensitive to the time-cost issue might overlook the fact that the time imposes real costs on society (such as physical productivity lost).

A second example of real costs that have escaped attention in health care CBA-CEAs is the value of volunteers' time. Indeed, we are unaware of a single health care CBA-CEA that has accounted for volunteer time, though in fairness we must note the limited number of studies in which the issue might have been important.

An unresolved cost assessment issue is whether analysts ought to assume efficiency in program operation or build in slack for likely inefficiencies. The former is appropriate for evaluating the ideal, while the latter seems more likely to reflect what will come to pass should the program be implemented. This issue has received virtually no attention in the empirical literature. Common practice has been to measure resources used in programs, rather than identifying efficient resource use, but relatively few studies suggest that the investigators have even contemplated the difference. Clearly, almost no one has consciously inflated costs to account for likely inefficiencies, cost overruns and the like (Wolf, 1978).

A technical cost issue of considerable importance in the literature derives directly from analysts' relative lack of attempts to distinguish marginal from average resource consumption. Most commonly, authors have used average total costs of existing programs to predict the costs of program expansion, modification, and so on. When capital costs are substantial, or marginal costs vary significantly, failure to distinguish marginal from average costs can produce, and often has produced, misleading cost estimates. Some analysts have demonstrated sensitivity to the distinction, but these have tended to be among the handful with some formal economic training. Direct extrapolation from average costs dominates the health care CBA-CEA literature.

In the preceding chapter, we noted that costs in a CEA can differ from those that would be included in the comparable CBA, since CEAs can include some economic benefit as negative costs. That is, all economic consequences are tallied in the cost column of a CEA, while they are divided between costs and benefits in a CBA. Several recent health care CEAs have incorporated negative costs in their cost assessments, for example the medical expenditures avoided by an intervention's having prevented later morbidity (Cretin, 1977; Deane and Ulene, 1977; U.S. Congress, Office of Technology Assessment, 1979; Stason and Weinstein, 1977). One related effort has introduced a cost-accounting procedure that we believe to be conceptually unsound, yet this procedure appears to have gained credence among scholars interested in health care CBA-CEA. We are referring to the concept of net health care costs, which includes a component adding in the costs of treating diseases that would not have occurred had patients not lived longer as a result of the original health care intervention. Thus, for example, a patient who avoids a premature death from stroke because of effective treatment of high blood pressure, but who late in life requires treatment for a cancer, would incur costs in this category. To us, the very concept of net health care costs is misleading. Presumably we are interested in net social costs, with health care constituting only one component. By the implicit logic of the net health care costs argument, *all* later health care costs should be included (periodic physicals, cosmetic surgery, and so on). More to the point, the comprehensive CEA ought to count as costs *all* future consumption that occurs because of the extension of life (that is, food, housing, entertainment, and so on). But including later consumption costs also necessitates including the individual's later productivity (earnings) as a benefit, which clearly might outweigh consumption. And including both consumption and earnings moves the analyst from the CEA mode toward the CBA mode. In short, net health care cost is not as meaningful as net social cost. In either case, to include later consumption costs that would not have existed in the absence of a medical intervention also requires the inclusion of later productivity, as reflected in earnings. Inclusion of consumption costs alone overstates costs in a CEA.

Availability of data and problems of quality hinder effective cost analysis in the health care literature, as well as in the CBA-CEA literature in other substantive areas. In the discussion of the use of hospital charge data, we observed that such data often provide an inaccurate picture of true opportunity costs. Charges, of course, are relatively accessible; many cost data are not, particularly when analysts wish (properly) to adjust market prices to reflect opportunity costs. The current interest in cost containment has promoted governmental efforts to acquire more and better cost information (for example, the National Medical Expenditures Survey), but the acquisition and appropriate use of cost data will linger as major problems in CBA-CEA for years to come.

The literature's handling of discounting and equity issues in cost analysis is discussed in separate sections below.

BENEFITS AND EFFECTIVENESS

Both conceptually and empirically, a central concern of many published health care CBA-CEAs is to adequately capture programs' health consequences. Only one such consequence lends itself to unassailable objective measurement—reductions in mortality—although even in this case, as we shall see below, variations in the kinds or quality of life saved introduce a note of subjectivity. Reduced days of morbidity or disability constitute a common, if not universally accepted, measure of health improvement. Of course, neither of these measures accounts for variations in the quality of the resulting days of less impaired health. As we will discuss below, analysts have adopted a few means of adjusting for this quality factor, but to date there has been nothing approaching consensus on specific methods of adjustment.

Other types of health benefits—distributional benefits, reassurance, and reduction in pain, for example—have never lent themselves to ready quantification or valuation in health care CBA-CEAs or, for that matter, in CBA-CEAs outside of the health care field. Much of the literature supports Fein's (1977, p. 752) contention that such "intangible" benefits are often acknowledged, sometimes in footnotes, and then ignored in formal calculations and ensuing discussion. We share Fein's concern that a sea of calculations may swamp unquantified considerations and thereby contribute to "a 'climate of opinion' [that] that which is measured is important and vice-versa." This risk places an extra burden on analysts to emphasize unmeasured benefits in presenting and interpreting their findings. Only a few analysts seem to recognize and effectively shoulder this burden.

The attempt to measure inherently subjective outcomes is an activity decidedly in its early infancy. Although there have been isolated attempts to employ health status indexes in CBA-CEAs, we are not aware of any CBA-CEAs that have used a direct measure of the most subjective health benefits. Nor have we found studies employing the indirect method of identifying net measurable costs (measurable costs minus measurable benefits) as the minimum value that would have to be assigned to an intangible benefit to make a program desirable. Indirectly, this "method" is implicit in several studies in which measurable net benefit was positive, implying that unmeasured health benefits would only increase the program's attractiveness and hence need not be valued explicitly. For example, Centerwall and Criqui (1978) demonstrated that thiamine fortification of alcoholic beverages to prevent Wernicke-Korsakoff syndrome in alcoholics produced sufficient health care resource savings that monetary valuation of health benefits was unnecessary to achieve positive net benefits. Some studies of CT scanning have found that it does not add to the nation's diagnosis bill, obviating the need to value less measurable benefits such as the procedure's noninvasiveness (Gempel et al., 1977).

The inability to quantify certain health benefits satisfactorily appears to be the primary reason for their exclusion from formal calculations. A secondary reason is a failure of analysts to recognize what patients want from health services. For example, recent criticisms of annual physical examinations have ignored the value of the reassurance associated with the physician's pronouncement that the patient is healthy (Spark, 1976). Similarly, comprehensive analyses of the tangible costs and benefits of treatment alternatives sometimes have ignored the emotional or psychological motivations leading patients to prefer one treatment over another. In their technically sophisticated CEA comparing hysterectomy and tubal ligation as sterilization alternatives, Deane and Ulene (1977) demonstrated how such factors can be incorporated qualitatively into an otherwise quantitative analysis, but only because the psychological factors supported the quantitative findings. Had the authors found hysterectomy more "efficient" than tubal ligation, they would have had difficulty incorporating the important nonpecuniary psychological costs of hysterectomy into the analysis. In any case, patients' objectives and values are not limited to measurable physical health improvement; and if patients' objectives do not represent social concerns, the very reason for considering a health program is challenged.[11]

Obviously, the significance of not being able to quantify certain benefits depends on their relative importance. In some cases, benefits have proven particularly difficult to measure objectively, yet their importance has prompted analysts to grapple with them in a CBA-CEA framework. Examples include mental retardation (Cohen et al., 1971), psychological problems (Saxe, 1981), and care of the terminally ill.[12] Without succeeding in quantifying the intangibles, the efforts of analysts to deal with problems such as these have contributed understanding of the nature of the problems and associated programs.

For many health programs, the principal health benefits are the more tangible, or quantifiable, reductions in mortality, morbidity, and disability. Nevertheless, even in these cases CBA-CEA assessment of benefits (effectiveness) is far from problem-free. How does one measure and value benefits (effectiveness) in units that are commensurable with each other, with costs, or both? For example, days of morbidity avoided are not directly comparable to days of mortality avoided.

There are three principal approaches to this problem in the health care CBA-CEA literature: (1) accepting it as unresolvable and selecting a single, presumably dominant, outcome as the index of benefit or effectiveness (implicit in this approach is the assumption, or hope, that nonmeasured benefits vary roughly proportionately and positively with the single outcome measure); (2) employing an index of health effects or of health status; and (3) valuing major outcomes in monetary terms. The first two of these provide effectiveness measures for CEAs, while the third yields the monetary benefit measurement needed for CBAs.

A Single Effectiveness Measure

The first approach is the most common one in the literature and the easiest to accomplish. It is also, however, the least conceptually appealing, for two reasons: Often it ignores certain benefits altogether and at other times it relies on the unsatisfactory (often implicit) assumption that decreases in mortality, for example, correlate highly with decreases in morbidity, pain and suffering, and so on. A prominent example, noted earlier, comes from the mid-1960s HEW disease control program analysis in which "lives saved" served as the proxy for all health benefits in the CEA comparison of programs. As the analysts observed, this effectiveness measure relegated arthritis to the bottom of the list of cost-effective programs. When the programs were compared by means of cost-benefit calculations, however, the ability to take into account reductions in arthritis-related morbidity and disability made the arthritis control program appear quite competitive with the programs that saved the most lives (Grosse, 1970).

The single-measure index of effectiveness continues to dominate health care CEAs, but modifications point the way toward more refined measures of health benefits. "Lives saved" is a gross but important index of effectiveness for many health programs. "Years of life saved" adds an element of quality to the nature of deaths averted.[13] This measure has been employed in several CEAs (Cretin, 1977; Luce, 1981). A further refinement involves adjusting the years of life saved to reflect the quality of those years. Klarman et al. (1968) provided an early example of quality adjustment in their CEA study of alternative treatments for kidney disease. They argued that a year of life with a well-functioning transplanted kidney was superior to a year of life on dialysis, given the time, inconvenience, and discomfort associated with the latter. Consequently, they arbitrarily valued a year of life on dialysis as equal to 0.75 years with a transplanted kidney. The arbitrariness of the value they chose might be a source of concern—why not 0.5 or 0.9?—except that they found that transplantation was more cost-effective than dialysis even if no quality adjustment was made. That is, the analysis was not sensitive to the specific value of the quality adjustment as long as one concurred with the basic assumption that life on dialysis was not preferable to life with a transplanted kidney.

Health Status Indexes

Over the past decade a substantial amount of research effort has been devoted to conceptualizing and testing a comprehensive measure of health, a measure we will label generically as a health status index. Designed to provide a snapshot of the health of an individual or group of individuals, the index can be used, theoretically at least, to measure the before and after effects of a medical or nonmedical intervention and, thus, provide the analyst with a comprehensive picture of the net health benefit gained. At least three major research groups are now refining this concept. The San Diego group pioneered health status index work with the first prominent methodological article in 1970 (Fanshel and Bush, 1970). They later coined the term "quality-adjusted life-year" in a paper that examined the cost-effectiveness of PKU screening (Bush et al., 1973). The health status index, as conceptualized by this group, consists of two basic components: a level of well-being at a particular time and a probability of progressing to different levels of well-being. The level of well-being consists of both a measure of functional level (for example, ability to work or walk unassisted) and a symptom-problem complex (for example, degree of pain or discomfort). The key to, and the most controversial aspect of, the overall index measure is the weighting schema. Through questionnaires, respondents are asked to weigh subjectively each health state on an absolute scale from zero to one, with zero being death and one being perfect health. The San Diego group has continually modified this complex process of calculating the health status index by simplifying the questionnaires and by validating the weighting schema (Kaplan et al., 1976, 1978, 1979).

In recent years, the health research and health policy communities have begun to use health status indexes in cost-effectiveness studies. Weinstein and Stason popularized the concept of quality-adjusted life-years in two prominent articles in the *New England Journal of Medicine* (Weinstein and Stason, 1977*b*; Stason and Weinstein, 1977). Two years later, OTA submitted a report to Congress describing the favorable cost per quality-adjusted life-year associated with funding pneumococcal vaccine for the elderly through Medicare (U.S. Congress, Office of Technology Assessment, 1979). The analysis played a major role in the development and enactment of the legislation that added such coverage to Medicare.

The second major group working on health status indexes is associated with the National Center for Health Services Research. This group has developed a sickness impact profile, which uses a questionnaire similar to that of the San Diego group but relies more heavily on the judgments of health professionals in weighting alternative health states (Bergner et al., 1976*a*, 1976*b*).

The third major research group, from the RAND Corporation, is developing the most comprehensive set of measures of health so far. This group rejects the concept of a single measure, preferring to characterize health status as consisting of three major components: physical, mental, and social health status (Brook et al., 1979). RAND is currently testing its health indexes in conjunction with its community-based national health insurance study.

Benefit Measurement

The third approach to valuing benefits in commensurable units is to translate all quantifiable outcomes into monetary terms—benefit measurement for CBA. In Chapter 3 we discussed the methodological issues of the various theoretical approaches to monetary benefit measurement. Here we note that, despite its conceptual appeal, the willingness-to-pay perspective has not yielded to efforts to develop consistent and meaningful empirical estimates. The literature includes very few attempts to apply willingness to pay in a CBA framework (Acton, 1975). By contrast, despite its conceptual limitations, the more manageable human capital approach has served as the cornerstone of health care CBAs. Analysts have been reasonably consistent in their use of the basic methodology of the human capital approach. That methodology is conceptually clear, and solid empirical assessment of the costs of illness has been performed (Cooper and Rice, 1976; Mushkin et al., 1978; Rice, 1966). A recent review of cost-of-illness estimates uncovered significant variations from one study to the next (Hodgson and Meiners, 1979), implying that the use of differing estimation procedures and data could compound spurious variations in benefit estimates introduced by the use of different sources of health-outcome data. The issue of the reliability and validity of cost-of-illness estimates has been addressed in a contract funded by the National Center for Health Services Research (Hu and Sandifer, 1981). In addition, analysts are working on conceptually new approaches to assessing the costs of illness (Hartunian et al., 1981; Policy Analysis, Inc., forthcoming).

We should emphasize that, while most CBA analysts have applied the human capital concept correctly, not all have. Benefits should be measured as the costs of illness avoided. Some analysts have used existing cost-of-illness estimates as direct measures of benefit, without recognizing that many of the illnesses avoided would have occurred years into the future and, hence, that benefits should be discounted. This has had the effect of inflating benefit estimates, in some cases considerably.

The literature demonstrates that choice of a benefit-valuation technique can influence significantly one's overall assessment of the positive side of a program. Furthermore, studies often find that indirect benefits, such as the value of productivity losses averted, dwarf direct medical care savings. For example, in examing worksite hypertension control programs, Hannan and Graham (1978) concluded that indirect cost savings generally equaled or exceeded program costs, but medical cost savings were only a fraction of program costs. This illustrates the profound impact that selection of the human capital approach can have on benefit valuation.

Beyond the choice of a basic approach to measuring benefits in any given study lies determination of the specific measure(s). In CEAs in the health care literature, the effectiveness measure often has been reasonably obvious, with different analysts selecting similar measures, thereby facilitating comparisons. Treatment of kidney failure is an example of different analysts' having selected the same measure of effectiveness—years of life saved—and, despite a difference of more than ten years in publication dates, their analyses having produced consistent results (Klarman et al., 1968; Stange and Sumner, 1978; Roberts et al., 1980). For some topics, however, effectiveness measures are less obvious, with the result that different investigators have selected qualitatively different measures and undertaken analyses that produced quite different and not directly comparable results. Earlier we reviewed some of the differences that have emerged in the CBA-CEAs on CT scanning. In fact, the problem of variable effectiveness measures seems generic in the area of diagnosis (McNeil, 1979). Its presence in the literature can be expected to grow if analysis of diagnostic procedures increases, as some observers believe it should (Weinstein, 1979). Resolution of the problem, if such is possible, may lie in imaginative efforts to identify multiple pathways from diagnostic accuracy to effects on patient management and health outcome (Wagner, 1981a). Of all the CT papers, only one attempted to relate scanning to such outcomes (Baker and Way, 1978); the other papers relied on intermediate outcomes, such as accurate diagnosis, as their measure of effectiveness. Baker and Way evaluated retrospectively the effects of body scanning on both patient management and health outcome. They measured the desirability of these effects by developing a scale ranging from one (for the case in which a scan was deemed to have saved a life) to eighteen (when a scan led to a patient's death). Although the scaling of effects involved arbitrary and subjective judgments, the authors' effort stands out as one of the few published attempts to bridge the gap between diagnosis and health outcome.

The literature includes relatively few examples of such efforts to grapple with challenging assessment problems. However, other approaches have been adopted. A few studies identify and array noncomparable measures of effects, such as that of Doherty and Hicks (1977) in comparing home care and day care programs for the elderly. The argument underlying the approach is that, if effects are important but cannot be measured in a common metric, decision-makers will find it more useful and less misleading to see them arrayed in an unfinished CEA (that is, one lacking a cost-effectiveness ratio) than to have one or more of them dropped for the sake of calculating a final cost-effectiveness ratio. Despite its incompleteness, the CEA contributes information and structure that can facilitate understanding of a policy issue. On the basis of their analysis, for example, Doherty and Hicks could not label home care as more or less cost-effective than day care. However, in the example they chose, they could conclude that day care was preferred on the basis of effectiveness criteria, while home care was less expensive.

The need for diverse effectiveness measures can reflect movement from one health care function to another. For example, mental retardation illustrates a substantive health problem for which assessments of prevention versus treatment necessarily involve quite different, noncomparable measures of effectiveness. Prevention of retardation, for example through PKU screening, has been valued in a cost-benefit framework for its ability to avoid the expenses of institutionalization and other care; that is, the benefits of the program are future costs avoided (Bush et al., 1973; Steiner and Smith, 1973; VanPelt and Levy, 1974). By contrast, many of the desired effects of programs providing care for an existing group of the retarded are less tangible and less economically oriented; the costs-avoided metric is clearly inadequate (Cohen et al., 1971). Obviously, the prevention-treatment effectiveness distinction is by no means universally applicable. Analysts have successfully relied on a consistent outcome measure in comparisons of prevention and treatment alternatives for kidney disease (LeSourd et al., 1968) and myocardial infarction (Acton, 1975; Cretin, 1977), among others. In these cases, preservation of years of life is a useful index of both prevention and treatment effectiveness.

As with cost analysis, benefit analysis suffers from a paucity of accessible, appropriate, high-quality data. We have the impression, however, that analysts devote more conscious attention to data issues concerning the benefit side of the equation, perhaps because the conceptual problems in benefit estimation are more obvious and interesting.

We close this consideration of the literature's treatment of benefits and effectiveness by noting two extremes that illustrate the point with which we opened this assessment: The rapid growth in the popularity of CBA-CEA in health care has produced a lot of mediocre and poor analysis, but it has also prompted useful methodological developments. Regarding the former, our review of the literature uncovered numerous examples of so-called CBA-CEAs that were devoid of effectiveness considerations; in essence, they were comparative cost analyses. At the other extreme, a few skilled analysts have incorporated CBA-like benefit measurements into sophisticated CEAs. As we noted in the previous chapter, traditional CEAs compared direct (and sometimes indirect) costs with effectiveness measures. It is possible, however, to include economic benefits in a CEA by subtracting them from costs, thereby deriving a net cost figure to compare with the effectiveness measures. Clearly this was Stason and Weinstein's (1977) intention in their analysis of optimal resource allocation in hypertension management. Ironically, the most direct evidence that this trend represents a merging of conventional CBA and CEA is the contrast between the title of a prominent analysis and its bottom line. Cretin (1977) labeled her study a "Cost-Benefit Analysis of Treatment and Prevention of Myocardial Infarction," yet she measured outcome as the dollar cost per year of added life, a CEA measure. Studies such as these demonstrate the potential for including both economic and noneconomic benefits in a single meaningful analysis.

DISCOUNTING

The discounting of costs and benefits realized over time is one of the more technical features of CBA-CEA and is consequently a principal source of confusion to the novice. This is reflected in the absence of appropriate discounting in papers written by persons, often health professionals, lacking training and experience in economic analysis. However, virtually all of the contributions published in journals in the forefront of health services research include discounting where appropriate.

Analysts who employ discounting generally handle the mechanics well. The single most common deficiency is the failure to test the sensitivity of findings (the bottom line of net benefit or cost-effectiveness) to the discount rate selected. Only a minority of the published studies employing discounting have included such sensitivity analysis. Yet, as several of these studies demonstrate, when significant realization of costs or benefits occurs well into the future, the discount rate selected and the method of discounting can play pivotal roles in determining a program's value (Stange and Sumner, 1978; Stason and Weinstein, 1977). For example, in her study comparing programs to treat or prevent myocardial infarctions, Cretin (1977) tested the sensitivity of her cost-effectiveness estimates to variations in the discount rate. The prevention program—the screening of school-age children for high concentrations of cholesterol—necessarily involved benefits deferred well into the future. With costs and benefits undiscounted, the net cost per year of life saved ranged from $2,441 to $2,855, depending on assumptions. Discounting at 5 percent produced a cost per year of life saved of from $9,353 to $12,640. At 10 percent, discounting caused the figures to leap to $66,660 to $94,460. These estimates compared with a range of $1,782 to $6,100 per year of life saved by the treatment alternatives, depending on the program and the discount rate. Cretin's article not only demonstrated the proper application of discounting, but it emphasized the dramatic effect that varying the discount rate can have on net cost estimation and hence on comparison of program alternatives.

A general CBA-CEA discounting question has received attention in the recent health care literature: Should effectiveness measures be discounted? Empirically, the question has been answered in the affirmative by Cretin (1977), Stange and Sumner (1978), and Weinstein and Stason (1976b), each of whom discounted effectiveness measures of mortality avoided in the future. The logic of discounting effectiveness is quite appealing, but the practice is relatively novel. We expect that both the logic and the examples set by talented analysts will increase the practice in the future.[14]

Changes over time in the discount rates used by health care CBA-CEA authors, as well as by government agencies, offer an ironic commentary on the times. As we explained in Chapter 3, discounting costs and benefits is independent of inflation, reflecting real opportunity costs, and analysts generally work in constant dollars (the value of money in a given reference year). Yet discount rates have crept upward over the period we studied, despite the fact that the real rate of return has remained basically unchanged. Historically, that real rate has run from 1 to 4 percent, occasionally higher. Yet since the early 1960s, discount rates employed by academic and government analysts have risen from that range to as much as 10 percent, a common figure today. We can only guess that an inflationary mentality has inappropriately injected itself into health care CBA-CEA. The importance of this development is that an unduly large discount rate introduces a negative bias in evaluations of programs in which benefits occur later than costs. This bias is felt most keenly in assessment of prevention programs, in which benefits are deferred well into the future, and hence are heavily discounted; this is well illustrated by Cretin's (1977) analysis of the effect of discounting on the cost per year of added life for prevention of myocardial infarction. Thus, other things being equal, analysis employing too high a discount rate can make prevention programs appear less economically desirable than they should. The literature, and policy analysis generally, will benefit from an appreciation of the appropriate range of rates for discounting.

ADDRESSING PROBLEMS OF UNCERTAINTY

The discount rate is but one of numerous potentially significant influences on the magnitude of cost and benefit estimates. As noted in the preceding chapter, it is a rare study that can be carried from conception to empirical conclusion without the necessity of the analyst's making assumptions to substitute for uncertainties, lack of data, conceptual problems, and so on. Despite this, it is not common practice in health care CBA-CEAs to test the significance of assumptions. Frequently, analysts even fail to carefully distinguish assumptions from sound empirical observations.

Several analysts deserve credit for sound, often imaginative means of dealing with uncertainty. Schweitzer's (1974) evaluation of prevention programs clearly illustrated the use of decision analysis to address the problem of alternative possible outcomes. In their assessment of the desirability and the structure of a national swine flu immunization program, Schoenbaum et al. (1976*b*) demonstrated how expert opinion could be utilized to produce necessary parameters unavailable elsewhere. The authors needed an estimate of the probability of an outbreak of swine flu and assessments of the impact of such an outbreak on health. Through use of the Delphi technique for soliciting a consensus among experts, they acquired the requisite estimates. Other authors have used probability theory to express expected values under conditions of uncertainty (Eddy, 1980*b*; Neuhauser, 1977*c*).

Of the possible uses of sensitivity analysis to address uncertainties, only one has been applied with some frequency in the health care CBA-CEA literature: the direct testing of findings to determine if they are sensitive to important assumptions. Even this most common application of sensitivity analysis has been used relatively infrequently, and, with a few notable exceptions, it has been used primarily for testing sensitivity to discount rates. The ability of sensitivity analysis to determine whether a major uncertainty precludes a definitive analysis does not appear to have encouraged analysts to tackle health care evaluation problems in which such uncertainties were obvious at the outset. Nor have analysts used measurable costs and benefits to establish minimum or maximum values for nonquantified variables in order for a program to appear worthwhile. As noted above, however, a few studies have approximated such uses of analysis. Centerwall and Criqui's (1978) assessment of thiamine fortification of alcoholic beverages allowed them to avoid valuing health benefits, since net cost savings were positive. And Gempel et al. (1977) found it unnecessary to attempt to value CT scanning's avoidance of invasiveness, since readily measurable cost considerations made scanning an attractive alternative to the diagnostic procedures it can replace.

Cretin's (1977) testing of the sensitivity of her findings to variations in the discount rate, discussed in the preceding section, illustrates the appropriate use of sensitivity analysis in its most common application. As Cretin's analysis demonstrated, program evaluation is highly sensitive to discounting when significant benefits (or costs) are deferred well into the future, a characteristic of many prevention programs. Discounting the costs of the cholesterol screening program by 10 percent instead of 5 percent increased costs per year of life by over 600 percent, while for the treatment alternatives, the benefits of which are more immediate, the corresponding increase was on the order of 50 percent. The potential for such dramatic differences explains why "responsible analysts usually offer the user of analysis a sensitivity analysis with respect to the discount rate used" (Weinstein, 1979, p. 59).

The authors of several good studies have also tested the sensitivity of findings to other uncertainties. For many health care programs, patient acceptance or compliance is a crucial variable— and an uncertain one—and hence a worthy candidate for sensitivity testing. The literature provides several examples. Schoenbaum et al. (1976b) examined the effect of acceptance on the optimal structuring of the national swine flu immunization program. Eddy's (1980a, 1980b) analysis of breast cancer screening also related such factors to program design. Weinstein and Stason's (1976b) study of hypertension control demonstrated how patient compliance can influence the outcomes of a CEA of disease management.

The literature offers relatively few examples of sensitivity analysis applied to other cost and benefit estimation, but those few are instructive. For example, LeSourd et al. (1968) found that the absolute magnitudes of individual benefit-cost ratios of kidney disease control alternatives were quite sensitive to variations in program size, target screening group, and so on, but that the relative rankings of the major programmatic alternatives (such as screening versus treatment and, within the latter, transplantation versus center dialysis versus home dialysis) were unaffected by the tested variations. In addition to testing sensitivity to the discount rate, Cretin (1977) included high and low direct cost estimates for the screening program. The analysis demonstrated less sensitivity to the direct cost estimation than to discounting. Geiser and Menz (1976) used sensitivity analysis extensively in examining how cost and outcome assumptions affected their analysis of public dental care programs.

The use of sensitivity analysis reflects a more sophisticated appreciation of CBA-CEA than that which characterizes most of the existing health care literature. At one level, inclusion of thoughtful sensitivity analysis multiplies the number of figures in an analysis and can add considerable complexity to the presentation and interpretation of findings. However, given both the logic and empirical evidence that assumptions can affect results significantly, the credibility and usefulness of CBA-CEA call for more frequent and judicious use of sensitivity analysis than is currently found in the literature. With the exception of a handful of high-quality studies, the existing health care CBA-CEA literature lacks credibility, in part because issues of sensitivity are addressed so rarely.

We note in closing this section that the use of sensitivity analysis carries with it a risk that many investigators may be unwilling to confront: A "solid" finding can dissolve under the scrutiny of sensitivity analysis, and nonresults are less exciting, and potentially less saleable, than definitive ones. Nevertheless, intellectually and from the perspective of the policymaker, accurate nonresults clearly are preferable to artificially definitive ones. The bulk of the existing literature does not permit us to distinguish these. Articles like Cretin's (1977), which make sensitivities clear, are the rare exceptions.

EQUITY

As we noted in Chapter 3, social programs generally entail a redistribution of resources. Sometimes this is intentional—Medicare and Medicaid are obvious examples—yet often it is inadvertent. The literature includes numerous examples of the latter, in which distributional implications are clear but not valued analytically. For example, the study by Schoenbaum et al. (1976b) showed that, although the swine flu immunization program was advertised as national in scope, high-risk-only strategies were considered and it was known that high-risk populations (such as the elderly) would benefit disproportionately from immunization in the advent of a serious epidemic.

Health care CBA-CEAs rarely have grappled seriously with equity issues. Obviously, selecting a topic to study is an implicit statement of concern with distributional issues, but as an objective rather than as an analytical variable in the CBA-CEA calculus (for example, the relatively large CBA-CEA literature on mental illness, geriatric services, and so on). Health care CBA-CEA should not be singled out for its failure to incorporate distributional considerations successfully. That failure reflects the general state of the CBA-CEA art and perhaps the inherent limitations of this form of analysis. But emphasis on this limitation is particularly important in the health care literature, where a readership unfamiliar with the techniques may be unduly impressed by formalism and its derivative conclusions, failing to place those conclusions in their proper distributional context. Many health care CBA-CEAs identify this concern, but it seems to get buried in the analysis that follows (Fein, 1977).

The most fundamental, perhaps intractable, equity problem is differentially valuing costs and benefits accruing to different groups of people. The literature offers few examples of attempts to address this problem directly. The issue is raised frequently, if implicitly, by authors' selections of benefit estimation methods. The most common CBA benefit estimation technique (the human capital approach) obviously values health benefits differentially, according to one's productivity. Less often recognized is that CEA effectiveness measures presumed to be value-free generally imply values. For example, a simple lives-saved measure of effectiveness implies that society (or the investigator) values the life of a ninety-year-old man the same as that of a ten-year-old child. Authors of studies employing such CBA and CEA measures rarely discuss the distributional implications of their selections, but the equity concern itself has produced a separate body of literature on the valuation of life (Acton, 1976; Rhoads, 1978; Zeckhauser, 1975; Zeckhauser and Shepard, 1976).

Early in this chapter we noted the apparent relative movement of the literature away from CBA and toward CEA. It is certainly plausible, as Weinstein (1979, p. 58) asserts, that this reflects growing distaste for explicit valuation of life or the belief that both conceptual and empirical limitations make the effort a "quixotic quest for a value of life." There is less conscious attention, however, to the potential distastefulness of implicit life valuation that CEA forces onto policymakers.

The appropriate handling of distributional issues remains one of the least developed features of CBA-CEA in the health care literature and elsewhere. While both theoretical and empirical progress can be anticipated (Weinstein, 1979), the major problems of dealing with equity concerns seem unlikely to be resolved in the foreseeable future. Perhaps the best that can be hoped for is increasing awareness of distributional concerns, achieved by increasing sophistication of the CBA-CEA readership and increasing emphasis on equity in written work, particularly in the presentation and interpretation of the results of analysis.

PRESENTATION AND INTERPRETATION OF FINDINGS

As we emphasized in the preceding chapter, two factors make it imperative that analysts present and interpret their findings carefully and clearly: (1) Technical limitations, inherent in analysis or in the abilities of particular analysts, often seriously restrict the possibility of arriving at unequivocal, definitive conclusions; and (2) the readership of health care CBA-CEA is generally unsophisticated about the techniques of this form of analysis. In addition, one must always recognize that numerous readers will focus on, if not limit their attention to, the abstracts and conclusions of articles.

An overall assessment of the health care CBA-CEA literature suggests that relatively few analysts have successfully addressed their responsibility to present and interpret findings carefully and clearly. Often, one suspects, this results from their own lack of insight. The exceptions, offering a thoughtful, useful conclusion to an analysis, are analysts who have produced technically and conceptually well-conceived studies. Examples abound. The analysis by Schoenbaum et al. (1976b) clearly identified factors that could influence the success and optimal structure of the national swine flu immunization program. Cretin's (1977) concluding analysis and remarks clarified the crucial role of discounting and demonstrated the need for and interpretation of sensitivity analysis. She made it impossible for the reader to conclude that there was an obvious best approach to reducing the toll of myocardial infarctions. Stason and Weinstein (1977) discussed how compliance and a variety of other factors could affect their conclusions about hypertension management, though Fein (1977) still found it necessary to emphasize limitations. Doherty and Hicks (1977) emphasized information organization and presentation in their assessment of health programs for the elderly; they refused to reduce their analysis to a bottom line. The authors of all such studies seem to be motivated by "the philosophy that it is not so much the *results* of a [CBA-CEA] that are likely to have an impact on policy as the *process* of structuring information in a systematic framework that brings to light the key uncertainties and the most important value trade-offs" (Weinstein, 1979, p. 53). This is inevitably reflected in these analysts' presentation and interpretation of their findings.

By contrast, most health care CBA-CEAs seem oriented toward the bottom line, generally the estimation of a benefit-cost or cost-effectiveness ratio. Aside from questions of measurement underlying the cost and benefit (effectiveness) components of these ratios, even this basic bottom line has been technically misinterpreted in numerous studies. At the extreme, at least one article with a title beginning with "cost-benefit ratio" does not contain a single cost-benefit ratio (Bennett, 1976).

Few analysts exhibit an awareness of the deficiencies of a benefit-cost ratio as compared with a measure of net benefits. The benefit-cost ratio clearly dominates in health care CBAs, yet the issue of the relative merits of the two measures is not even addressed in methodology articles directed to a health care audience. On the contrary, several methodology articles uncritically present the benefit-cost ratio as the appropriate measure of relative program desirability.

Cost-effectiveness ratios, and simply the term cost-effective, are employed even more uncritically than benefit-cost ratios in CBAs. In many articles, "cost-effective" refers to one of the two words but not both. That is, some authors have employed the term when they mean that a program or technology is effective, irrespective of cost; for others, "cost-effective" connotes "cheap," irrespective of effectiveness. There are several instances of purported CEAs in which only a single program or technology is examined and is then adduced to be cost-effective, despite the absence of an alternative with which to compare it.

Subtleties of technical interpretation of CBA-CEA bottom lines largely have escaped attention in the health care literature. We found not a single study which recognized that a lack of either comparable costs or effectiveness can prohibit meaningful comparison of the cost-effectiveness ratios of alternative programs. Only a few analysts have demonstrated an awareness that cost-effectiveness per use of a technology need not imply overall cost-effectiveness. For example, in certain delivery settings an automated EKG is more cost-effective than a manually read EKG, but if the ease and availability of the former lead to excessive use, the national EKG bill might actually rise without necessarily contributing to improved health (Arthur D. Little, Inc., 1976). A similar phenomenon followed the introduction of the automated, multichannel chemistry analyzer, which caused a sharp drop in the cost per test but produced a large increase in the numbers of tests performed (Weinstein and Pearlman, 1981). Perhaps the most dramatic demonstration of the difference between average and marginal cost effectiveness was Neuhauser and Lewicki's (1975) estimation that the cost per additional case of colon cancer found by repeated stool guaiacs rose from under $1,200 for the first stool guaiac to $47 million for the sixth.

Even when a ratio or net benefit measure is used correctly technically, the assumptions that underlie it and the intangible or unmeasured costs and effects that are excluded from it get lost. A few studies presented results in a manner that makes these factors clearer. As discussed above, the most common strategy has been careful discussion of how the bottom line could be affected by such factors. Some authors have presented ranges of results reflecting sensitivity to assumptions (LeSourd et al., 1968; Cretin, 1977). A third approach, less commonly adopted, has been to step back from the bottom line and provide a tabular display of programs and their (noncommensurable) effects. This approach does not yield a conclusion as to which of several competing programs is the best, but it does array alternative sets of consequences effectively and thereby can aid decision-makers by clarifying trade-offs (Doherty and Hicks, 1977). It also allows nonquantifiable effects, such as equity issues, to be accorded the prominence they deserve.

Such methods of presentation cannot compensate for analysts' misinterpretation of their own studies. A common error in health care CBA-CEA is the unwitting, inappropriate use of ex post facto (retrospective) analysis of existing health care programs as the basis for policy proposals. Analysts assess the costs and benefits of isolated existing programs and then directly infer implications for a regional or national expansion of the program. We have discussed the numerous problems inherent in this mixture of retrospective analysis and future policy prescription. Yet this approach appears to be common in the health care CBA-CEA literature.

FROM ANALYSIS TO IMPLEMENTATION

In health care studies, as elsewhere, the chasm between CBA-CEA and policy formulation and implementation is almost invariably bridged by the heroic assumption that a theoretically technically desirable program can be translated readily and directly into an operational one. Health care CBA-CEAs always have had a policy orientation, but the literature is nearly devoid of empirical attempts to make the adjustments needed to reflect political and cost realities (but see Luft, 1976; Wolf, 1978). Health care CBA-CEA should not be faulted for this lack; the implementation literature is simply too new.

Luft (1976) used two health care examples in his contribution to the implementation literature: development of freestanding surgicenters and use of work evaluation units to test functional work capacity to supplement the conventional information about the health status of patients who have recently had myocardial infarctions. Through these examples, he demonstrated how differing interests can block implementation of socially desirable programs and how analysts can use recognition of differing interests and influence to develop predictive CBA. Empirical application of Luft's important conceptual contribution could increase the realism and usefulness of CBA-CEA.

While not formally employing Luft's approach, a few other studies have observed how interests might be expected to block or inhibit implementation of socially desirable programs. For example, one study concluded that, in certain large delivery settings, automated EKG may represent a cost-effective alternative to the traditional manual readings. The investigators noted, however, that diffusion of this technology might be inhibited by cardiologists, to whom it could represent a threat to reading fees and a change in referral patterns (Arthur D. Little, Inc., 1976).

Another proposal in the implementation literature is that analyses build in consideration of the sensitivity of basic findings to unanticipated cost overruns (Wolf, 1978). We are not aware of any health care CBA-CEAs that have done this, though there are numerous instances in which it might have been done. For example, Schoenbaum et al. (1976*b*) could not have been expected to anticipate the Guillain-Barré syndrome—and its costs—that accompanied the national swine flu immunization program. Also, of course, the program experienced significant additional production and distribution costs. The analysts might have explored the implications of unanticipated cost overruns. Certainly any future analysis of proposed public health programs should do so.

The policy usefulness of health care CBA-CEAs awaits concerted efforts to incorporate into analysis the barriers to and costs of implementation. The general absence of such considerations reflects the state of the art in CBA-CEA in general. Its impact is felt acutely in social service program analyses, where these barriers and costs are potentially great.

In assessing the quality of the health care CBA-CEA literature we have relied primarily on judgments of how the practice of analysis compares with a set of theoretical standards, discussed in Chapter 3. Two caveats related to this approach must be recognized. One is that some authors have used terms such as "cost-effective" much more freely than they should have. Nevertheless, we have felt it appropriate to include their articles in a review of CBA-CEA since they contribute to the health care community's perception of the meaning of terms and uses of analysis.

The second caveat is that several of the standards of ideal (or idealized) analysis may be unobtainable. If so, any review of the literature will have a critical flavor to it. Many of the flaws of the health care CBA-CEA literature reflect inherent, or at least common, analytical problems. Examples include difficulties incorporating distributional concerns into formal analysis and deficiencies of data accessibility, quality, and consistency. Some common CBA-CEA problems impose unusually severe burdens on health care studies. The difficult and often controversial valuation of less tangible costs and benefits, such as lifesaving and reduction of physical suffering and emotional distress, is often central to the health care analyst's chore. Even more basic, the estimation of production relationships seems particularly challenging in health care, where the difficulty of attributing health outcomes to health care inputs has led many scholars to rely for evaluation on intermediate measures such as structure and process (Donabedian, 1969). Technical change occurs with such extraordinary rapidity that forward-looking health care CBA-CEAs are particularly handicapped. And even some commonly accepted second-best CBA-CEA practices are hard to justify in health care CBA-CEA, for example the use of market prices as measures of true opportunity cost.

Not all of the flaws in the health care literature are attributable to inherent difficulties. The relative novelty of health care CBA-CEA seems to account for the exaggerated importance of several errors. Representative are the absence or mishandling of discounting and the presentation of purported CEAs that examine only one program (that is, there are no alternatives) and conclude that it is cost-effective. More significant is the tendency of investigators to use purely retrospective evaluation of existing programs to develop policy proposals for the future, with little or no regard for the changes that will transform the structure and functioning of such programs. Many studies are plagued further by the black box approach to ascertaining production relationships: the identification of inputs and outputs proceeds without devoting sufficient attention to the efficiency of production, or even to basic questions of causation versus correlation.

By contrast, the best of health care CBA-CEA makes the novelty of the literature a source of encouragement. A handful of skilled analysts are breaking methodological and substantive ground, working on evaluative techniques, and producing informative, thought-provoking analyses. In recent years, investigators have demonstrated how analysis can yield insight into the nature of timely policy issues (Schoenbaum et al., 1976b),[15] contribute to efficient program planning (Eddy, 1980b), grapple with technical evaluation problems (Weinstein and Stason, 1976b), and apply to understudied technical aspects of medicine such as diagnosis (McNeil, 1979; Wagner, 1981a). Such work augurs a variety of interesting, and, one hopes, useful, developments in a field in which novelty provides a set of wide-open methodological and substantive opportunities.

A recent methodological development of considerable promise is the growing analytical comprehensiveness of CEAs and the consequent narrowing of the gap between CBA and CEA. Early health care CEAs tended to compare direct program costs with single-outcome measures of effectiveness such as lives saved. Recent efforts to incorporate indirect costs and develop more inclusive indexes of effectiveness (for example, quality-adjusted life-years) have begun to transfer a major virtue of CBA—its comprehensiveness—to CEA, without the accompanying problem of explicitly valuing noneconomic health benefits. Several studies demonstrate comprehensive cost accounting, with both positive costs and negative costs (indirect economic benefits) aggregated on the cost side of the CEA equation. The remaining noneconomic values constitute the programs' effectiveness. In some instances, the remaining effectiveness measure is a simple, single outcome—sterilization, for example (Deane and Ulene, 1977)—while in others it is a more complex index, such as Weinstein and Stason's (1976b) quality-adjusted life-years from hypertension control. In still others, effectiveness measurement or valuation is made irrelevant by the fact that complete cost accounting indicates a positive net benefit before remaining effectiveness is taken into account (Centerwall and Criqui, 1978). The narrowing of the gap between CBA and CEA is vivid in this last case. And recall that Cretin (1977) labeled her study a CBA, yet she did not place a dollar value on years of life saved and she presented results in terms of costs per added year of life—a typical CEA bottom line. While one might be tempted to dismiss this as a case of mislabeling, the growing economic sophistication and comprehensiveness of CEAs introduce a healthy ambiguity in terms.

A second example of promising developments is reflected in the work of Eddy (1980*b*), Neutra (1977), Schoenbaum et al. (1976*b*), Weinstein and Stason (1976*b*), and others who have used mathematical techniques to explore optimal program or decision design. Rather than simply evaluate a given configuration of inputs (that is, a defined program), these analysts have investigated how variation in several parameters, and hence in the input mix, influences optimal program structure. This is similar to sensitivity analysis in that the latter tests the robustness of a finding, while the former shapes the finding. In future research, related imaginative developments in, and uses of, sensitivity analysis should be considered equally important.

While our assessment of the quality of the literature has relied on comparison of practice and a set of theoretical standards, we should note that there are other bases for assessment of quality. For example, if one believes that quality is best reflected in the validity and reliability of results, one might seek internal or external measures of validity and reliability. An example of an internal measure is comparison of findings across studies of the same topic. To be sure, one must be wary of one study's replicating the methodology of earlier studies, or of the use of the same sources of data leading to a shared bias (consistent, but not valid, results). But in the absence of a shared bias, consistency of results is certainly suggestive of meaningful findings.

The literature provides a few cases of multiple analyses of a single subject, studies of treatment of renal disease being an excellent example. Two early contemporary analyses ranked treatment alternatives in the same order, transplantation being most cost-effective in one study (Klarman et al., 1968) and cost-beneficial in the other (LeSourd et al., 1968), followed in both studies by home dialysis, and, last, center dialysis. These results were confirmed in studies published ten and twelve years later and thus using more recent data (Stange and Sumner, 1978; Roberts et al., 1980). Similarly, three separate studies of PKU screening concluded that it is a socially desirable medical practice (Bush et al., 1973; Steiner and Smith, 1973; VanPelt and Levy, 1974). By contrast, analyses of CT scanning have produced widely discrepant findings, reflecting differences between head and body scanning, technical changes (realized and anticipated) over the period of time covered by the studies, and differences in investigators' perspectives as to what constitutes effectiveness in scanning or, more generally, in diagnosis (Abrams and McNeil, 1978; Baker and Way, 1978; Gempel et al., 1977). We have not attempted a systematic comparison of analyses on single subjects, but this might prove to be an enlightening approach to evaluating the literature.

Assessment of the quality of individual contributions to the literature has received primary attention in the last section of this chapter. In the first sections, we examined the overall composition of the literature, but judgments about quality were limited to observation of the conspicuous absence of certain substantive concerns, such as important diseases and medical techniques. Here we note that an interesting indication of the overall composition of the literature is the mix of CBA-CEAs with positive and negative findings. If some medical practices are socially and economically desirable and others undesirable (or of questionable desirability), one might expect a balanced literature to include a good mix of positive and negative findings. A lack of balance certainly need not reflect poorly done individual studies. Rather, it might result from analysts having a systematic bias in favor of studying desirable or undesirable programs. For example, if CBA-CEA were applied primarily to analyzing programs whose worth had been challenged, one might anticipate a preponderance of negative findings in the literature. A preponderance of positive findings could follow from medical professionals' analyzing (or commissioning analyses of) pet projects whose diffusion into practice they favor. Dominance of positive or negative findings could reflect systematic underestimation or overestimation of either benefits or costs. For example, as discussed above, few analyses include a realistic assessment of the costs of getting a policy implemented and of the possible dilution of benefits that may follow. These factors should produce overly optimistic results—that is, they introduce a distinct bias toward positive findings. However, many health care programs are characterized by important intangible benefits, the value of which frequently is not incorporated into analysis. This factor introduces a bias toward unduly negative findings.

We have found a dominance of studies having positive findings. To be sure, there are notable exceptions, with some analyses producing distinctly negative findings (Baker and Way, 1978; McNeil et al., 1976; Neuhauser and Lewicki, 1975; Weinstein and Fineberg, 1978). Surprisingly few studies have produced equivocal results.[16] Further, there may be a shift taking place, with movement from the positive toward the negative. This could reflect the general questioning of medical technology and the growth of cost-consciousness, both of which emerged in the 1970s.

At the beginning of this book, we explained our restriction of substantive attention to personal health care services. In concluding our review of the literature, it seems appropriate to observe that the community of health care CBA-CEA analysts has strongly established a similar border. Unless we remain cognizant of the existence of that border and its implications, this parochialism can mislead technical aspects of analysis and, more importantly, reinforce a social myopia about health resource allocation. A prominent example of a technical problem is the recent emphasis on measuring net health care cost in CEAs. As we discussed earlier, the socially relevant concept is net *social* cost, of which net health care cost is but one component.

Social myopia about health resource allocation results from failure to explore the possibility of cost-effective alternatives to personal health services. In the battle to reduce mortality and disability due to motor vehicle accidents, how might highway safety efforts—technical (such as safer road surfaces and shoulder barriers), legal (increased law enforcement), and so forth—compare with improved emergency medical services? To reduce hypertension-related mortality and morbidity, what is the appropriate mix of medical interventions and community health education on avoidance of risk? While there are separate studies of the costs and benefits of each such strategy, there is a paucity of comparative analyses crossing the medical-nonmedical or personal health-public health border. A noteworthy exception is comparison of community water fluoridation with a variety of individual treatment approaches to preventing dental caries (Burt, 1978). Our concern is not meant to reflect adversely on either existing or future individual contributions to the health care literature; the quantity and importance of analyses of specific medical problems and technologies is sure to grow, a development to be desired. Rather, we conclude that high-level policymakers, health planners, and individual health practitioners would benefit from the widening of perspective that some border-crossing analysis would offer.[17]

NOTES

1. The empirical analysis presented in this section derives from counts and classification of over 500 references on health care CBA-CEA. The development of the bibliography and classification of the references are described in Appendix A. For reasons explained in the appendix, the analysis in this section covers references dated from 1966 through 1978, although the bibliography includes a few references from years prior to 1966 and many references for 1979, 1980, and 1981.
2. See table 4.1, which summarizes the findings discussed in this section. Breaking the period into the early years (those before 1974) and recent years (1974–1978) represents an arbitrary decision based on our observation of trends. Nevertheless, it is interesting to note that this dividing line or one year earlier seemed appropriate for all of the phenomena of interest. Detailed data from which table 4.1 and figures 4.1 and 4.2 were derived are presented in Appendix B.
3. In the data illustrated in figure 4.2, we merely distinguished medical and nonmedical journals. Here we are subdividing the latter into health care journals and nonhealth journals. Nonhealth journals' share of the literature has receded as interest in economic issues has spread rapidly among all the health care professions.
4. The observation that physicians are making relatively more contributions to the literature in recent years is based on our impression. We made no attempt to formally categorize authors by degree or profession.
5. In a recent review, Weinstein (1979, p. 60) observed that "Diagnostic procedures, apart from screening tests, have received little attention." Our attribution of nearly a quarter of the codified literature to diagnosis is not necessarily at variance with this observation, since we include many screening programs in the diagnosis category.
6. The technical economic problem is one of significant externalities: these diseases are public health problems because they are communicable and because preventing them (for example, through immunization) benefits many members of society rather than just the recipient of the prevention measure.
7. In no year did we manage to categorize more than 40 percent of the references in other than "miscellaneous," with 20 percent being more typical.
8. The literature discussed in this section includes over 400 references published from 1966 to 1981. Rather than cite them here, we have prepared topic-specific reference lists in Appendix C.
9. CBA-CEAs on CT scanning emerged after the diffusion process was well under way. Even if they had been published earlier, effective policy levers were not in place throughout the country. Indeed, al-

though certificate-of-need programs existed, much subsequent policy and procedure evolved as a result of experiences in dealing with CT applications.

10. That people value such lost time is demonstrated by the willingness of many individuals to accept significant charges from private physicians in lieu of waiting a long time in low-cost medical clinics. The waiting-time mechanism of rationing medical services is highly socially inefficient, producing a deadweight loss—that is, patients lose their free time and no one gains directly from that loss.

11. There are instances in which the patients' objectives and values may be considered irrelevant, or at least secondary to society's values. Care of the severely mentally ill patient represents an extreme example. Externalities and paternalism provide more common justifications. A good example is the requirement that children receive certain immunizations prior to enrolling in school.

12. The VA is conducting a study, including a CEA, of a pilot hospice program at Wadsworth VA Hospital Center in Los Angeles.

13. "Years of life saved" is not clearly preferable to "lives saved." Everyone would agree that more years saved per death averted is preferable to fewer (other things being equal); but are ten years saved for one person preferable to four years saved for each of two people? Clearly the answer is inherently subjective.

14. Some analysts have argued that society's interests in intergenerational equity, and in the future in general, imply a social rate of time preference lower than the opportunity cost of capital, and hence that the former (lower) rate should be used to discount benefits (effectiveness) and the latter (higher) rate costs. This conceptual issue has not arisen in the empirical studies in the health care CBA-CEA literature. However, it is interesting to note that both individual and public decisions suggest that we may behave in quite the opposite manner. For example, conscious decisions to continue smoking imply a heavy discounting of the future relative to immediate gratification. At the societal level, public decisions to fund renal dialysis, rather than kidney disease research, screening, and prevention, suggest a high social rate of time preference. Of course, this logic assumes that, individually and collectively, we can interpret the abstraction of a future death averted by prevention as the same "commodity" as postponement of the death of a visibly ill individual. Obviously, we cannot do this. Nevertheless, our behavior and decisions are far from consistent with a low social rate of time preference.

15. The analysis of the national swine flu immunization program (Schoenbaum et al., 1976*b*) was conceived of, in part, as an experiment to see whether a formal analysis, relying heavily on concurrence of expert opinion (through use of a Delphi), could be accomplished quickly—prior to a policy decision—and still produce useful information. Despite its limitations—failure to anticipate social, legal, and medical problems and their economic sequels—the analysis served to inform and put issues into perspective for much of the health care community.

16. It can be argued that it takes a strong constitution to present equivocal findings. There is a common perception that the publication market

prefers "definitive" to ambiguous findings. This is reflected in the CBA-CEA literature, in which equivocal results seem to be much more rare than probabilities would lead one to expect. That is, while we observed a preponderance of studies with positive findings, there are probably many more studies with negative than with ambiguous findings. The latter tend to be competent analyses, the ambiguity often reflecting allowance for variation in uncertain parameters (for example, Cretin, 1977).

17. A budgetary pragmatist might argue that medical and nonmedical resource allocations are bureaucratically independent, with border-crossing reallocations extremely unlikely, and hence that border-crossing analysis is not worthwhile. While we concur about the resource allocation process in the short run, relative resource allocation does change eventually, and it might be responsive to analytical input. Clearly, this has been occurring in federal government prevention initiatives within the Department of Health and Human Services (U.S. Department of Health, Education, and Welfare, 1979). More to the point, however, our concern derives from the belief that the strength of analysis lies in its ability to affect thinking about problems—perspective—and not in the making of explicit resource allocation decisions.

5

Potential: Health Policy Uses and Usefulness of CBA-CEA

IN THE PRECEDING chapter we observed that an assessment of the technical quality of the literature was not the same as an assessment of its usefulness, its relevance to the thinking and behavior of health care providers and policymakers. Clearly the motivating force behind the growth in the CBA-CEA literature is the potential usefulness of analysis, not inherent interest in the theory or methodology. As we indicated in Chapter 1, the health care cost "crisis" has prompted a wide variety of efforts to deal with escalating costs. CBA-CEA is one such effort; to some observers it is viewed as a front-line soldier in the war on cost inflation. Indeed, the potential of CBA-CEA for contributing significantly to cost containment and improved resource allocation seems to be an article of faith in much of the health policy community. In the first and second chapters we noted several expressions of such faith emanating from government agencies, private insurers, medical professional organizations, and academic health policy centers. Yet the fact remains that both the potential significance and nature of CBA-CEA contributions to health care resource allocation have yet to be established.

The purpose of this chapter is to explore both of these factors— the nature and the potential significance of CBA-CEA in health policy—in the context of two additional dimensions: institutional setting and time. With regard to the former, we evaluate differences in the uses and usefulness of analysis across a variety of health care professions and organizations, some concerned with delivering health services, others charged with financing or monitoring their provision. As we explain below, the different incentives of and constraints on these groups will cause significant variations in their desires and abilities to employ CBA-CEA. With regard to the time dimension, we differentiate uses of analysis to date from possible uses. As we will demonstrate, belief in the policy usefulness of analysis represents a faith in the future. Direct applications of analysis to policymaking have been extremely limited. And that holds across all health care professions and organizations.

This chapter is structured in accordance with the above dimensions. However, to add perspective to our intent, we note that the purpose of the chapter is to address questions such as the following:

— In what ways might CBA-CEA contribute to health care cost containment?

— How might CBA-CEA contribute to improved resource allocation?

— Has CBA-CEA made significant contributions to date? If so, what and how?

— What are the factors that shape and limit the role of CBA-CEA?

— How might changes in the health care environment alter the nature and extent of the potential of CBA-CEA for affecting resource allocation in the future?

— What is the prognosis for the health care economy, given aggressive CBA-CEA therapy?

We identify alternative influences that CBA-CEA might have on health care resource allocation. Decision-making is only one—and perhaps not an important—role of CBA-CEA in a spectrum of potential uses and impacts. The uses and potential usefulness of analysis are explored in the context of four categories of possible users: (1) individual providers of health care (primarily physicians) and organizations devoted to serving them (professional associations and medical schools); (2) institutional providers of care (hospitals, health maintenance organizations, and local public health agencies); (3) organizations financing care (public and private third-party payers and organized consumer groups such as big business and labor unions); and (4) organizations involved in monitoring or otherwise regulating the quality of care (PSROs, health planning organizations, the Food and Drug Administration, and health care research organizations). In each of these four categories we examine both the use of CBA-CEA to date and its likely use in the future.

In selecting institutions to be explored, we were guided by their importance in health care resource allocation and by a desire to represent adequately the major functions indicated by the categorization (individual provision of care, institutional provision, financing, and monitoring). Clearly we have not included all significant elements of the system. Table 5.1 lists those elements, including several that we do not discuss explicitly in this chapter.

Following categorical examination of uses and usefulness, we drop the user-specific focus and turn our attention to some general considerations defining the potential usefulness of CBA-CEA. In part, this discussion serves to summarize key points from the preceding sections. However, its purpose is to reframe the examination of policy uses of analysis: to move from a positive examina-

Table 5.1: Partial List of Individuals and Groups Making or Influencing Resource Allocation Decisions

Individual physicians and other health care professionals
Individual patients
Medical professional societies and boards
Consumer groups
Health industry representatives and organizations
Hospitals, clinics, and other health care institutions
Labor organizations
Businesses
Health maintenance organizations
Medicare and Medicaid
Other governmental health care programs
Health planning organizations
Professional Standards Review Organizations
Blue Cross and Blue Shield associations
Other health care insurers and third-party payers
Other quality assurance or utilization review groups
Food and Drug Administration
Rate-setting commissions
Voluntary health organizations
Public health departments
Other state and local health agencies
U.S. Congress, executive agencies, and state legislatures
Health care systems, such as those of the Veterans Administration
    and the Department of Defense
Medical schools
Biomedical and health services researchers
Other health-related associations

Source: U.S. Congress, Office of Technology Assessment, 1980*a*.

tion—that is, an assessment of what is (and is likely to be)—to a normative evaluation—that is, an assessment of how CBA-CEA *should* be used in health policy making. This evaluation derives from both technical and social considerations.

POTENTIAL USES OF ANALYSIS

The potential uses of analysis are as heterogeneous as the potential users, yet relatively few discussions of CBA-CEA explicitly identify and differentiate among alternative uses. This is regrettable, because an assessment of the usefulness of analysis inevitably must rest on the standard against which performance is measured. For example, many detractors of CBA-CEA argue that it has not proved to be an effective decision-making technique. But criticizing analysis on this ground assumes that producing decisions is the proper role of analysis, a premise far from universally accepted.

Analysis as a decision-making technique—a common lay perception of CBA-CEA shared by some analysts—represents one extreme on the spectrum of potential policy uses or impacts. According to this popular view, a well-done analysis should produce the socially optimal answer to a policy question, and only bureaucratic intransigence or political factors will impede or prevent its implementation. At the other end of the spectrum is the view of CBA-CEA as a pernicious or sinister force, an assault on equity and the democratic ethos. A slightly less negative characterization of CBA-CEA is as a method whose technical and ethical limitations preclude useful output and whose formalism obfuscates, rather than clarifies, issues and intimidates the analytically unsophisticated. Furthermore, proponents of this view argue, the false precision and increasing popularity of CBA-CEA divert physical resources and intellectual effort from genuine analytical and policy needs in the health sector, needs such as system-wide reforms in reimbursement mechanisms.

A more positive perception of CBA-CEA is as a consciousness-raising exercise. That is, CBA-CEA is not expected to have direct influence on policy decisions, but its presence in the literature and in policy debates serves to raise the general awareness and understanding of the economic side of health care, particularly among members of the medical profession. In this view, individual CBA-CEAs are unlikely to have a significant influence on either specific medical practices or policy, but as contributions to a growing body of literature they may have a subtle, incremental impact on medical practice as medical professionals become gradually more conscious of costs.

The predominant view among leading health care CBA-CEA practitioners and methodologists is, as Weinstein writes (p. 53), "[I]t is not so much the *results* of a cost-benefit analysis that are likely to have an impact on policy as the *process* of structuring information in a systematic framework that brings to light the key uncertainties and the most important value trade-offs." Weinstein has also observed (p. 66) that "The greatest value of a formal analysis may be that it can force the various interested parties to agree what it is that they disagree about" (Weinstein, 1979). According to this view, individual analyses can have specific policy impacts by shaping the nature and direction of the policy debate, rather than by providing any direct answers. Thus, CBA-CEA is seen as a technique for *assisting* in decision-making. It feeds information (data) and perspective into a decision-making process that is, in many cases, inherently political.

Clearly, no fine lines demarcate each of these positions on the spectrum of potential policy impacts of CBA-CEA. However, by way of summary, figure 5.1 presents the variety of perceived impacts.

The next four sections examine the positions on this spectrum of each of the four categories of potential analysis users, in each case distinguishing between current and probable future positions. In essence, these sections examine the interaction of three dimen-

Figure 5.1: Range of Potential Impacts of CBA-CEA

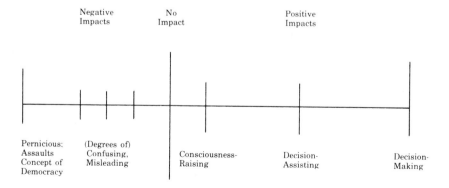

sions: user category, use and impact of analysis, and time (that is, present versus future). We differentiate between use and impact because the use of analysis need not be followed by the intended impact. For example, a third-party insurer might commission CBA-CEAs to be used in making reimbursement policy decisions; yet the resulting analyses might prove an inadequate technical basis for formulating a decision, or political factors might impede implementation of a technically sound, analytically grounded nonreimbursement decision.

At the outset, we should emphasize that virtually no experts would characterize the overall impact of CBA-CEA on health care practice and policy as being substantial. However, whether one assesses the record as encouraging or dismal may rest as much on one's basic attitudes toward analysis as on anything substantive. For reasons suggested below, the same characterization seems likely to hold in the future.

PAST AND FUTURE USES OF CBA-CEA BY INDIVIDUAL PROVIDERS AND THEIR ORGANIZATIONS

The growth of the CBA-CEA literature in medical journals, the introduction of health economics instruction in medical school curricula, and the formation of cost-containment committees in dozens of national, state, and local medical societies are all illustrative of the growing interest among the medical community in cost-effectiveness in health services. Clearly, much of the recent health care CBA-CEA literature has been directed at individual medical practitioners with the intention of contributing to an internal resolution of the cost "crisis." Whether analysts expect to serve more than a consciousness-raising function is unclear, but certainly they hope to encourage physicians to practice more cost-effective medicine.

DIRECT IMPACTS ON PHYSICIAN BEHAVIOR

Conversations we have had with academic physicians suggest to us a strong consensus that CBA-CEA has had little direct impact on individual physician behavior.[1] However, the consensus dissolves at that point. There is disagreement as to whether, or how much, CBA-CEA has significantly affected physicians' consciousness of economic issues. Explanations for the lack of impact on practice are numerous, varying significantly from one observer to the next. And the consensus on current practice impact does not translate into agreement on the future role of CBA-CEA in directly influencing individual physician behavior: Opinion seems to be split roughly in half between those who believe that CBA-CEA will cause many physicians to alter their medical practices and those who anticipate continuation of the current absence of significant effect.[2]

The principal explanations for the lack of impact to date can be grouped under two headings: The novelty of CBA-CEA in health care and the irrelevance of much of CBA-CEA to medical practice decision-making.

As we demonstrated in the preceding chapter, until very recently the literature on health care CBA-CEA was sparse, particularly the medical literature. Since few physicians read the non-medical health care literature, their exposure to the concepts and practice of CBA-CEA was minimal prior to the last few years. Needless to say, lack of exposure correlated highly with (and presumably caused in part) a lack of understanding of the techniques and meaning of CBA-CEA.

The novelty of CBA-CEA in health care also accounts for some of the quality problems in the published literature. However, while poor analytical quality certainly could be a barrier to application of the results of analysis, few observers cite it as a significant factor in the failure of physicians to apply findings to their practices. The readers' naiveté about CBA-CEA limits their appreciation of technical problems.

In a similar vein, the uncertainties in analysis frequently prevent determination of an unequivocal conclusion. Even when a firm bottom line is presented (program A is more cost-effective than program B), nonquantified factors (for example, the distribution of costs and benefits) can make the conclusion far from definitive. Thus, one could argue that even high-quality analyses frequently do not produce findings that can or should be translated directly into changes in practice by individual physician decision-makers. This seems an attractive explanation for physicians' nonresponse to analysis, particularly combined with whatever bewilderment they may feel as a result of their unfamiliarity with CBA-CEA. It is not, however, an explanation often noted in discussions on the subject. The explanation presupposes that other, preliminary barriers to application of analysis have been surmounted; the evidence is to the contrary. Thus, one might anticipate that such inherent technical limitations of analysis will grow in importance as other barriers fall. The significance of such limitations is considered in detail later in this chapter.

If the novelty of CBA-CEA in the health care literature—and hence physicians' unfamiliarity with both the methods and findings of analysis—is identified as the principal explanation for the lack of medical practice application, it follows that the increased presence of CBA-CEAs and related articles in the medical literature should inform and educate members of the medical profession and then possibly lead to changes in medical practice. This emphasis presupposes the potential for significant behavioral impact.

There are two basic sources of CBA-CEA irrelevance to medical practice decision-making—one substantive, one structural. In the substantive category, many CBA-CEAs have involved assessments of the desirability of social programs, and thus social, not individual, decision-making was at issue. Examples include the several studies of communicable disease control programs (Albritton, 1978; Schoenbaum et al., 1976a, 1976b), community- or industry-based screening programs (Eddy, 1980b; Hannan and Graham, 1978; Schweitzer, 1974; Weinstein and Stason, 1976b), and fluoridation of municipal water supplies (Newbrun, 1978). The subject matter of such studies precludes a direct practice response by individual physicians.

While this may serve as a useful partial explanation of the absence of significant behavioral response by individual practitioners, it cannot explain the observed degree of nonresponse, since much of the health care CBA-CEA literature is clearly relevant to decision-making in individual practice. Nor is this an often-cited explanation. A more cogent argument concerns structural irrelevance: according to a strict economic interpretation, most physicians' interests in cost-effective care deviate significantly from those of society. All physicians share an interest in understanding the effectiveness of medical procedures—procedures involving risks that outweigh medical benefits are undesirable—but concerns with the economic side of cost-effectiveness are either nonexistent or dependent on the physicians' economic environment. In general, as one physician describes it, "Cost data are psychologically remote. [The physician's] one-on-one relationship with the patient is not in the context of the cost to society."[3] However, the physician's economic circumstances can often produce a subsconscious reaction to costs. To a fee-for-service physician whose patients are well-insured, the cost of a procedure may be irrelevant, at best; at worst, if higher cost is associated with higher income, a finding that a procedure is not socially cost-effective could reflect its being a cost-effective means for the physician to increase his or her income. If the physician is salaried and the patients are well-insured, the economic factor is a curiosity, a social problem of no direct importance to the individual practitioner. Only if the physician works within the context of prepayment—that is, if he or she bears financial liability for the use of resources—does the professional concern with cost-effectiveness begin to approach the social concern. In any case, the patient's economic wherewithall often will be a major consideration: In an environment of prepayment or substantial insurance coverage, high costs of procedures do not translate into direct economic burdens on patients; hence the high costs are something of an abstraction to both the patient and physician.

This economic interpretation, emphasized by many knowledgeable observers, attributes the lack of effect of CBA-CEA on medical practice to its irrelevancy and even inconsistency with medical norms, irrespective of the quality or quantity of the literature. Accordingly, unless the reimbursement rules of the game were changed, this argument suggests that the future would auger little change in the application of CBA-CEA to individual decision-making. Note that this explanation need not rely on physicians' selfish monetary interests, nor simply on their indifference to economic considerations. Rather, nonresponse to CBA-CEA can reflect physicians' properly fulfilling their roles as agents of their patients. A physician's primary responsibility is to weigh all the costs and benefits of a procedure *to the patient*. If a particular test has a small probability of improving a diagnosis that could affect case management, the physician's responsibility to the patient is to compare that potential benefit with the cost to the patient—out-of-pocket costs, time lost, pain, and so on. In the case of a quick, noninvasive laboratory test, the nonmonetary cost of the procedure may be miniscule. If the patient's insurance covers the monetary cost, then, from the perspective of both physician and patient, the probability of benefit (to the patient or to management of the case) need not be great to warrant use of the test. From society's perspective, social costs may exceed expected social benefit; but asking the physician to adhere to the social standards of desirability requests him or her to deviate from the patient's best interests. In effect, the physician is placed in the untenable position of violating either the patient's or society's interests. Tradition, and perhaps even logic, favor serving the patient's interests.

The differences between social and individual economic and ethical considerations constitute the only frequently advanced explanation that does not imply a brighter future for the ability of analysis to directly alter individuals' medical practice policies. Only system-wide changes in the economic environment, such as growth of HMOs or major reimbursement reforms, could more closely align the practice of medicine with the precepts of analysis. The strength of the explanation does not depend on technical ignorance of CBA-CEA within the medical community; hence anticipated increases in familiarity with analysis need not promote the direct application of findings. Accordingly, barring external pressures, the economic incentives and ethical norms of medicine will continue to preclude widespread application of the findings of health care CBA-CEAs, except in cases where a procedure is demonstrated to be both more effective and less costly than an alternative. However, external pressures could increase the demand for and use of analysis. In addition to forces already in motion, proposed system-wide changes could increase medical interest in CBA-CEA. For example, a ceiling on national health care expenditures, with providers free to adapt to it as they saw fit, might lead the medical and hospital administration professions to identify unnecessary costly procedures and to police themselves to reduce their frequency.

Growth in the health care CBA-CEA literature should complement other efforts to raise the medical community's economic consciousness. Combined with institutional efforts to promote cost containment, CBA-CEAs may make some physicians sensitive enough to encourage either specific practice changes or a general cost-consciousness in their patterns of resource consumption. Thus, the effects of analysis may be real and desirable yet very subtle. Several indications of physicians' concern about costs support the plausibility of this line of reasoning, although the important question is how much practice will change in a cost-effective manner.

It should be emphasized that, when pressed, many of the academic physicians who believe that their medical colleagues can and will respond to CBA-CEA concur that they actually have in mind a response solely to the effectiveness side of the analytical equation. That is, a sophisticated analysis of sequential testing for purposes of diagnosis might conclude that the nth test was not cost-effective because it produced too many false positives. However, the grounds for physicians' responding to this would be the lack of medical effectiveness or, in fact, the potential for health damage. In essence, the medical mind-set is one of *medical* benefits and risks, with economic costs generally of limited concern.

Other health care providers, such as nurses and dentists, might also be interested in analysis, with their respective practice changes a function of similar factors, as well as the individual's autonomy in determining the scope of his or her work. As we observed in Chapter 4, however, few CBA-CEAs have been directed toward providers other than physicians. This is one reason that we limit attention here to physicians' reactions to analysis. Other reasons include the following: given the reimbursement and decision-making systems, physicians play the central role in the medical resource allocation process; they possess the requisite expertise to interpret the effectiveness side of medically technical CBA-CEAs; much of the recent CBA-CEA literature in health care has been directed at a physician audience; and physicians possess the professional autonomy to implement practice changes.

PROFESSIONAL ORGANIZATIONS AND CBA-CEA

Intended to represent their members' interests and serve their communities, several medical societies have initiated efforts to promote cost-consciousness among their members and cost-effectiveness in the delivery of services. Certainly much of the involvement of these groups reflects a genuine concern about the social implications of inefficient medical resource allocation. Their involvement also reflects the belief that, if the health care community does not get control of cost inflation, government regulators will do the job for it. But regardless of the motivation, the demonstrated interest suggests a receptivity to the kind of learning CBA-CEA can promote. This interest extends well beyond the medical community. For example, the American Dietetic Association has recently completed a study of the costs and benefits of nutrition care services (1979), and dentists have discussed the relative efficiency of alternative methods of preventing and treating caries and periodontal disease (Burt, 1978; Burt and Warner, forthcoming; Scheffler and Rovin, 1981). Whether the findings of such investigations will ever translate into significant changes in practice remains to be seen; we would expect technical professional considerations (that is, the effectiveness side of the equation) to continue to dominate practice decisions. But the consciousness-raising function of CBA-CEA seems well served by such efforts.

Many observers believe that the best way of promoting cost-effective practice is through medical education, the entry point into the world of practice. As we observed in Chapter 1, health economics is joining anatomy and physiology in the curriculums of the nation's medical schools (Hudson and Braslow, 1979). A variety of instructional efforts focused on cost-effectiveness in the practice of medicine is entering residency education (Kridel and Winston, 1978). Medical faculties are exhibiting an unprecedented openness to health economics education, and newly licensed physicians seem to be emerging with greater sensitivity to the need for cost-effective care.

The value of these efforts remains to be established. The specific contribution of CBA-CEA is even more ambiguous. Nevertheless, the educational atmosphere suggests a receptivity to the kind of understanding CBA-CEAs can transmit. We expect that CBA-CEA will contribute to the emerging cost-consciousness in the medical community, although other considerations, noted above, seem likely to continue to dominate much of the decision-making in individual practices. To the extent that reimbursement or regulatory policy is influenced by analysis, CBA-CEA can have an indirect effect on such decision-making. The roles of analysis in reimbursement and regulation are considered later in the chapter.

PAST AND FUTURE USES OF CBA-CEA BY INSTITUTIONAL PROVIDERS

Many institutional providers of care have a strong incentive for seeking cost-effective provision of services: They must operate within a budget. Health maintenance organizations are a good example of this in the private sector, and local health agencies are their counterparts in the public sector. Until recently, the most significant institutional providers of care, hospitals, rarely confronted explicit budget constraints.[4] However, increasing restrictions on reimbursement, including systems like prospective reimbursement, have greatly increased hospitals' interest in enhancing efficiency.

The need to operate within a budget increases the potential salience of CBA-CEA. This is particularly true for an organization possessing considerable discretion as to which services it will provide. Thus a local health department might be very interested in analyses comparing the costs and benefits of alternative programs for the community. With their services better defined, hospitals and

HMOs might have greater interest in efficiency analyses—that is, in determining the least costly means of delivering a given service.

HEALTH MAINTENANCE ORGANIZATIONS

Despite the apparent potential relevance of CBA-CEA to institutional providers, we are aware of only a few instances in which CBA-CEAs have been consulted by such organizations with an eye toward decision-making. In a recent survey of eleven HMOs, the OTA found that only the very largest HMO had conducted a formal CBA-CEA, and that effort had received some federal financial support (U.S. Congress, Office of Technology Assessment, 1980a). For years researchers associated with Kaiser Permanente have studied the cost-effectiveness of multiphasic health checkups, with the intent of seeking efficient means of protecting their members' health (Collen et al., 1977; Dales et al., 1979). Recently, Collen assessed the cost-effectiveness of biofeedback in order to help determine whether it should be covered by the Kaiser HMO (Collen, 1980). Analysts at several other HMOs report that they have consulted the health care CBA-CEA literature, but only one HMO has used the literature as a basis for decision-making. That exception involved a decision to eliminate routine chest X-rays and to modify adult physical examinations, pediatric prevention schedules, and indications for CT scans. The same HMO had investigated the literature on electronic fetal monitoring and coronary bypass surgery but found the results too equivocal to influence institutional policy decisions (U.S. Congress, Office of Technology Assessment, 1980a).

The barriers to use of CBA-CEA seemed reasonably similar from one HMO to the next. The organizations lacked the resources to perform in-house analysis—the requisite time, money, and expertise[5]—and several did not possess expertise appropriate to fully comprehend the published literature. HMO analysts noted that pressures to conform to the practice standards of the predominant fee-for-service system reduced many of their resource allocation problems to questions of efficiency; that is, how can the HMO provide service X inexpensively, yet in a manner that will look satisfactory to the membership (that is, in a manner that will mirror fee-for-service practice)? The political and marketing forces precluded decisions to withhold demanded services solely on the grounds of cost-effectiveness.

The HMOs also noted the irrelevance of much of the published literature, which focuses on all-or-nothing evaluations of medical procedures and technologies. The issue for many administrators is not whether they should acquire a CT scanner, but which indications are appropriate for scans and what volume and frequency produce cost-effective scanning (U.S. Congress, Office of Technology Assessment, 1980*a*).

Finally, the HMO analysts who were surveyed drew a clear distinction between the direct use of formal, sophisticated CBA-CEAs and an awareness of the basic issues underlying CBA-CEA. The latter was viewed as essential to HMO resource allocation decision-making, while the former was considered unnecessary and even inappropriate. Most HMO resource allocation decisions involve relatively narrow parameters (for example, how often to provide service X, or how to provide service Y inexpensively), and analysts felt that informal cost calculations generally would yield needed information.

Evidence from the OTA survey suggests an important prediction about the future role of CBA-CEA in HMO decision-making: unless the analytical capabilities of HMO staffs are upgraded significantly or the published literature is much simplified, formal CBA-CEA seems unlikely to play a direct or significant role in HMO policymaking. However, if CBA-CEA analysts were to move from sophisticated analyses to simpler ones focusing on the cost side of the equation, HMOs might find such input directly applicable. This conclusion echoes a general theme in many writings on CBA-CEA: The utility of analysis is a function of how directly it addresses a client's (or reader's) needs (Quade, 1975). As the HMO survey shows, the gap between decision-makers' perceived information needs and what published CBA-CEAs provide is substantial.[6]

HOSPITALS

We are not aware of studies of CBA-CEA use by other provider organizations; however, it seems probable that many of the above findings would generalize to hospitals. Many hospitals have staff analysts capable of understanding CBA-CEA, but political factors play a major role and the parameters of resource allocation decisions may be relatively narrow. Also, the speed required for many hospital resource allocation decisions certainly will not permit the time required to perform a careful CBA-CEA. Thus only those published analyses that directly address a given allocation question are helpful to the decision-makers. Such analyses undoubtedly represent only a small subset of those published in the literature.

Increasing pressures on hospitals to live within budgets should increase the salience of CBA-CEA. Nevertheless, we would expect significant use of CBA-CEA to be limited to those hospitals having the staff and the inclination to devote resources to long-term planning and consideration of alternative configurations of facilities and services. All such planning will invariably be seriously constrained by the politics of hospital administration.

LOCAL HEALTH DEPARTMENTS

CBA-CEA may be most relevant to local public health departments. These agencies generally operate within a budget, and many have a degree of latitude in planning their programming. They offer a mix of personal health services and public health activities, and directors have some discretion in deciding which of the efforts deserve emphasis. Given the community, or social, orientation of health departments, CBA-CEA seems an appropriate tool for providing information for program planning. The principal limitation on the use of analysis in local health departments seems to be the basic analytical expertise required. The political factor is germane here, as it is in HMOs and hospitals, but the set of acceptable activities seems less narrow in the health departments. Thus, although we do not expect it to be extensive, we recognize a potential for creative use of analysis in planning the work of local health departments. Our skepticism reflects doubts that many health departments will acquire the requisite analytical expertise, but the potential for impact is evident.

We caution that institutional providers may be forced (or strongly encouraged) to alter services or policies in response to reimbursement decisions or regulations resulting from analysis. Such effects of CBA-CEA must be considered indirect, since the provider is responding to explicit economic or legal cues rather than to the analysis that influenced those cues. We now turn to the potential roles of analysis in the areas of reimbursement and regulation.

PAST AND FUTURE USES OF CBA-CEA
BY ORGANIZATIONS FINANCING CARE

The financers of medical care have an obvious interest in assuring that the care delivered is cost-effective. To those who bear the cost burden directly—the consumers of care—that interest amounts to value for money. To private third-party payers, the ability to sell insurance is dependent on offering an attractive package of services with a competitive premium structure. To public third parties such as Medicare, the potential to contain costs rests to a significant degree on their ability to control charges and reimbursable services. As major financers of the costs of illness, each of these organized groups has not only an interest in promoting cost-effective care, but also the market power to translate a judgment concerning cost-effectiveness into a meaningful change in health care practice. Individual resource allocation decisions of the typical physician might effect a cost savings of thousands or even tens of thousands of dollars, but a single policy established by any of these institutions could have cost implications in the hundreds of millions of dollars.

With motivation such as this, it is not surprising that much of the enthusiasm and support for CBA-CEA derive from the community of health care bill-payers. Officials from the national Blue Cross and Blue Shield associations have expressed their interest in applying the findings of CBA-CEAs to reimbursement recommendations, and federal officials have stated a similar interest for purposes of determining Medicare reimbursement policies. A few private corporations have commissioned CBA-CEAs to assess the advisability of providing certain prevention programs for employees (Hannan and Graham, 1978).

BUSINESS AND LABOR

The interest of big business and labor in health care cost containment is a growing phenomenon. In the past, a variety of factors, especially favorable tax treatment of health insurance as a fringe benefit, has encouraged the expansion of health care benefits in employment contracts. Only recently has business begun to perceive a significant potential for controlling business costs by constraining the costs of health insurance and by improving employee health. Similarly, labor unions are beginning to view increases in health care costs as cutting into their members' benefit packages, consuming resources that might otherwise provide additional benefits.

Business and labor are convening increasing numbers of conferences to address industry health care cost and cost-effectiveness issues. For example, in June 1980, Health America, a firm that bills itself as "a national coalition for health promotion," organized a conference called "The First Executive Conference: The Corporate Commitment to Health." Topics discussed included screening, physical fitness, smoking cessation, alcohol and chemical abuse, nutrition and weight control, and stress and hypertension. A few months later, *Business Week* held a conference on "Cost-Effective Strategies for Corporate Health Care," at which the subjects examined included changing employee life-styles, counseling employees on the use of health services, reviewing claims, utilizing in-house medical personnel, self-insuring for employee health care, and promoting systematic economic changes through competition in health care services.

Industry trade journals are also devoting attention to cost-effectiveness issues. For instance, two successive issues of one journal featured articles reporting successful business programs to reduce health care costs (Taking Action to Contain Health Care Costs, 1980). The programs included IBM's voluntary health screening, reported to have significantly decreased its population of uncontrolled hypertensives; Blue Cross's estimated savings of $1,000 per case in Philadelphia by placing patients in a home care plan; and General Motors' alcohol rehabilitation program, reported to have saved nearly $10,000 in disability benefits and over $10,000 in lost work hours simply by treating twenty-five employees.

Still another indicator of corporate interest and action in cost-effectiveness is a report that major firms are increasingly contracting independently with PSROs to review admissions and treatment patterns for their employees. Reportedly, as many as fifty PSROs are performing this so-called private review on a contractual basis.[7]

Clearly, there is increasing interest within the private sector in decreasing health care costs by both promoting health and delivering care more efficiently (or cost-effectively). This interest, to a large extent, stems from powerful financial incentives that are finally becoming large enough to the private sector to warrant action (Luce, 1979). Nevertheless, the amount of interest exhibited in formal CBA-CEA to date remains small, though not nonexistent (Hannan and Graham, 1978). We anticipate that analysis oriented directly toward business and labor's perspective will increase.

THIRD-PARTY PAYERS—GENERAL

The ability of the major third-party payers to benefit from use of CBA-CEA is less obvious. Unlike individual health care practitioners and professional associations, third-party payers can realize only very limited benefit from the consciousness-raising function of analysis. Clearly these institutions possess the analytical capacity and the economic incentives to pay serious attention to CBA-CEAs, yet the question remains whether, and if so how, such institutions will use formal analysis. The ability of a good CBA-CEA to clarify issues and collect and organize information could assist planning and decision-making within many of these organizations. However, whether the findings of studies could be applied directly to general reimbursement decisions remains unclear. Some kinds of findings would lend themselves neatly to policymaking. For example, a clear-cut determination that a certain diagnostic procedure is both more expensive and less accurate than an alternative procedure would serve as grounds for nonreimbursement or nonacquisition of the former, though the medically decisive factor probably would be the technical accuracy of the procedure alone. A large cost differential between two equally effective procedures might also serve as support for a use-constraining policy decision, though opposition might be substantial if significant elements of the medical community questioned the equality of effectiveness. Indeed, CBA-CEAs seem unlikely to overcome significant opposition from the medical community to any policies recommended on the basis of analysis, possibly excepting the case of a truly dramatic cost difference.

This point deserves emphasis because of a major implication: clear-cut, unobjectionable CBA-CEA findings will be the exception, not the rule. Furthermore, such findings seem likely to reflect reasonably obvious differences between the alternatives being studied. When a CBA-CEA is undertaken out of genuine interest in evaluating alternatives, without significant prior expectations as to the outcome of the analysis, that outcome is unlikely to be definitive. As we have discussed in the preceding two chapters, analytical uncertainties and technical problems in CBA-CEA often produce equivocal results. Competing professional opinions on technical issues exacerbate the problem. Thus, definitive CBA-CEAs may support policy decisions, but their potential to *shape* such decisions seems limited by technical and political factors.

BLUE CROSS AND BLUE SHIELD

A few reimbursement decisions have been based on cost-effectiveness criteria. For example, the national Blue Cross and Blue Shield associations have recommended that member plans not reimburse automatically for batteries of laboratory tests on admission to a hospital, on the grounds that the very limited yield of the tests does not warrant their cost. Early in the CT era, some payers decided to withhold reimbursement for body scans until such time as their efficacy could be established. Safety and efficacy have long been criteria for reimbursement, but in this instance the importance of establishing efficacy seemed to rest on cost implications.

More recently, an excellent CEA contributed directly to development of a cancer screening program when the National Cancer Institute contracted with Blue Cross-Blue Shield to develop a model prepaid health service benefit package for cancer screening (Eddy, 1978a). Blue Cross-Blue Shield's medical necessity program, begun in 1977, was an approximation of cost-effectiveness logic for making coverage decisions; however, the program's emphasis on reducing the use of outmoded and redundant procedures places the weight of a nonreimbursement recommendation on the effectiveness side of the equation. Regardless of the motivation, the program has led Blue Cross-Blue Shield to recommend discontinuation of routine payment for approximately seventy surgical and diagnostic procedures, as well as the admissions tests mentioned earlier. It has been estimated that full implementation of these recommendations could save $300 million annually (U.S. Congress, Office of Technology Assessment, 1980a).

California Blue Shield is one of the few member plans that have formally adopted cost and relative efficacy as considerations in making coverage decisions. As in most plans, stage of development and general medical acceptance remain their principal criteria, but they have denied routine payment in a few cases in which a new procedure has been demonstrated to cost more than, and achieve the same result as, an existing procedure. Clearly this represents an application of CEA logic, though the nonreimbursement decisions represent the simple CEA cases, ones in which there is no trade-off between lower cost and higher quality (U.S. Congress, Office of Technology Assessment, 1980a).

FEDERAL GOVERNMENT

Instances of nonreimbursement decisions based on CBA-CEA are few and far between in the federal government. The government's coverage recommendations traditionally have derived from four criteria: safety, efficacy, stage of development, and acceptance by the medical community. To date, cost has not been used as an explicit criterion, nor, generally, has relative efficacy. The cost issue has arisen in certain dramatic cases in the past. The most notable was the debate over public funding of renal dialysis for end-stage kidney disease. Though not a conventional reimbursement decision (the population in question was not merely the elderly suffering from renal failure), the dialysis issue forced both bureaucrats and legislators to face a dramatic trade-off between cost and preservation of life. As we discussed in Chapter 2, CBA-CEAs convinced the bureaucrats to back off from support of a national dialysis program, given its short-term annual price tag of $1 billion and the greater estimated cost-effectiveness of kidney disease prevention strategies, but legislators were persuaded to enact funding legislation. Indeed, the case is quite instructive. Regardless of the technical quality of the studies, cold analysis could not capture a highly emotive factor: Existing victims of kidney disease, their relatives, and others who learned of their woes constituted a much more powerful political constituency than did the individuals, obviously ignorant of their plight, who would develop kidney disease in later years in the absence of an effective prevention program. In essence, Congress, presumably representing the wishes of society, did not equate years of life saved by avoiding onset of a disease with years of life saved for those who are visibly ill (Weinstein, 1979). This is not necessarily irrational behavior. Rather, it is an indication that the rationality of analysis is not the only rationality to be considered.

The current atmosphere in health policy circles—dominated by concern about cost and skepticism about the value (or relative value) of many procedures—has opened the door to the possibility of adding cost, or cost-effectiveness, as a coverage criterion. The Health Care Financing Administration has explored means of introducing cost as a criterion in Medicare coverage decisions. In 1980, the HCFA began an examination of whether the "reasonable and necessary" language in the Social Security Act, combined with other references to "reasonable cost," might permit inclusion of cost as a criterion.[8]

Notwithstanding the unresolved issue of including cost in the coverage formula, at least one precedent has already been set. In the spring of 1980, the Health Care Financing Administration rescinded an earlier decision to reimburse selectively for heart transplants (Reiss et al., 1980). The decision was based, in large part, on a staff estimation that costs for the procedure could reach as high as $500 million.[9] The HCFA argued that costs of this magnitude would prevent it from paying for other procedures that may be more cost-effective. In cooperation with the former National Center for Health Care Technology, the Health Care Financing Administration initiated in 1980 an eighteen-month study of heart transplants that will include a cost-effectiveness component. Its future coverage decision will be based on the resulting evaluation.

One should not misinterpret enthusiasm and activity as suggesting that cost-effectiveness will soon emerge as a dominant or even important factor in coverage decisions. Many analysts and officials have expressed reservations about the state of the art in measuring cost-effectiveness. They point out the difficulty of adequately measuring either of the two sides, cost and effectiveness, and anticipate a less than congenial reception to the technical limitations of analysis in a policy arena unfamiliar with it. The recent OTA report found that, although "Performing an analysis of costs and benefits can be very helpful to decision-makers ... [CBA-CEA] ... exhibits too many methodological and other limitations ... to justify relying solely on the results of [such] studies in making a decision" (U.S. Congress, Office of Technology Assessment, 1980*a*, p. 5). Again we conclude that, even if cost or cost-effectiveness is adopted as a coverage criterion, only the most clear-cut instances of excessive or unnecessary cost will be candidates for noncoverage decisions. It is important to note that even that small subset of practices will be limited further by the reluctance of officials to reexamine earlier coverage decisions. That is, attention will be focused on new technologies and procedures, those for which reimbursement precedents have not been established.

A corollary is that the need for and role of formal, sophisticated CBA-CEA will be very limited. Academic analyses may serve to support cost-effectiveness thinking—the consciousness-raising function—but except for a handful of technical studies, such as Eddy's work on optimal cancer screening (1980*b*) and OTA's analysis of pneumococcal vaccine (U.S. Congress, Office of Technology Assessment, 1979), formal analysis seems unlikely to serve as the direct basis for coverage decisions.

Finally, we note that the demise of the National Center for Health Care Technology in 1981 reduces much of the bureaucratic thrust toward incorporating cost-effectiveness into coverage criteria. Legislated by Congress in 1978 to assess the safety, efficacy, and cost-effectiveness of medical technologies, the Center was expected to serve as an integral component of the federal reimbursement decision-making process. Discontinuation of the Center, with its technology assessment activities transferred elsewhere in the Public Health Service, seems to have resulted from concern that the Center's activities would stifle medical technology innovation. It does not appear to represent repudiation of analysis per se.

PAST AND FUTURE USES OF CBA-CEA BY ORGANIZATIONS MONITORING OR REGULATING THE QUALITY OF CARE

Economic forces and public choices have moved health care further and further outside the boundaries of the conventional market. In place of the market's discipline, a wide variety of organizations and agencies have evolved to oversee, and often control, the workings of the health care system. These organizations share an interest in promoting the quality and efficiency of health care, but their specific charges, resources, and modes of operating vary significantly. In this section we examine the relevance of CBA-CEA to each of four such organizations: PSROs, health planning agencies, the Food and Drug Administration (FDA), and the federal agencies engaged in research on health and health care.[10]

PROFESSIONAL STANDARDS REVIEW ORGANIZATIONS

Established by federal law in 1973 (Public Law 92-603), the PSRO program is intended to help improve the quality and control the costs of medical services reimbursed by federal payment programs. Individual PSROs consist of medical professionals who function as a local peer review group. The federal program sets standards and criteria for the desired quantity and quality of medical services, and the PSROs evaluate the services actually provided against these standards. Payment for services is made only when the services are deemed medically necessary.

It is clear that PSROs are viewed in part as mechanisms for controlling health care costs. The legislative emphasis was placed on the other side of the coin—assuring the quality of care—but the objective of avoiding payment for unnecessary services was explicit. The perceived economic role of PSROs has been highlighted recently by attempts to assess their cost-effectiveness. A 1977 study by HEW concluded that no reduction in unnecessary hospital days resulted from PSRO activities (U.S. Department of Health, Education, and Welfare, Health Services Administration, 1978), but a 1978 HEW study on Medicare rates found a small net resource savings attributable to a 1.5 percent utilization reduction ($4.6 million more than the review costs of $45.9 million) (U.S. Department of Health, Education, and Welfare, Health Care Financing Administration, 1979*b*). The Congressional Budget Office has reexamined the same data and concluded that review costs exceeded utilization savings by about 30 percent (U.S. Congress, Congressional Budget Office, 1979, 1980). Regardless of which study better portrays the truth, the studies collectively denote an implicit federal concern with the cost-effectiveness of PSROs.

In addition to these national studies, analysts have examined the cost-effectiveness of several individual PSROs, again focusing on their cost-containment achievements. But what is the role, if any, of CBA-CEA in the work of PSROs? To date, we are aware of only one kind of application of analysis, and that one has been used only infrequently. A few PSROs use analyses similar to CBA-CEA to determine where they might best invest their review resources— for example, which diagnoses deserve the most attention in terms of potential reductions in unnecessary days of hospitalization. In effect, CBA-CEA thinking contributes to internal program planning and management.

We are aware of no instances in which CBA-CEA has been applied to PSROs' reviews of services. This lack of use of CBA-CEA reflects not only the mandate of the organizations but also the resources available to them. Although we cannot rule out the possibility that PSROs will use CBA-CEA in the future, we do not anticipate it, since development of standards based on CBA-CEA would be very difficult, as would development of a willingness and capacity within PSROs to apply such standards. The barriers to PSRO use of CBA-CEA include the following:

— PSROs focus on eliminating unnecessary care—that is, care that is of no value to the patient. In essence, PSROs restrict their attention primarily to instances in which effectiveness is zero. By definition, such care is not cost-effective. The more difficult questions, when effectiveness is positive, generally are not addressed by PSROs.

— CBA-CEA is best used as a comparative tool—for example, in comparing one treatment to an alternative, given a diagnosis or illness problem. PSRO reviews, however, take the therapy as the given, without beginning with a diagnosis and without asking which of several alternative treatments might be more cost-effective.

— PSRO standards derive from the prevailing patterns of

practice within the medical community. These patterns generally are not derived from consideration of relative social costs and benefits.

— The medical professionals constituting PSROs have neither the training nor, often, the disposition to think in terms of cost-effectiveness.

— PSRO staffs also lack the requisite analytical expertise. Though the latter can be remedied, it is unclear whether or how trained staff could work with a medically-oriented group to incorporate CBA-CEA into the review process.

Continued emphasis on cost containment in the health policy arena, and hence continued growth in cost-consciousness in the medical community, can be expected to push PSROs toward CEA-like thinking. Movement in that direction will be more rapid if individual PSROs are subjected to examinations of their own cost-effectiveness. But barring a major change in the law and in the composition of PSROs, these organizations cannot be expected to emerge as leaders in the application of CBA-CEA to health care regulation.

HEALTH PLANNING ORGANIZATIONS

In contrast to PSROs, health planning organizations seem logical consumers and perhaps producers of CBA-CEAs. The most recent principal organizations in the planning system, local Health Systems Agencies (HSAs) and state health planning and development agencies, have had a mandate to consider cost-effectiveness in their work and to strive for cost containment. In addition, many of these agencies have begun to employ analysts who can understand and even perform analysis. The 1974 law creating the agencies required them to employ individuals possessing analytical training and skills, and it reinforced the agencies' analytical capacities by providing for the use of consultants, establishing regional centers for health planning in order to supply technical assistance, and creating a National Health Planning Information Center. Despite these factors, the history of CBA-CEA in health planning is less than illustrious, and its future is clouded by the transitional status of organized health planning at the present time. Congress has decided to deemphasize the national health planning system. As a result, some of the states can be expected to increase their support of organized planning activities. Thus, unlike the case of the

PSROs, the future of CBA-CEA in health planning is not clearly negative.

Although health planning has existed in various forms for centuries, modern efforts are only a decade and a half old. In 1966, Congress enacted legislation establishing comprehensive health planning agencies and the regional medical program. With planning and compliance purely voluntary under law, legislators perceived these agencies as acting as catalysts for fostering cooperation among the pluralistic and fragmented elements of the health care system.

It soon became apparent that voluntary compliance was not effectively constraining or directing the growth of the system. Thus, in 1972 Congress passed Section 1122 of the Social Security Act, which permitted federal funds for capital expenditures to be withheld if substantial capital projects were not approved by state planning agencies. Beginning with New York in 1964, several states enacted certificate-of-need laws empowering planning agencies to deny reimbursement to hospitals for large capital expenditures unless the agency determined that there was a need for the service.

Two years after the passage of Section 1122, Congress enacted the National Health Planning and Resource Development Act (Public Law 93-641), which required all states to legislate certificate-of-need laws as a condition for receiving federal health care funding. The Act demonstrated a definite concern that cost considerations be integrated into the planning process, and, through its ability to deny certificate-of-need applications, the law provided health planning agencies with unprecedented potential muscle to effect resource allocation decisions.

Until passage of amendments to the Act in 1979, the principal theme of planning was need. Cost and cost-effectiveness were treated as being secondary to or derivative from need. Thus a planning agency concerned about cost-effectiveness had to subsume its interest under need. The 1979 amendments, however, clearly specified cost-effectiveness as a criterion in reviews of the appropriateness of health services. The amendments included numerous references to cost-effectiveness, efficiency, and the like. It is clear from the language of the amendments that Congress envisioned planning agencies as weighing the economic factors against the health outcome—the costs against the benefits—although there is no evidence that Congress intended the agencies to perform formal CBA-CEAs.

The barriers to the use of analysis, however, were greater than the new mandate might have suggested. These barriers included the following:

— The analytical capability of many agency staffs remained limited.

— Appropriations for planning had fallen well below the level of authorized funding.

— The entire certificate-of-need review process had to be completed within ninety days, which restricted the potential for reasoned, analytical deliberation.

— The planning agencies were precluded by law from gathering data, and much of the data they needed for cost-effectiveness assessments were simply unavailable.

— At its base, health planning remains fundamentally a political process. Analytical input may not be irrelevant to planning decisions, but it will rarely serve as the driving force in agencies' arriving at decisions. To the extent that analytical input challenges the objectives of the dominant political powers, analysis may be suppressed or fought.[11]

The federal health planning bureaucracy has demonstrated a realistic grasp of the desirability of and constraints on direct application of CBA-CEA to planning at the state and local levels. On the one hand, consideration of costs and benefits has been urged, even required, of the planning agencies. On the other hand, the mandate did not extend to the performance or even use of formal CBA-CEAs. Thus, the government had been attempting to foster cost-consciousness and gradually to build an analytical capability within health planning agencies, but officials recognized both the limitations of that capability and the inherent limitations of the state of the art in CBA-CEA.

One might expect to find numerous instances of health planning agencies' having used formal CBA-CEA despite these limitations. To the contrary, a recent study found no evidence of HSAs' having used formal CBA-CEA to assist in making resource allocations (U.S. Congress, Office of Technology Assessment, 1980a). In its investigation of the issue, OTA discovered one example of an HSA's using CBA for the majority of its recommendations in its annual implementation plan. The Miami Valley (Dayton, Ohio) HSA included fifty-four CBAs in its 1980 plan. Generally, the staff contrasted the costs and cost savings of a given health program with the productive value of the estimated years of life saved by the program (the human capital method of valuation discussed in Chapter 3). Analyses were done quickly and included no discussion of assumptions, levels of uncertainty, and so on. After reviewing the CBAs, OTA concluded (p. 76) that "It was clear that the HSA staff had neither the time, the resources, nor the expertise to carry out valid CBA studies ... This example is indicative of the bind in which the planning agencies find themselves. They are encouraged, and even mandated, to do more than they are perhaps capable of doing. The skills, data, and funds that the agencies need to perform high-quality CEA/CBA-type studies are not available." The OTA also observed that there was no evidence that the Miami Valley or any other HSA had used or intended to use CBA in resource allocation decision-making.

While the future of formal analysis in the planning process does not appear significant, it cannot be ruled out. More to the point, the basic receptivity of much of the health planning community to cost-effectiveness thinking, combined with the previous federal mandate establishing cost-effectiveness as a basic planning criterion, suggest that informal comparisons of costs and effectiveness will play increasing roles in planning activities. This may be dependent on individual states' increasing their support of planning functions as the federal government decreases its support of health planning.

FOOD AND DRUG ADMINISTRATION

Through a series of laws, the FDA has been assigned increasing authority to monitor and regulate the marketing of drugs and medical devices. Federal involvement in drug regulation dates from the Pure Food and Drug Act of 1906, intended in part to help prevent adulteration and misbranding of drug products. Six years later, the Sherley amendment was passed, prohibiting false and fraudulent curative or therapeutic claims on product labels. The legislation creating the FDA was passed in 1927.

A landmark piece of legislation in the history of drug and device regulation is the 1938 Food, Drug, and Cosmetic Act. The Act established labeling requirements for drugs and prohibited interstate commercial shipment of new drugs prior to federal determination of their safety under the conditions of use listed on their labels. The Act also authorized the FDA to remove from the market any drug it proved to be unsafe. The agency's regulatory power was increased further in 1951 under the Durham-Humphrey Amendment, which defined criteria and categories, based on levels of drug safety, for restricting a drug to prescription use only.

Following the thalidomide tragedy, Congress enacted the Drug Amendments of 1962, which required drug manufacturers to provide "substantial evidence" that their products were efficacious as well as safe. The amendments included a requirement for prompt reporting to the FDA of safety and efficacy information on marketed products and increased the authority of the FDA to remove from the market drugs determined to be unsafe or ineffective. Finally, the amendments initiated the investigational new drug process used by FDA to regulate drug studies in human beings.

Regulation of medical devices lagged behind drug regulation; the 1938 Food, Drug, and Cosmetic Act provided only minimal regulatory authority over devices. The Medical Device Amendments of 1976 (Public Law 94-295) greatly increased this authority, instructing the FDA to require manufacturers to demonstrate acceptable levels of safety and effectiveness for their products. Controls vary according to the classification of a device in one of three categories. The most restrictive category includes invasive devices, those playing a central role in sustaining life, and those posing significant potential for causing injury or illness. The amendments permit the FDA to restrict the use of specified devices to professionals with specific training or to special facilities.

The activities of the FDA have had profound impacts on American medical care, both direct and indirect. Directly, FDA actions have kept certain presumably inefficacious or unsafe drugs off the market through the evaluation process. Other drugs, currently available in Europe and elsewhere, remain unlicensed in the United States because they are being scrutinized by the FDA. Indirectly, according to many observers, the time and expense associated with the review and approval process have significantly slowed the rate of new drug innovation in this country. In effect, these observers argue, FDA regulation has had the unanticipated and undesirable effect of deterring the search for useful new pharmaceutical products because of the increased costs of research and development and the uncertainty of receiving eventual market approval (Grabowski, 1976; Peltzman, 1974; Wardell et al., 1980).[12]

Since its inception, the FDA has restricted its attention to issues of drug and device safety and efficacy. The Food, Drug, and Cosmetic Act does not authorize the FDA to use economic criteria in evaluating drugs and devices, but neither does it prohibit it.

Thus the legality of employing cost-effectiveness in evaluation remains untested. Certainly precedent argues against it. In only a few instances of FDA analysis have economic considerations even received mention (U.S. Congress, Office of Technology Assessment, 1980*a*). Nevertheless, an argument can be made for including cost-effectiveness considerations in the review process. The use of an economic criterion might encourage manufacturers to search for efficiency-oriented innovations, for example the development of less expensive but comparably effective alternatives to existing treatments. Application of a cost-effectiveness criterion might assist public and private third-party payers in containing costs.

The arguments against incorporating the economic factor into FDA evaluation are at least equally compelling. Indeed, we find them more compelling. Inclusion of an economic criterion would exacerbate technical, managerial, and philosophical problems in regulating drugs and devices. The following illustrate the nature of probable difficulties:

— Data problems would be magnified: The FDA would have to either develop a new economic data-gathering capacity or rely on the paucity of existing data. The first alternative suggests significant costs with no assurance that the end product will be valid, reliable data. The second alternative reverses the relative importance of these problems: Questions of reliability and validity would be paramount, and costs could be substantial.

— Inclusion of cost-effectiveness would represent an additional regulatory hurdle for manufacturers to clear, with the associated implications for investment of time and resources. At minimum, this extra investment could increase the consumer cost of approved products. In addition, the new regulatory burden might exacerbate the purported "drug lag" and an anticipated "device lag"—that is, additional regulation could decrease the incentive to innovate, with a potential consequent loss of new and useful products.

— Disapproval of a new drug (or device) on cost-effectiveness grounds would remove the possibility of exploring other uses of the drug in actual medical practice. The ultimate uses of pharmaceutical products occasionally end up quite different from the uses for which they were developed; in fact, some of the ultimate uses may never have been anticipated before marketing and years of clinical experience.

— Cost-effectiveness information before marketing cannot translate directly into price-effectiveness data after marketing. Unless the FDA (or another agency) were to get into the business of controlling prices, the FDA review process would offer no assurance that potential cost-effectiveness would translate into realized cost-effectiveness.

— Experts believe that many of the cost-effectiveness differences among related drugs, for example, will be small and therefore not subject to unequivocal ascertainment through CEA. By contrast, in a comparison of a drug and a related device, costs may differ significantly, but assessment of relative effectiveness may be difficult.

— Many people believe that choices regarding economic considerations are best left to consumers and providers. Despite its flaws, the medical marketplace will prove a more efficient regulator of drugs and devices than will a regulatory agency.

Traditionally, the FDA's mandate has been to protect the public from inefficacious and unsafe drugs and devices. Adding cost-effectiveness review to the existing responsibilities would take FDA into an entirely different regulatory realm. To be sure, we anticipate that, in a political environment preoccupied with cost containment, gross disparities in the cost-effectiveness of medical alternatives will raise FDA eyebrows and perhaps eventually influence approval decisions. However, institutionalizing cost-effectiveness in FDA review, in whatever guise, strikes us as inefficient and inappropriate.

FEDERAL HEALTH RESEARCH AGENCIES

Support of research on health and health services is distributed among literally dozens of agencies in the various departments of the federal government. However, the vast majority of research dollars are channeled through the Department of Health and Human Services, and a handful of its agencies manage the bulk of its research funds. A minute portion of these funds supports much of the formal CBA-CEA performed in the United States. Indeed, this funding represents the most visible linkage of formal CBA-CEA to federal health policy.

The largest share of federal health research dollars is devoted to basic and applied biomedical science, centered in the NIH. The uncertainties surrounding such research, particularly basic research, severely restrict objective evaluation of its effectiveness; this virtually precludes the possibility of undertaking meaningful CBA-CEA. In addition, biomedical research appears to be well served by an effective resource allocation mechanism already in place: the peer review and evaluation system. The relative lack of need for applying CBA-CEA in this area, as well as the technical problems of doing so, explain the absence of CBA-CEA activity. These conditions, and hence the role of analysis in biomedical research, should persist well into the future.

The spirit of CBA-CEA has been represented at NIH in recent years in a series of "consensus development exercises." Though these vary in structure, all can be considered technology assessments intended to evaluate and estimate the pros and cons of emerging technologies. Most of the exercises have focused on scientific issues of efficacy and effectiveness, but a few have examined a full range of medical, economic, social, political, legal, and ethical issues.[13]

The bulk of the limited support for formal CBA-CEA comes from two of the Department's organizations, one devoted exclusively to health services research—the National Center for Health Services Research (NCHSR)—and the other funding research relevant to its reimbursement and management functions—the Health Care Financing Administration (HCFA)—which administers Medicare and Medicaid and the PSRO program. The NCHSR supports a number of CBA-CEAs covering a wide variety of health services issues (U.S. Department of Health, Education, and Welfare, National Center for Health Services Research, 1979). Two of NCHSR's five research priority areas—health care costs and cost containment, and planning and regulation—specifically identify CEAs as desirable in researching pertinent issues (U.S. Department of Health, Education, and Welfare, National Center for Health Services Research, 1978a). The HCFA's research support also includes several efforts focused on cost-effectiveness issues (U.S. Department of Health, Education, and Welfare, Health Care Financing Administration, 1979a).

The NCHSR is solely a research arm of the health bureaucracy. As such, use of the findings from NCHSR-supported research falls outside its control. Our impression is that NCHSR-funded CBA-CEAs have not played much of a role in health policymaking. By contrast, the HCFA is structured in a way that should facilitiate application of CBA-CEA findings. The HCFA can tailor research projects to its administrative needs, as it has been doing in the heart transplant case, and it should be able to employ the findings in its policy-making process. Nevertheless, it is difficult to pinpoint specific examples of HCFA-supported CBA-CEA leading to Medicare or PSRO policy in the past. This is not to say that there has been no relationship, but rather than whatever impact CBA-CEA has had on policy has been indirect and thus difficult to identify. Structurally, HCFA is the prototype of an agency that should have the organizational ability to fund and use CBA-CEA. If direct use of CBA-CEA emerges in the near future, the HCFA seems a plausible place for it to happen.

Support of CBA-CEA constitutes only a small fraction of the research resources of these two agencies. Their health services research funds totaled only $50 million in fiscal year 1980. However, health services research focused on medical technology, and specifically CBA-CEA, briefly had an ally in the National Center for Health Care Technology (NCHCT). Established by Congress in 1978, the NCHCT was designed to "undertake and support assessments of health care technologies." The NCHCT was expected to set priorities for technology assessment. In this capacity, one of its specific charges was to undertake and support CBA-CEAs of current and developing technologies. The NCHCT developed CEAs of such technologies and practices as intraocular lenses, estrogen use by postmenopausal women, and antenatal diagnosis.

The NCHCT was intended to serve other agencies that request policy direction on medical technology issues. For example, the HCFA asked the NCHCT for advice on the appropriateness of reimbursing through Medicare for certain technologies. In 1980, NCHCT responded to over fifty such requests. As we noted above, in the discussion of the role of analysis in reimbursement, the criteria for Medicare reimbursement do not currently include cost-effectiveness. But if efforts to alter this situation succeed, a successor to NCHCT might acquire the ability to incorporate cost-effectiveness into its reimbursement recommendations. Several factors, especially the abbreviated history of NCHCT, preclude an assessment of likely future use of CBA-CEA in coverage decisions.

POTENTIAL USES AND USEFULNESS OF ANALYSIS: GENERAL CONSIDERATIONS

Three themes have pervaded this chapter: (1) the direct use of CBA-CEA has been extremely limited, (2) interest in analysis has been growing within most of the major groups concerned with medical decision-making, and (3) we have concluded that policy applications of CBA-CEA in the near future will be indirect and limited, regardless of the inclinations of the potential user groups. Limited use to date can be attributed in part to the novelty of CBA-CEA in health care. But another explanation, applicable to both current experience and our reading of the future, focuses on inherently restrictive characteristics of analysis and decision-making. As noted above, the explanation has two principal components: technical problems in analysis and environmental, or incentive, problems associated with use of analysis. Because this explanation applies to all of the potential user groups in the health care arena, we feel it deserves emphasis here. We note, too, that this explanation of why the use of analysis has been so limited has a normative analog: it helps us to determine how analysis *should* be used.

TECHNICAL PROBLEMS

Technical problems in CBA-CEA are of two types, one reflecting the practice of analysis, the other inherent limitations. There are relatively few examples of technically high-quality analysis. While the need for technically complete studies is not always obvious (see Chapter 6), such problems as inappropriate specification of production relationships; inadequate identification, measurement, or valuation of costs or benefits; lack of discounting of future costs and benefits; and failure to examine sensitivities pervade the literature and restrict its applicability to policy. Though one should never play down the difficulty of producing a technically high-quality study, many such problems can be resolved: the practice of analysis can and should improve over time. Thus, this current restriction on the usefulness of CBA-CEA seems likely to recede in importance. It certainly should be responsive to increased analytical training of students in schools of medicine, public health, public policy, and the like.

Of greater consequence in the long run are the inherent limitations of analysis. These include the inability to predict with precision the outcomes or costs, or both, of programs still on the drawing board, fundamental problems in quantifying or valuing certain important but less tangible health benefits, controversy over the appropriate discount rate, inadequate data bases, the inability of analysis to adequately incorporate considerations of equity, and significant uncertainties in many perfectly managed studies. The rapidity and profundity of technical change in medicine exacerbate analytical difficulties; the point at which an analysis might have the most significant impact on health resource allocation—before a procedure or technology has become widespread in medical practice—is also the point at which evaluation uncertainties are most dramatic. Sensitivity analysis sometimes can demonstrate that inherent technical analytical problems do not affect qualitative conclusions, but frequently these difficulties preclude a definitive assessment of the desirability of competing programs. Ultimately, research may resolve some of these problems, but, for the foreseeable future, most such limitations seem likely to remain inherent. In particular, the uncertainties that pervade analysis severely restrict the potential of a study, however high its quality, for resolving definitively the cases in which alternative programs are similar in both cost and effectiveness.

ENVIRONMENTAL PROBLEMS

Even if technical analytical problems did not exist, environmental factors, or incentives, would limit the potential direct application of CBA-CEA findings. As emphasized above, the economic environment of the provision of most health care services in the United States does not encourage attention to cost-effectiveness in individual provider-consumer interactions. In many situations, the economic incentives produce indifference; in certain fee-for-service contexts, the economic incentive actually may run contrary to cost containment, with socially cost-ineffective care being lucrative, or cost-effective, for the provider. The small but growing prepaid segment of the health care market is a noteworthy exception to the standard economic incentive. According to one HMO physician, "In an HMO setting, physicians *are* sensitive to cost. You hear them talk about it ... there are specific discussions about, for example, the cost of coronary artery bypass."[14] In this environment, CBA-CEAs will find a more receptive audience. In general, however, the fee-for-service system seems a likely illustration of how the failure to tailor analysis to the interests and needs of potential users can translate into nonuse.

The economic barrier to physicians' responding directly to CBA-CEA may be partially surmounted, short of requiring participation in HMOs, by an indirect method: if third-party payers choose not to reimburse for a specific procedure, pressure is applied on practitioners to limit their use of it. Hence, a major question is whether governmental and nongovernmental insurers will apply the findings of CBA-CEAs to reimbursement policies. The economic interests of such institutions are generally consonant with the spirit of CBA-CEA, but another environmental barrier looms large in their consideration of directly applying findings: the political opposition of organized medicine, the medical technology industry, and even the well-insured consumer. Some officials of third-party payers have expressed confidence in their ability to transcend political considerations, but, in the face of the technical limitations of analysis, political pressure will remain a powerful obstacle in all but the most clear-cut, least controversial cost-effectiveness decisions.

APPROPRIATE USE OF CBA-CEA

Direct policy applications of CBA-CEAs are likely to be few in number because of the political and economic barriers to them. The technical limitations of analysis provide a strong intellectual rationale for concluding that this is as it should be. A negative assessment of the policy usefulness of analysis is not, however, a general condemnation of the potential for CBA-CEA to make a useful contribution in the health care arena. The consciousness-raising potential of analysis in the medical and health policy communities has been partially realized already, with further contributions almost assured. While this contribution is relatively intangible, its potential importance should not be underestimated. It may contribute to the creation of a milieu in which both attitudes and behavior change constructively. On a more tangible level, analyses can be undertaken with the intention of confirming expectations (making the obvious more obvious) in order to support policy decisions. This use of analysis, not unknown in the past, seems a legitimate one if the intention is made explicit. Finally, another less tangible use of analysis appears to have the potential for playing a growing role in deliberations on health policy: Analysis can serve to frame appropriate questions, identify issues requiring resolution, and, by contributing both specific information and a broader perspective, generally inform a policy debate. This is the decision-assisting function of analysis, quite distinct from decision-making.

Several steps can be taken to facilitate the use of analysis in all of these dimensions. Experts concur that analyses should be tailored to potential users' self-perceived needs. Some believe that analyses must have a client at the outset. Where possible, decision-makers (clients) should be integrally involved in the structuring and performance of analysis. While CBA-CEAs should explore the potential of alternative programs under optimal circumstances, they should also assess the costs of implementation realistically, allowing for the possibility of cost overruns, political barriers to implementation, and so on (Luft, 1976; Wolf, 1978). Clearly, the use of analysis can be facilitated by somewhat more coercive means, such as a legislative mandate requiring its use (by health planning agencies, for example). Note, however, that use does not imply usefulness: A significant improvement in health care resource allocation need not result from increased performance of analysis.

A number of questions remain as to how to enhance the cost-effectiveness of CBA-CEA. For example, can we identify the characteristics of a useful analysis that is not exorbitantly expensive? Is support of CBA-CEA a rational use of scarce health care evaluation resources, or might alternative investments yield greater dividends in improved health care resource allocation (for example, more funds for traditional medical efficacy studies)? We do not possess the information, or insight, necessary to answer such questions. However, in Chapter 6 we suggest ideas and research efforts that might facilitate understanding of the uses and usefulness of analysis.

Conclusion

The application of CBA-CEA to problems of health care resource allocation is a relatively new endeavor, particularly within the medical community. As a result, the inherent technical problems of CBA-CEA are matched by presumably avoidable technical errors of commission and omission. In addition, analyses generally have been performed in a policy vacuum: practical implementation concerns have been overlooked, and analysts have not tailored their work to the needs of specific clients. The political, economic, and knowledge barriers to application of analysis, combined with the technical problems, account for the limited direct use of analysis to date. Of course, future experience may diverge significantly from current experience. Conditions favoring increasing usefulness and use of analysis should emerge, but expectations can be anticipated to rise also. We guess that the important benefits from analysis, both currently and in the future, will be relatively intangible indirect effects on medical practice and policy—effects that are exceedingly difficult to observe and value.

This illustrates the complexity involved in assessing the usefulness and use of analysis. In large part, a summary assessment rests on the standard against which analysis is judged. Measured against the conception of CBA-CEA as a decision-making technique, analysis must be judged a failure to date, with a similar prognosis for the future. Measured against the less demanding standard of indirect policy impact—clarifying issues, providing data, contributing perspective to a policy debate—analysis rates a qualified positive verdict, with the outlook for the future brighter than experience to date. Only a handful of analyses have been designed for or introduced into previous policy debates, but it is the apparent intent of public and private sector officials to reverse this situation. Many experts seem to concur that high-quality CBA-CEA has considerable potential for contributing in this less evident but nevertheless meaningful fashion (Weinstein, 1979). As stated by a committee studying decision-making in a nonmedical arena (Committee on Principles of Decision Making for Regulating Chemicals in the Environment, 1975):

> There is no objective scientific way of making decisions, nor is it likely that there ever will be. However, use of the techniques developed by decision theory and benefit-cost analysis can provide the decision maker with a useful framework and language for describing and discussing trade-offs, noncommensurability, and uncertainty. It can help to clarify the existence of alternatives, decision points, gaps in information, and value judgments concerning trade-offs. Furthermore, it should facilitate communication between the decision maker and his staff of analysts, and between the decision maker and the public.

Analysis scores highest, in both its accomplishments and potential, when measured against a yardstick of education. The economic incursion into the medical literature appears to have contributed to a heightening of physicians' and health policymakers' cost-consciousness. The concept of resource scarcity, of competing demands on the pool of resources, is gaining familiarity and credibility within a profession in which, until recently, social economic concerns were rarely even contemplated. While it would be unreasonable to attribute significant behavioral change to existing health care CBA-CEA efforts, many health care experts believe that analysis is contributing to a milieu that is having a significant influence on thinking. These experts regard scattered efforts to convert thinking into practice as being in the vanguard of significant cost-effective changes in medical practice. Whether or not significant changes occur (and these may be difficult to observe), there would seem to be virtue in having health care professionals think systematically and fully about resource allocation problems. This general process may ultimately prove more useful than any specific association between analysis and changes in behavior.

NOTES

1. The distinction between CBA-CEA and its components is critical here and in later discussion. Many physicians make practice decisions on the basis of new knowledge of the effectiveness of procedures, weighing risks and medical benefits, but apparently relatively few have altered their practices in response to knowledge that a procedure is medically effective but more expensive than a comparably effective procedure—the kind of finding a CBA-CEA might produce.
2. Here we are referring to voluntary physician response. Obviously, if CBA-CEAs are used by third-party payers to make reimbursement decisions, the community of medical practitioners will respond. However, they will be responding to the economic factor—the reimbursement policy—and not, separately, to the CBA-CEAs.
3. Richard Watkins, personal communication.
4. This refers to the majority of hospitals in the private sector. Many public hospitals, including state and county hospitals and the VA system, have long been subject to annual budgets.
5. In its study of the implications of CBA-CEA of medical technology, OTA examined the resource costs required to conduct an analysis. In Appendix C of their study, they report typical professional and support staff needs, data and data sources, and the range of total costs required to perform an analysis (U.S. Congress, Office of Technology Assessment, 1980a).
6. As technical complexity is often perceived to be a selling point in academic papers, this raises the question of whether potential CBA-CEA users, such as HMOs, will ever find their real needs addressed in the published academic literature. It may well be that we need another forum for the conducting of relatively simple analyses and a vehicle for disseminating their findings. This is not to suggest that the academic literature is failing in its mission, but rather that its mission may be other than directly changing specific medical practices.
7. Personal communications with PSRO officials.
8. "Reasonable and necessary" has never been defined explicitly. However, its interpretation in practice has been limited to the four criteria listed above; cost has never been included.
9. Reiss et al. later revised the estimated costs to vary anywhere from $146 million to $4.5 billion.
10. For additional discussion on each of these four organizations, see chapters 6–9 of the OTA report (U.S. Congress, Office of Technology Assessment, 1980a).

11. The politics of local planning decision-making are not solely narrow interest groups competing with one another for the spoils of planning largesse. The agency itself is caught in a conflict of interest: on the one hand it is supposed to represent the interests of the immediate community; on the other it is intended to represent the interests of the broader society. The potential conflict is evident in considering approval of a new CT scanner, which will serve (provide benefits to) members of the immediate community but whose costs will be spread over a larger region, the state, and even the nation as its costs are diffused throughout the public and private insurance systems.

12. The effects of FDA regulation of medical devices are excluded from this discussion because implementation of the 1976 Medical Device Amendments has been too recent for other than anecdotal observations. Conceptually, effects similar to those experienced with drugs seem probable.

13. For example, in 1979 the National Eye Institute sponsored a consensus development exercise on intraocular lens implantation and the Division of Research Services sponsored one on the use of microprocessor-based "intelligent" machines in patient care. Each of these investigated a variety of cost and benefit issues. All told, from September 1977 through November 1980, NIH's Office for Medical Applications of Research held twenty-eight such forums.

14. Richard Watkins, personal communication.

6

Summary and Agenda for the Future

IN THE PRECEDING three chapters we have examined the principles, practice, and potential of CBA-CEA in health care. In this
concluding chapter we review the main points related to each of
these three phases of our investigation and reiterate the circumstances that have brought CBA-CEA into the health policy lime-
light. We later map out an agenda of researchable questions, the
resolution of which could foster improvements in the art and
science of analysis and in the effectiveness with which analysis is
applied to health policy problems. The potential value of CBA-CEA
may be limited by inherent analytical and environmental problems, but, given the novelty of CBA-CEA in health care, it would be
illogical to suggest that it has already realized its full potential.

SUMMARY

GROWTH OF INTEREST IN ANALYSIS

In Chapters 1, 2, and 4 we documented the rapid growth of interest
in CBA-CEA in the medical and health policy communities. In part
this documentation had an empirical flavor: numbers of health
care CBA-CEAs, particularly those in medical journals, increased
exponentially through the 1970s. Yet the growth of interest is
equally well reflected in such nonquantitative indicators as physicians' expressions of interest, informally and formally through
medical association committees; the introduction of health economics material into medical education curriculums; and study of
the subject by national government and private sector organizations.

The growth of interest seems to stem from concern about the
high and rapidly escalating costs of health care. Many members of

both the medical and health policy communities view CBA and CEA as front-line soldiers in the developing war on cost inflation. To interested medical professionals, CBA-CEA has the potential for helping the medical community to get its own house in order, to control costs from within. Health policymakers perceive in CBA-CEA a basis for restricting the flow of resources into the health care system, with CBA-CEAs contributing to decisions to constrain capital investment and to withhold reimbursement for inefficient medical practice. In both cases, CBA-CEA is perceived to be relatively nonthreatening. The intention is to use this tool in the existing structure of the delivery and financing of care. By contrast, many other approaches to health care cost containment rely on fundamental changes in the basic system (for example, expenditure ceilings or an HMO-based national health insurance program).

The growth of interest in analysis is so recent that neither the potential nor the limits of CBA-CEA have been realized. The apparent enthusiasm for analysis reflects the widespread perception of a cost "crisis" and suggests that both the potential and limits of CBA-CEA will continue to be explored.

PRINCIPLES

Cost-benefit and cost-effectiveness analysis are conceptually simple. They are no more nor less than a formalization of common sense in considering alternative means of addressing a problem. Yet, while they are simple in concept, they are often exceedingly difficult in execution. Analysts have found no uniformly satisfactory approach to incorporating intangibles, such as physical pain and suffering and distributional values, into the quantitative calculus that dominates analysis. The need to predict the inputs and outcomes of hypothetical programs taxes the imagination of the most skilled analyst and serves as a major source of the uncertainty that pervades CBA-CEA. Identifying and acquiring appropriate data are commonly difficult and not infrequently impossible.

Throughout this book we have treated CBA and CEA as essentially a single mode of analysis. They have a similar set of analytical steps, and each results in a comparison of the positive and negative consequences of alternative means of achieving an end. The principal difference between them lies in the valuation of the positive consequences of programs. As we saw, however, even this distinguishing feature is losing its sharpness. Recent sophisticated health care CEAs are incorporating some dollar-valued benefits into the cost side of the equation (as negative costs), and increasing recognition of the meaning of CBA in health care is bringing it closer to CEA. The human capital approach to measuring indirect benefits in CBA values livelihood, not life itself; thus a CBA is really a net dollar benefit for some nonmonetized health outcomes. The newer more sophisticated CEA seems to be a significant step forward in that it combines the best of both CBA and CEA.

The steps in CBA-CEA are the following:

— Defining the problem and objective(s): This step defines the scope and character of an analysis.

— Identifying alternatives: This step determines the range of options to be considered, given the constraints imposed by the definition of the problem and objectives.

— Describing production relationships: This is the most technically demanding aspect of analysis, as well as one that often requires considerable creativity; specification of a production function directly determines quantities of input and outcome and, hence, provides the raw material for cost and benefit assessment.

— Identifying, measuring, and valuing costs: These activities, for both costs and benefits, make up the heart of analysis; it is here that one encounters esoteric questions about the nature of costs and mundane issues concerning acquisition of needed data.

— Identifying, measuring, and valuing benefits and effectiveness: Similar to cost analysis, benefit and effectiveness assessment brings to the fore problems of measurement and valuation. Analysts must decide how to deal with benefits that are clearly important but hard to quantify. The valuation of benefits for CBAs has involved a long-standing value-of-life controversy, particularly regarding the human capital approach to valuing averted productivity losses.

— Discounting: This technical procedure, a source of much confusion to the nonanalyst, serves to make present and future dollars (or units of effectiveness) commensurable. It permits analysts to summarize a stream of costs or benefits occurring over a period of years in a single number—the present discounted value of costs or benefits. Although

discounting is a purely technical step in analysis, it is not
devoid of controversy; debate has centered on issues such as
selection of an appropriate social discount rate and whether
nonmonetary effectiveness units should be discounted.

— Addressing problems of uncertainty: Most CBA-CEAs are
pervaded by uncertainties. Sensitivity analysis, a basic
approach to dealing with many uncertainties, adds great
power and potential to analysis because it permits determination of the importance of uncertainties; unfortunately,
sensitivity analysis is used all too infrequently.

— Dealing with issues of equity: A major weakness of CBA-
CEA is its limited ability to incorporate distributional
concerns. Particularly in areas in which redistribution, or
equity, is a central concern, such as in health services,
analysts must develop means of according these considerations the prominence they deserve.

— Presenting and interpreting findings: The art of summarizing the findings of an analysis represents the step in
which communication skills are foremost. It is in the conclusion of a CBA-CEA that analysts succeed or fail in
conveying what they have done and learned. This can
profoundly influence the impact an analysis has on policy
and practice decision-making. To maximize effective communication, analysts must use conventional communication skills and develop novel means of presenting findings
(such as the array method). Misinterpretation of empirical
results is a risk if analysts are not thoroughly familiar with
the uses and limitations of measures such as net benefit and
the cost-effectiveness ratio.

— Facilitating the transition from analysis to implementation: Analysts should be realistic in structuring and performing analyses in order to maximize their usefulness in
policy decisions. Analysts should work closely with prospective users throughout the analytical process, and they
should be conscious of how political and economic interests
will view the costs and benefits they have been studying.

The state of the art in CBA-CEA methodology has passed the
primitive stage, but analysis is far from a mature science. Several
significant improvements in the methodology of CBA-CEA as it is
applied to health care problems have taken place in the last decade;

continued improvements loom on the horizon. Nevertheless, many deficiencies appear unlikely to be addressed successfully in the near future, whereas others seem to be inherent in the analytical process. CBA-CEA may always remain a mix of science and art. It seems to us today that the skillful artist has a greater chance of producing analytical breakthroughs than does the competent technician.

PRACTICE

The most striking characteristics of CBA-CEA in health care are its rapid growth and its adoption and application by members of the health care community in the 1970s. In the 1960s, the practice of CBA-CEA was the province of a small cadre of health economists. Throughout the 1970s, CBA-CEA diffused to a diverse group of health services researchers, including several physicians who have lacked formal training in analysis. Two apparent results have been an increase in medical professionals' awareness of analysis and a decrease in the technical quality of the average published analysis. Particularly in the medical specialty journals, one finds dozens of articles with fatal and often flagrant technical or conceptual flaws. At the other end of the quality spectrum, the growth of analysis has spawned a group of analysts who have combined medical and economic expertise, often through collaboration, to advance health care CBA-CEA in terms of both methodology and substance.

The growing medical interest in CBA-CEA accounts for several trends that we observed. The traditional emphasis on prevention has yielded to greater concern with diagnosis and treatment, the principal interests of physicians. The shift in emphasis has been substantial: From 1966 through 1973, more CBA-CEA contributions (44.7 percent) dealt with prevention than with either diagnosis or treatment; yet from 1974 through 1978, prevention accounted for a smaller share of contributions (22.0 percent) than either of the other two categories. Similarly, the medical focus of the literature accounts for a relative shift in the orientation of articles from an organizational to an individual (practitioner) perspective.[1]

The substantive concerns of health care CBA-CEA articles generally reflect the significance of health (particularly medical) problems, with some notable exceptions. The nation's number one killer, cardiovascular disease, is the disease category that has captured the most attention in the CBA-CEA literature. The nation's most feared killer, cancer, is represented by numerous articles on cancer screening, but, to our surprise, during the period we studied (1966–78), we found not one contribution related to cancer treatment. Other medical conditions that were well represented in the literature include mental illness, drug abuse and alcoholism, communicable diseases, birth defects, a variety of surgeries, and dental care.

The most overrepresented substantive focus, relative to its overall health importance, is kidney failure. The striking and well-publicized economic issues and policy prominence surrounding treatment of end-stage renal disease undoubtedly account for the extensiveness of its coverage. Other diseases, such as diabetes, have received little attention in the literature. Also underrepresented are certain major nonmedical health problems such as accidents and smoking-induced illness.[2] Individual capital-intensive medical technologies have not been studied as frequently as their recent policy prominence would suggest. The one exception, CT scanning, is one of the most intensively analyzed subjects in the CBA-CEA literature. Drugs, the epitome of scientific progress in medicine, have rated only implicit and tangential interest (as a component of hypertension management, for example).

In Chapter 4 we examined specific technical strengths and weaknesses of contributions to the literature. Rather than attempt a thorough review here, we will simply note prominent examples of both categories. Regarding weaknesses, a typical structural problem is that the growing practice-specific orientation of health care CBA-CEA has reduced the breadth of analyses. Many recent analyses, perhaps even a majority, examine the cost-effectiveness of only a single program or practice; the lack of alternatives other than nothing or the status quo means that the potential strength of analysis in comparing alternatives is not being realized.

A variety of technical and conceptual deficiencies pervade the literature. A common one is extrapolation from black box production relationships to hypothetical future programs differing significantly in terms of size, location, and so on. In general, conceptualization of production relationships is one of the most difficult components of analysis. Some technical analytical steps are handled poorly or not at all—for example, discounting—while others are utilized too infrequently—for example, sensitivity analysis. Incomplete or inadequate identification and measurement of both costs and benefits diminishes the usefulness of many analyses. Finally, even the bottom lines of CBA-CEAs are presented or interpreted inaccurately. Use of a benefit-cost ratio rather than net benefit is a common example. And misinterpretation of ratios—benefit-cost and cost-effectiveness—may be more frequent than correct interpretations.

The numerous, pervasive weaknesses found throughout the literature should not diminish our awareness and appreciation of several excellent contributions to the recent literature. These studies have produced meaningful substantive output—at least one has had a direct and substantial impact on policymaking (Eddy, 1978, 1980a)—and they have advanced the methodological frontiers of health care CBA-CEA. Weinstein and Stason's work on hypertension policy (1976b) has helped to define and clarify many aspects of CEA, including the elements of the cost-effectiveness formula, lending prominence to the idea of adjusting health outcomes for quality and illustrating the use of sensitivity analysis. Cretin's (1977) study of prevention and treatment alternatives for myocardial infarction also demonstrated the effective and appropriate use of the techniques of discounting and sensitivity analysis. Together, work such as that of Weinstein and Stason and Cretin has helped to redefine and expand CEA, narrowing the conceptual gap between it and CBA.

Eddy's (1980b) analysis of optimal cancer screening programs stands out as a sparkling example of imaginative, technically sound application of mathematical modeling to resolution of a problem of national significance. The thoroughness of his work and his attention to presenting and interpreting his results in an intelligible manner contributed to decisions by Blue Cross-Blue Shield and the American Cancer Society to alter their recommendations on screening practices. Both in terms of its technical competence and its policy impact, Eddy's work remains a distinct deviation from the norm. It demonstrates what can be accomplished with the appropriate expertise, resources, and cooperation between analysts and potential users.

In contrast to Eddy's mathematically sophisticated analysis, the study of swine flu immunization by Schoenbaum et al. (1976b) illustrates that technical simplicity in a sound conceptual framework can produce meaningful findings. The authors set out with a pragmatic goal—to perform an analysis quickly enough to inform an impending policy decision—and they succeeded in providing useful insights. This analysis and Eddy's illustrate radically different types of analysis that share the characteristics of technical soundness and potential policy usefulness.

Acton's work (1973, 1975) represents the striving for methodological progress through applied example. Acton's research on the costs and benefits of circulatory disease programs included investigation of the feasibility of using willingness-to-pay measures to value the benefits of programs. While the willingness-to-pay approach is laden with problems, Acton's research represents a contribution to a methodological debate that transcends its health care origins.

There are several other high-quality analyses that approach or extend the potential of CBA-CEA. Assuming that analysts continue to produce such work, we expect that both the state and practice of the art will improve in the 1980s.

POTENTIAL

Regardless of the technical quality of a CBA-CEA, ultimately it must be evaluated in terms of its relevance to and impact on the thinking and practice of health care professionals and policymakers. Technical virtuosity does not necessarily translate into policy relevance. In Chapter 5 we examined the factors that influence the policy potential of analysis in a variety of settings, and we noted the range of impacts analysis can have. Obviously the perceived effectiveness of analysis will be a function of what one expects from it.

The perception that CBA-CEA should produce policy decisions—that it is a decision-making technique—is a common but misguided one. It is also an expectation that dooms analysis to failure. The technical limitations of analysis and the fact that policy decisions rarely occur in a political vacuum preclude most analyses from coming up with policy-defining conclusions. At best, CBA-CEA can inform policy decisions; it can serve as one of several inputs into a complex decision-making process.

The view of CBA-CEA as a decision-making technique is a policy perspective, as well as a theoretical notion. As we discussed in the preceding chapter, officials of both public and private third-party payers have expressed an interest in using CBA-CEAs to make reimbursement decisions. We pointed out the difficulties of putting this into practice, in other than a trivial manner (that is, in a situation in which one medical practice is dramatically more cost-effective than another, especially when the former dominates the latter in both cost and effectiveness). Thus, in this context we believe the policy potential of CBA-CEA is extremely limited. Similarly, the notion that individual physician decision-making can be swayed significantly by cost-effectiveness information strikes us as naive and unrealistic, especially in a fee-for-service system with insured patients; in this situation, the relevance of social cost-effectiveness information becomes questionable. It also begs the question of the physician's technical ability to appreciate the limitations and strengths of CBA-CEAs.

For a variety of reasons, the potential for direct application of CBA-CEA to policy in a number of other organizational contexts seems to be more limited than advocates would like to believe. In particular, we perceive very little potential for use of CBA-CEA in such regulatory agencies as the FDA and PSROs. Even in seemingly likely users of CBA-CEA, such as HMOs and health planning organizations, a variety of political and resource constraints will impose severe restrictions for many years into the future.

If one's perception of the role of analysis is more modest, its potential for affecting policy appears much greater. Exposure to CBA-CEAs in the medical literature may alter decision-making in physicians' practices in a general manner, however subtly. Similarly, health planners may incorporate notions of cost-effectiveness into needs assessments, possibly unconsciously. Third-party payers may evolve concepts of reimbursable services that include an economic component, even while specific CBA-CEAs may prove insufficient to justify individual reimbursement decisions. In short, the policy potential for CBA-CEA lies in the ability of analysis to raise the cost-consciousness of those who make decisions concerning the allocation of health care resources.

Toward a Research Agenda

The enthusiasm that much of the health services research and policy communities have for analysis has produced strong recommendations for significant additional resources devoted to the performance of CBA-CEAs and related forms of social analysis of health care resource consumption (Wagner, 1979). These recommendations are based on the linking of CBA-CEA to cost containment, but that linkage rests on assumption rather than empirical evidence. The presumed utility of CBA-CEA has yet to be demonstrated, and a rational approach to analysis has not been mapped out. The call for an expansion of CBA-CEA is not necessarily premature, but, given the state of knowledge, the mix of basic and applied CBA-CEA research appears to us to be unduly biased toward the latter. That is, both analysis and health policy might benefit from some basic research on the techniques, uses, and usefulness of CBA-CEA. The National Center for Health Services Research and other agencies concerned with medical technology assessment are logical focal points for the support and direction of such research.

The following are researchable questions related to the methodology and value of analysis; the discussion is intended to be suggestive rather than comprehensive.

RESEARCH ON ENVIRONMENTAL ISSUES

Our knowledge of potential users' receptivity to CBA-CEA is very limited and largely theoretical. Empirical studies seem to be warranted both to assess the current state of receptivity and to determine ways of enhancing it. This holds for both individual and institutional potential users of analysis.

There is considerable tangible evidence that physicians are being exposed to the language and concerns of economics, but how has this exposure affected the medical community? The recent survey on the cost-of-care issue by the American College of Physicians, with its 45 percent response rate, suggests that awareness and interest are high. But how knowledgeable are physicians about the meaning of cost-effectiveness? And how receptive are they to changing their behavior in a socially cost-effective direction? Our assessment, deriving from an experiential base, is that few physicians understand what cost-effectiveness means. They tend to perceive cost-effectiveness as referring to low cost *or* high effectiveness. Many appreciate the comparative perspective implied by the term, but their experience is generally limited to instances in which one procedure dominates another in both cost and effectiveness. Relatively few physicians are attuned to the difficult cost-effectiveness issues—those in which one procedure costs more than, and is at least as effective as, another procedure, or those in which society's cost-effectiveness interests differ from those of the individual (insured) patient.

This assessment reflects only two observers' impressions. There is a real need to pursue efforts to study physician awareness of, interest in, and understanding of CBA-CEA. Research ought to address such questions as:

— What is the amount (intensity) and nature of physician awareness of and interest in medical care cost issues?

— What is the amount of interest in and understanding of articles in the medical literature that relate to cost issues?

— What is the amount of interest in and understanding of CBA-CEAs in the medical literature?

— How do physicians perceive that they respond to their awareness of cost concerns in general and specific CBA-CEAs?

— How do they actually respond? That is, what response is suggested by empirical evidence on changes in behavior?

— What changes in the literature might facilitate use of published CBA-CEAs?

— What changes in physician education might facilitate use of CBA-CEAs? What might or should be done along these lines in undergraduate medical education (Hudson and Braslow, 1979), residency training (Kridel and Winston, 1978), and continuing education?

— How, if at all, do answers to the above questions vary by such dimensions as the economic nature of the practice (fee-for-service versus salaried versus prepaid physicians)?

This last question deserves particularly careful attention, as it is possible that economic incentives play a highly significant role in determining interest in and response to cost-effectiveness information. This seems logical and is consistent with evidence that economic incentives affect the provision of certain types of medical procedures (Luft, 1978).

To study questions such as these, surveys should be complemented by more objective explorations of knowledge and response, including experiments. For example, a random group of physicians might be provided cost data on laboratory tests (for example, prices of procedures or the physician's individual expenditure patterns relative to his or her colleagues); their subsequent test-ordering behavior would be monitored and compared with that of a control group (Grossman, 1981). Ongoing efforts to convey principles of cost-effective care to medical students and practitioners should be evaluated carefully. Despite the polarized views of observers on the likelihood of inducing changes in behavior, physician awareness, interest, understanding, and behavior should be measured in terms of how much response there is, not whether or not there is a response.

A related set of questions concerns potential institutional users of analysis. Officials of several governmental and nongovernmental organizations have indicated considerable knowledge of and interest in the use of CBA-CEA. The extensiveness of such knowledge and interest ought to be determined across a variety of types of agencies and the nature of intended uses of analysis carefully assessed. The influence of environmental factors such as politics on current and expected uses of analysis needs to be explored much more deeply than it has been to date. For example, third-party payers' reimbursement policies are subject to close scrutiny by several politically influential interest groups. Thus the question arises as to whether, and under what circumstances, insurers might be able to base decisions not to reimburse on CBA-CEAs. Could a decision not to reimburse rest on an analytical finding that a procedure was safe and effective but more costly than another procedure? How great would the cost difference have to be to justify such a decision? How would different views of the relative effectiveness of the procedures affect the insurer's ability to make a nonreimbursement decision? At the extreme, will decisions not to reimburse be possible for cases other than demonstrably ineffective or unsafe procedures, or for cases in which one procedure clearly dominates another on the grounds of both cost and medical effectiveness?

Research should explore institutional mechanisms for increasing the usefulness of analysis. As noted above, institutional use can be mandated, a somewhat extreme but effective means of creating a role for analysis in policy. In settings that might be naturally receptive to analysis, such as HMOs, mechanisms for increasing awareness and communication of CBA-CEA findings could be examined. For example, an analyst or analysis ombudsman might be employed to keep track of developments and communicate them to the appropriate medical and administrative personnel.

RESEARCH ON TECHNICAL ANALYTICAL ISSUES

Research on such environmental issues can enlighten the health policy community as to the nonanalytical factors that influence the use of CBA-CEA, but another set of technical questions remains unanswered. These center around the basic issue of the technical potential of analysis to be useful. That is, given common and inherent problems in analysis, how, if at all, can CBA-CEA contribute to policy decision-making?

Two principal questions are of concern. The first relates to the implications of the uncertainties that seem to be inherent in CBA-CEAs: Are these such as to rule out definitive bottom-line conclusions in all but the most obvious cases? The sense that important uncertainties pervade analysis is not based on a specific study of the issue, but it seems to be a researchable question. The more important question is whether such pervasive uncertainties result in pervasive inconclusiveness. Are the findings of careful studies of genuinely controversial issues usually sensitive to unresolvable uncertainties? If so, the implication for policy applications of analysis is direct and strong: In general, CBA-CEAs by themselves will not answer a basic policy question. They may contribute data, perspective, and insight into the nature of the question, but decision-makers will have to rely on additional inputs to arrive at their policy choices. If sensitivity analysis frequently can handle analytical uncertainties, decision-makers should be able to rely more heavily on the findings of CBA-CEAs.

This issue is a crucial one, for two reasons. First, there is a need to determine the technical limitations on direct application of CBA-CEA findings. Second, if inevitable, confounding uncertainties severely restrict direct bottom-line application of CBA-CEA findings, how sophisticated do studies need to be? Several experts have argued that simple, informal analyses can contribute most of the insight of a sophisticated, expensive, detailed analysis, while consuming many fewer resources. In essence, the question is one of finding the most cost-beneficial level of effort to put into CBA-CEAs. One experienced analyst and research administrator has observed that "Methodological issues are of secondary importance. Simplicity is generally perfectly adequate."[3] Another has defined good analysis as "finding the minimum amount of information necessary to get the right answer."[4] Thus the question is, what is that minimum necessary amount of information?

In part, the amount of information and analytical sophistication needed is a function of the subtlety of the cost-effectiveness question at issue. Several knowledgeable health care experts argue that the major cost problems in medicine derive from medically ineffective or inappropriate care and hence that improvements in the quality of medicine practiced would also conserve health care resources. Many other observers disagree; they perceive cost containment as the antithesis of improving the quality of care. This is itself an important researchable question, because if health system cost problems reflect primarily medically inappropriate care, rather than medically acceptable but socially expensive care, society's approach to cost containment might emphasize the more traditional analysis of medical effectiveness and its communication and translation into practice. Fewer resources would need to be directed toward the newer and more complex analysis of cost-effectiveness.

Raising issues such as these may displease the purist. In part, they sound anti-intellectual and threaten to retard methodological progress. Such concerns warrant attention, but the policy question of how government agencies might best allocate their research resources rests on determination of cost-effective analytical procedures and projects. A given amount of resources can be spread over any number of CBA-CEA efforts and medical effectiveness studies; the question is ascertaining the best value for the money.

Value for the money is a function not only of the technical sophistication of CBA-CEA but also of the substantive focus of analysis. Among medical technologies, expensive equipment-embodied technologies have drawn the most policy attention in recent years (for example, through the certificate-of-need process); as we noted in Chapter 4, CT scanning has been the single most studied equipment-based procedure in the CBA-CEA literature. Yet there is a growing body of evidence indicting low-cost but frequently utilized technologies (such as laboratory tests) as a major source of medical care cost inflation (Fineberg, 1979; Maloney and Rogers, 1979; Redisch, 1974; Scitovsky and McCall, 1976). Should CBA-CEA attention be turned to assessing appropriate use patterns for such technologies? Similarly, can CBA-CEA be directed more productively toward, say, surgical procedures than equipment-based technologies? In short, to determine the most cost-effective uses for CBA-CEA, we must determine where considerable inefficiency now prevails and where such inefficiency might be susceptible to analysis-induced correction.

These are only a few of the questions about analysis whose resolution might direct and expedite effective production and dissemination of CBA-CEA findings. We now have an experiential base of understanding of the inherent potential uses. If traditional economic resource allocation mechanisms continue to disappear from medicine, if technology-specific policy continues to evolve, and if interest in and support of analysis grows, it would seem prudent to direct research strategy toward basic questions.

CONCLUSION

While the long-term role of CBA-CEA is unclear, analysis could be a growth industry over the next few years. This would be consistent with recent intellectual trends in health services research and federal government initiatives to promote medical technology assessment. Of course, if bureaucratic support is withdrawn, the impetus for analysis to grow would be lessened. Growth and interest should be particularly strong in the medical community, given the novelty of CBA-CEA and concern about cost inflation. Interest in the nonmedical health services research community will be sustained by the medical profession's involvement with analysis, but one might anticipate some diminution in the current level of enthusiasm as the problems and limits of analysis become understood.

We noted earlier that some of the enthusiasm for CBA-CEA in the medical and health policy communities reflected the fact that, as an intervention, CBA-CEA tends not to threaten the status quo. Indirectly, this same fact may explain, in part, why many health services researchers have embraced CBA-CEA as a worthwhile scholarly endeavor: They perceive it to be the only game in town. Many scholars have concluded that a piecemeal, technology-specific approach to problems of resource allocation—such as that embodied in CBA-CEA—is relatively ineffectual. It may have small marginal benefits, but, by failing to address underlying structural problems, it cannot have a significant and sustained impact. The desirable alternative, major system-wide reform, appears highly unlikely in the foreseeable future. Hence we find the inclination to jump on the CBA-CEA (or, more generally, technology assessment) bandwagon.

Should CBA-CEA be promoted? Again, the question of standards—of expectations—arises. CBA-CEA is no panacea. It will not solve the health cost inflation problem. It will not rectify the general problem of health resource misallocation. Indeed, some analysis risks exacerbating the problems because it emphasizes measurable costs and benefits, and consequently deemphasizes considerations of equity and the like. Analysis has the potential for contributing to marginal improvements in resource allocation and cost inflation, but the most likely vehicles for its realizing success— through educating and informing health care decision-makers— will remain the least tangible in terms of our ability to evaluate its achievements. Thus we must recognize and accept the frustration that we probably will never accomplish a definitive assessment of the value of analysis: It may be considerable, but it will not be wholly measurable.

Do the incremental benefits of analysis exceed its costs, or is analysis an "Incidious Poison in the Body Politick"? (Williams,

1972). While the benefits of analysis are often incremental or intangible, the direct costs are generally low. As a result, even some of the more cynical analysts believe that the potential benefits justify most investments in analysis. If the problem addressed by analysis is large—say, involving the allocation of millions of dollars—an inexpensive CBA-CEA need have only a marginal beneficial effect to be worthwhile. Alternatively, only one out of dozens of such analyses need have a significant positive effect in order to justify the total investment in all of the analyses.

The real question is not the direct costs of analysis, but rather the total opportunity costs. Emphasis on CBA-CEA diverts attention from other efforts. Is CBA-CEA the most cost-effective way to increase the cost-consciousness of the medical community? It is certainly conceivable that less expensive, easier to understand cost studies might better serve that function. Does the focus of many members of the health policy community on CBA-CEA divert intellect and energy from the more challenging effort of developing and selling rational system-wide reforms?

As with so many other evaluation problems, the relative novelty of health care applications of CBA-CEA precludes any definitive forecasts of its future roles and implications. The inclination is to want to praise or damn CBA-CEA, but neither option seems reasonable. The nature of these techniques and their practitioners' use of them suggests two conclusions: Analysis is unlikely to achieve the prominence and policy effect advocates envision, but neither will detractors' negative assessments be fully realized. In short, the analytical cup is one-quarter full. The question is whether it will ever be less then three-quarters empty.

NOTES

1. A societal perspective continues to dominate. The relative shift from organizational to individual reflects the proportions of articles not having a societal orientation.
2. We recognize that the boundaries drawn around our literature search undoubtedly caused us to miss dozens of contributions on such non-medical public health issues. For example, the literature on highway safety includes CBA-CEAs. Our point is that subjects such as this are underrepresented in the literature read by those who deal with their health implications.
3. Jeffrey Weiss, personal communication.
4. Comment by Stuart Altman at the December 13, 1978, meeting of the Advisory Panel on Cost Effectiveness, Office of Technology Assessment, U.S. Congress.

Appendix A

Development of Health Care
CBA-CEA Bibliography and
Classification of References

In Chapter 4 we presented an empirical analysis of the growth and content of the health care CBA-CEA literature. The analysis derived from counting and classifying over 500 references in a bibliography covering the years 1966–1978 and including CBAs and CEAs on personal health services topics, reviews and comments on such literature, and discussions of CBA-CEA methodology directed specifically toward health care professionals; these references constitute most of this book's bibliography.[1]

Excluded from the counts and analysis are scores of CBA-CEAs on nonmedical but health-related subjects (for example, traffic safety and control of environmental pollution), as well as dozens of general books and articles on CBA-CEA methodology. Thus, certain articles that have had a profound impact on health care CBA-CEA were not included in the analyses because they were not directed exclusively toward an audience concerned solely with personal health services. The seminal work of Rice on measuring the cost of illness is a case in point (Rice, 1966; Cooper and Rice, 1976), as is the related work of Acton and others on measuring the value of life (Acton, 1976; Jones-Lee, 1976; Zeckhauser, 1975; Zeckhauser and Shepard, 1976). These studies are at the heart of a long-lived CBA intellectual debate. Each has formed the basis of attempts to value the health benefits of programs, but the issues and techniques transcend categorization as personal health care methodologies; they are equally relevant to numerous human welfare programs outside the personal health services arena. Studies that examine only the cost of health programs are

---

1. The bibliography also includes many CBA-CEA references from 1979, 1980, and 1981, as well as all of the non-CBA-CEA references cited in the text. The latter are preceded in the bibliography by asterisks. The empirical analysis of trends in the CBA-CEA literature runs only through 1978 because we did not strive for the same comprehensiveness of coverage in later years that we did for those in 1966–1978. Most of the CBA-CEA references for 1979–81 were identified in the *Index Medicus* and *Journal of Economic Literature* or were brought to our attention individually by colleagues. We did not scan reference lists in the most recent articles, consult abstracts in conference programs, and so on. Consequently, we have undoubtedly missed many appropriate references for these most recent years, possibly including some high quality analyses.

also excluded from the analysis. Similarly, several excellent studies of the social costs of specific illnesses are excluded because they are not CBA-CEAs.

We were liberal in classifying a reference as a CBA or CEA. Although we have not read many of the included references, we have read a limited number at random. Our reading suggests that some of the studies which purport to be CBAs or CEAs are not. At least one article whose title says it presents a cost-benefit ratio does not include any comparison of economic costs and benefits (Bennett, 1976). More commonly, articles have a clear CBA-CEA intent but approach analysis in a technically unsound manner.

We included such references because even if we had had the time to read each of the 500-plus articles with great care, a consistent inclusion-exclusion rule would have been difficult to design; and, more important, because our objective was to identify and characterize the literature that is introducing health care professionals to the ideas and analysis of cost-effectiveness in health care delivery. Whether an article is of high or low quality, it serves this function. In several fields, such as nursing administration and certain medical specialties, conceptually inaccurate articles appear to constitute the bulk of the CBA-CEA literature.

References included in the bibliography were obtained from four sources: computer-assisted searches of the literature, published indexes of professional literature, reference lists of individual articles, papers, and books, and communication with leading health services researchers. Two computer-assisted searches provided numerous references. MEDLARS covered relevant citations from *Index Medicus*. For the years 1966 through 1975, this search covered the subject heading "cost and cost analysis" (which, until 1976, included CBA and CEA). From 1976 through 1978, the search was limited to the *Index Medicus* subject heading "cost-benefit analysis," which was introduced in 1976 and which includes both CBA and CEA. The second computer-assisted search was conducted by the National Health Planning Information Center, using the key words "cost-benefit analysis" and "cost-effectiveness analysis." For the period after the MEDLARS search, *Index Medicus* was consulted directly. Published indexes also supplied many relevant economic studies not included in *Index Medicus*. Beginning with the 1966 editions, two indexes of economic literature were searched: the *Index of Economic Articles* and the *Journal of Economic Literature* (entitled the *Journal of Economic Abstracts* before 1969).

After compiling the bibliography, we classified each 1966–78 CBA-CEA reference according to the following:

- Year (1966–78)
- Type (CBA, CEA, general or unknown)
- Publication vehicle (medical journal; journal intended primarily for non-physician health care professionals, administrators, or health services researchers; nonhealth journal; other)
- Medical function of program or technology (prevention, diagnosis, treatment)
- Physical nature of program or technology (technique, drug, procedure, equipment, personnel, system)
- Decision orientation—that is, whose decision-making the paper is intended to assist (individual practitioner, organization, society)
- Subject matter (a specific program or technology, review article, methodology)

Classification involved numerous arbitrary judgments. Many of the assignments depended on the content of abstracts or even the wording of titles. Where available information suggested that each of two (sometimes three) categories was appropriate, half (or one-third) credit was assigned to each. For example, in the "medical function" category, certain screening programs were recorded as half prevention and half diagnosis. (A comprehensive blood pressure control program was counted as one-third for each of prevention, diagnosis, and treatment.) "Unknown" or "other" categories were used liberally when we lacked confidence in our ability to categorize references accurately.

While the possibility remains that numerous assignments were not optimal, we are unaware of any significant sources of bias. Thus, at the least, our quantitative analysis should provide an accurate qualitative characterization of the size, nature, and contents of the literature.

Appendix B

Detailed Counts and
Classification of
CBA-CEA References

In the first section of Chapter 4 we examined empirical trends in the size and character of the CBA-CEA literature. In addition to the discussion in the text, we presented a table summarizing these trends (table 4.1) and two graphs, one illustrating the overall growth of the literature (figure 4.1) and the other showing the growth of articles in medical and nonmedical journals (figure 4.2). In this appendix we present the detailed annual counts and classification from which the analysis in Chapter 4 was derived. Appendix tables correspond to subjects discussed in the text as follows: diffusion, B.1; publication vehicles, B.2; mix of CBAs and CEAs, B.1; medical function, B.3 and B.4; decision orientation, B.5.

Table B.1: CBAs and CEAs by Year

Year	CBAs*	CEAs†	CBAs Plus CEAs	Other‡	Total (CBA-CEAs Plus Others)
1966	4.5	0.5	5.0	0	5.0
1967	4.0	1.0	5.0	0	5.0
1968	5.5	4.5	10.0	4	14.0
1969	2.0	1.0	3.0	2	5.0
1970	2.5	8.5	11.0	3	14.0
1971	9.5	10.5	20.0	5	25.0
1972	13.5	5.5	19.0	6	25.0
1973	24.5	16.5	41.0	2	43.0
1974§	18.5	16.0	34.5	6	40.5
1975§	17.0	21.5	38.5	12	50.5
1976	39.5	36.5	76.0	13	89.0
1977	31.5	45.5	77.0	18	95.0
1978	32.0	38.0	70.0	21	91.0
Total	204.5	205.5	410	92	502

*All papers identified as CBAs in title or otherwise known; 0.5 indicates half CBA and half CEA.

†All papers identified as CEAs in title or otherwise known; 0.5 indicates half CBA and half CEA.

‡All other papers, including those the title of which does not state CBA or CEA, general methodology papers, and so on.

§Fractional entries for 1974 and 1975 are due to one article in a journal with the publication date Dec. 1974–Jan. 1975.

APPENDIX B

232 APPENDIX B

Table B.2: CBA-CEA Literature by Type of Publication and Year

Year	Medical Journals*	New England Journal of Medicine	Nonmedical Journals†	Other‡	Total§
1966	0	0	1.0	4	5.0
1967	0	0	1.0	4	5.0
1968	4	2	6.0	4	14.0
1969	2	1	2.0	1	5.0
1970	4	1	5.0	5	14.0
1971	10	0	7.0	8	25.0
1972	6	0	14.0	5	25.0
1973	11	1	19.0	13	43.0
1974#	22	1	7.5	11	40.5
1975#	20	7	14.5	16	50.5
1976	43	4	30.0	16	89.0
1977	44	5	24.0	27	95.0
1978	41	8	25.0	25	91.0
Total	207	30	156	139	502

*Journals read primarily by physicians; excludes nursing, dental, public health, hospital journals, and so on; includes psychiatric journals.
†All other journals, including nonphysician-oriented health journals, economic and policy analysis journals, and so on.
‡Books, chapters in books, unpublished papers, and so on.
§Literature listed under the *"New England Journal of Medicine"* column is excluded here; it is included under the "Medical Journals" column.
#Fractional entries for 1974 and 1975 are due to one article in a journal with the publication date Dec. 1974–Jan. 1975.

Table B.3:   CBA-CEA Literature by Medical Function and
Year

Year	Prevention	Diagnosis	Treatment	Other*
1966	0.0	0.0	0.0	5
1967	0.0	0.3	1.7	3
1968	2.5	3.0	3.5	5
1969	1.5	0.5	2.0	1
1970	2.0	1.0	3.0	8
1971	6.5	3.5	4.0	11
1972	7.0	2.0	3.0	13
1973	14.5	4.0	10.5	14
1974	2.5	5.0	13.0	20
1975	5.0	10.0	14.5	21
1976	14.5	16.0	27.5	31
1977	10.5	15.5	36.0	33
1978	18.0	24.5	17.5	31
Total	84.5	85.3	136.2	196

*Includes mixes of all three functions, administration, general, and unknown.

Table B.4:   Treatment Functions by Year*

Year	Cure	Rehabilitation	Maintenance	Total
1966	0.0	0.0	0.0	0.0
1967	1.3	0.3	0.0	1.7
1968	1.0	1.0	1.5	3.5
1969	1.5	0.0	0.5	2.0
1970	0.5	1.0	1.5	3.0
1971	2.0	1.0	1.0	4.0
1972	1.5	1.5	0.0	3.0
1973	4.5	3.5	2.5	10.5
1974	5.0	6.5	1.5	13.0
1975	6.5	3.0	5.0	14.5
1976	10.0	6.5	11.0	27.5
1977	24.5	4.5	7.0	36.0
1978	8.0	3.5	6.0	17.5
Total	66.3	32.3	37.5	136.2

*Palliation is not included, because there were no relevant articles.

Table B.5: Decision Orientation by Year

Year	Individual	Organization	Society	Unknown
1966	0.0	0	3	2
1967	0.0	0	5	0
1968	0.0	4	8	2
1969	0.0	2	2	1
1970	1.0	3	6	4
1971	4.0	2	14	5
1972	2.0	5	12	6
1973	2.0	7	26	8
1974*	5.5	2	21	12
1975*	2.5	11	24	13
1976	12.0	4	48	25
1977	13.0	4	48	30
1978	8.0	7	49	27
Total	50	51	266	135

*Fractional entries for 1974 and 1975 are due to one article in a journal with the publication date Dec. 1974–Jan. 1975.

Appendix C

CBA-CEA Literature by Subject

The following publications are divided into a variety of health care topics. Publications are identified by author and year; full citations can be found in the bibliography. Bibliographic entries not included in these lists fall into the "miscellaneous" category. The following topics are included:

—alcoholism
—birth defects and genetic counseling
—breast cancer detection
—cancer screening (other than breast cancer)
—cardiovascular disease
—communicable diseases
—computerized tomography
—dental care
—diagnostic procedures (not included elsewhere)
—drug abuse
—emergency medical services (not included under cardiovascular disease)
—family planning
—fetal monitoring
—geriatric services
—health manpower
—hospital services and systems (not included elsewhere)
—hypertension
—institutional versus home care (not included elsewhere)
—maternal and child health services
—mental illness
—nutrition
—occupational health and rehabilitation
—pharmaceutical services
—prevention (not included elsewhere)
—renal disease
—rheumatic fever

—screening and early detection (not included elsewhere)
—surgery (specific)
—surgery (nonspecific)
—therapy (not included elsewhere)

ALCOHOLISM

Hertzman et al., 1977
Johns et al., 1976
Mulford, 1979
Rundell et al., 1979
Schramm, 1977
Swint et al., 1977a, 1977b, 1978

BIRTH DEFECTS AND
GENETIC COUNSELING

Akehurst and Holterman, 1978
Angle et al., 1977
Bush et al., 1973
Chapalain, 1978
Committee for the Study of Inborn
    Errors of Metabolism, 1975
Conley and Milunsky, 1975
Glass, 1975
Hagard et al., 1976a, 1976b
Inman, 1978
Layde et al., 1979
Mikkelsen et al., 1976

Nelson et al., 1978
Sarna et al., 1979
Scriver, 1974
Steiner and Smith, 1973
Swint et al., 1979
VanPelt and Levy, 1974

BREAST CANCER DETECTION

Bailar, 1976
Christie, 1977
Doberneck, 1980
Gravelle, 1976
Holler, 1976
Kodlin, 1972
Kristein and Arnold, 1978, 1980
Moskowitz and Fox, 1979
Moskowitz et al., 1976
Seidman, 1977

CANCER SCREENING
(OTHER THAN BREAST CANCER)

Cromwell and Gertman, 1977
Dickinson, 1972
Eddy, 1978, 1980*a*, 1980*b*, 1981
Foltz and Kelsey, 1978
Galliher, 1976
Kagan and Skinner, 1978
Kristein, 1978, n.d.
Luce, 1981
McNeil, 1978
Neuhauser and Lewicki, 1975, 1976
Schweitzer and Luce, 1979
Smith, 1977
Spratt, 1978

CARDIOVASCULAR DISEASE

Acton, 1973, 1975
Bennett and Winchester, 1977
Berwick et al., 1976
Bloom and Peterson, 1973
Bryant et al., 1974
Charles et al., 1978
Cretin, 1977
Criley et al., 1975
Emlet et al., 1973
Fabricius, 1978

Feigenson, 1979
Feigenson et al., 1978
Flagle, 1976
Gorry et al., 1977
Grande et al., 1980
Havia and Schuller, 1978
Hiatt, 1977
Krause et al., 1977
Lubeck and Bunker, 1981
McGregor and Pelletier, 1978
Martin et al., 1974
Marty et al., 1977
Mather et al., 1971
Mustard, 1977
Pauker, 1976
Preston, 1977
Reiss et al., 1980
Reynell and Reynell, 1972
Rios et al., 1978
Russell et al., 1976
Stason and Fortess, 1981
Urban et al., 1981
Weinstein et al., 1977

COMMUNICABLE DISEASES

Abel-Smith, 1973
Albritton, 1978
Ambrosch et al., 1979
Axnick et al., 1969
Blount, 1973
Brodsky and Scherzer, 1976
Cohn, 1972, 1973
Collis et al., 1973
Ekblom et al., 1978
Elo, n. d.
Farber and Finkelstein, 1978
Feingold, 1975
Fenwick 1972
Grab and Cvjetanovic, 1971
Keith et al., 1975
Klarman and Guzick, 1976
Koplan et al., 1979
Menz, 1971
Moulding, 1971
Ponnighaus, 1980
Porro de Somenzi, 1979
Ramaiah, 1976
Saunders, 1970

Schoenbaum et al., 1976*a*, 1976*b*
Stilwell, 1976
Waaler, 1968
Weisbrod, 1971
Witte et al., 1975

COMPUTERIZED TOMOGRAPHY

Abrams and McNeil, 1978
Bahr, 1978
Baker and Way, 1978
Banta and McNeil, 1978*b*
Bartlett et al., 1978
Carrera et al., 1977
Evens and Jost, 1976, 1977, 1978
Evens et al, 1977*a*, 1977*b*, 1979*a*, 1979*b*
Gempel et al., 1977
Knaus and Davis, 1978
Knaus et al., 1981
Laguna et al., 1977
Swartz and Desharnius, 1977
Thomson, 1977
U.S. Congress, Office of Technology Assessment, 1978*b*
Wagner, 1981*a*
Wortzman and Holgate, 1979
Wortzman et al., 1975

DENTAL CARE

Berman, 1971
Boggs, 1973
Burt, 1978
Burt and Warner, forthcoming
Cuzacq and Glass, 1972
Davies, 1973*a*-1973*f*
Doherty and Powell, 1974
Field and Jong, 1971
Geiser and Menz, 1976
Godfrey, 1980
Grainger, 1973
Horowitz et al., 1979
Jong and Gluck, 1974
Lewis et al., 1972
McCombie, 1979
Nelson et al., 1976
Scheffler and Rovin, 1981
Stephen et al., 1978

DIAGNOSTIC PROCEDURES
(NOT INCLUDED ELSEWHERE)

Adelstein and McNeil, 1978
Arthur D. Little, Inc., 1976
Bennett et al., 1978
Fineberg, 1979
Gelfand et al., 1978
Goldhaber et al., 1974
Hur et al., 1979
McNeil, 1979
Pole, 1971*a*, 1971*b*, 1972
Showstack and Schroeder, 1981
Sonnenburg et al., 1979
Wagner, 1981*b*
Weinstein and Pearlman, 1981
Weiss, 1971
Werner et al., 1973

DRUG ABUSE

Backhaut, 1973
Fernandez, 1972
Goldschmidt, 1976
Hannan, 1975, 1976
Holahan, 1970, 1973
Hu et al., 1978
Jeffers and Johnson, 1973
Leslie, 1976
Leveson, 1973
McGlothlin et al., 1972
Retka, 1977
Scanlon, 1976
Sirotnik et al., 1975

EMERGENCY MEDICAL SERVICES
(NOT INCLUDED UNDER
CARDIOVASCULAR DISEASE)

Gill, 1974
Hallstrom et al., 1981
Savas, 1969

FAMILY PLANNING

Bertera et al., 1979
Blumstein and Cassidy, 1973
Catford and Fowkes, 1979

Deane and Ulene, 1977
Jaffe et al., 1977
Osteria, 1973
Robinson, 1979
Sugar, 1978

FETAL MONITORING

Banta and Thacker, 1979a, 1979b
Cohodes, n.d.
Quilligan and Paul, 1975
Rabello and Paul, 1976

GERIATRIC SERVICES

Doherty and Hicks, 1977
Doherty et al., 1975
Kane et al., 1974, 1976
Lashof, 1977
Rathbone-McCuan, et al., 1975
Ruchlin and Levey, 1972
Schultz and McGlone, 1977
Stanford Research Institute, 1978
Starr, 1975
Weiler, 1974

HEALTH MANPOWER

Allanson, 1978
Alter et al., 1979
Crabtree, 1978
Dhillon and Bennett, 1975
Knapper and Dungy, 1978
Kushner, 1976
Leroy and Solkowitz, 1981
Marram, 1976
Marram et al., 1975
Martin and Newman, 1973
Morrow et al., 1976
Romm et al., 1978
Spitzer et al., 1976a, 1976b
Sussna and Heinemann, 1972
Wingert et al., 1975

HOSPITAL SERVICES AND SYSTEMS
(NOT INCLUDED ELSEWHERE)

Aikawa, 1974
Bendixen, 1977

Berry, 1974
Brian et al., 1976
Budetti et al., 1981
Coyne, 1980
Finkler, 1979
Fofar, 1979
Green, 1970
Griffith and Chernow, 1977
Hamilton, 1968
Heagarty et al., 1970
Hohn et al., 1980
Lucas, 1979
Matlack, 1974
Norling 1975
Penner, 1978
Smith, 1973
Sullivan and Thuesen, 1971
U.S. Congress, Office of Technology
  Assessment, 1977
Weinstein and Fineberg, 1978

HYPERTENSION

Bertera and Bertera, 1981
Bryers and Hawthorne, 1978
Fein, 1977
Feldstein, 1974
Ferguson, 1975
Foote et al., 1977
Gillum et al., 1978
Hannon and Graham, 1978
McNeil, 1976
McNeil and Adelstein, 1976
McNeil et al., 1975a
Shepard et al., 1978
Stason and Weinstein, 1977
Stokes and Carmichael, 1975
Strong, 1977
Walworth et al., 1977
Weinstein and Stason, 1976a, 1976b,
  1977a

INSTITUTIONAL VERSUS HOME CARE
(NOT INCLUDED ELSEWHERE)

Creese et al., 1977
Hurtado et al., 1972
Jackson and Ward, 1976
Lavor et al., 1976
Leitch, 1968

MATERNAL AND CHILD
HEALTH SERVICES

Geller and Yockmowitz, 1975
Levin, 1968
Reid and Morris, 1979
U.S. Department of Health, Education,
and Welfare, 1966c

MENTAL ILLNESS

Banta and McNeil, 1978a
Bernard, 1979
Foley et al., 1973
Ginsberg et al., 1977
Glass et al., 1977
Guillette et al., 1978
McCaffee, 1969
May, 1970a, 1970b, 1971a, 1971b
Michels et al., 1976
Murphy et al., 1976
Mushkin and Cotton, 1967
National Institute of Mental Health,
1975
Panzetta, 1973
Saxe, 1981
Sharfstein et al., 1976
Sheehan and Atkinson, 1974
Solomon, 1979
Weisbrod et al., 1978

NUTRITION

American Dietetic Association, 1979
Popkin et al., 1980
Spears, 1976
Tunbridge and Wetherill, 1970
Yates, 1978

OCCUPATIONAL HEALTH AND
REHABILITATION

Atherley et al., 1976
Bond et al., 1968
Briggs et al., 1979
Chung et al., 1980
Conley, 1975
Desimone, 1974-75
Fast, 1978

Hughes, 1974
Moore and Hoover, 1974
Phillips and Hughes, 1974
Thrall and Cardus, 1974

PHARMACEUTICAL SERVICES

Ashmole et al., 1973
Bishop, 1979
Gumbhir and Brown, 1975
Hefner, 1979
McGhan et al., 1978
Speight, 1975
Wolfe, 1973
Yorio et al., 1972

PREVENTION
(NOT INCLUDED ELSEWHERE)

Hilbert, 1977
Kristein, 1977a, 1977b
Kristein et al., 1977
Lave and Lave, 1977
Merck, Sharp, and Dohme, n.d.
Rogers et al., Forthcoming
Rowe and Bisbee, 1978
Scheffler and Parringer, 1980
Sencer and Axnick, 1975
Shapiro, 1977
Shepard, 1977
Terris, 1980
U.S. Congress, Office of Technology
Assessment, 1979
U.S. Department of Health, Education,
and Welfare, 1979
Warner, 1979b

RENAL DISEASE

Barnes, 1977b
Buxton and West, 1975
Dodge, 1977
Klarman et al., 1968
LeSourd et al., 1968
McNeil, 1976
McNeil and Adelstein, 1975
McNeil et al., 1975a
Mani et al., 1976
Menz, 1971

Pliskin, 1974
Pliskin and Beck, 1976
Rettig, 1981
Roberts et al., 1980
Salvatierra et al., 1979
Schippers and Kalff, 1976
Stange and Sumner, 1978
Stewart et al., 1973
U.S. Bureau of the Budget, 1967
U.S. Department of Health, Education, and Welfare, 1967b
U.S. General Accounting Office, 1975

RHEUMATIC FEVER

Giauque, 1972
Pantell, 1977
Robinson, 1971
Saslaw et al., 1965
Tompkins et al., 1977a

SCREENING AND EARLY DETECTION
(NOT INCLUDED ELSEWHERE)

Bay et al., 1976
Chadwick et al., 1970
Chamberlain, 1978
Clayman, 1980
Collen et al., 1969, 1970, 1973, 1977
Dales et al., 1979
Dawson et al., 1976, 1979
Felch, 1976
Forst, 1973
Gelman, 1970
Greenwood et al., 1979
McNeil and Adelstein, 1976
Pole, 1968, 1971a
Schweitzer, 1974
Simmons, 1976
Siu, 1976
Teeling-Smith, 1975

SURGERY (SPECIFIC)

Bennett, 1976
Bredin and Prout, 1976
Bredin et al., 1977

Brown, 1975
Cole, 1976
Fitzpatrick et al., 1977
Glass and Russell, 1974
Holmin et al., 1980
Jackson et al., 1978
Korenbrot et al., 1981
Neuhauser, 1977c
Neutra, 1977
Patiala et al., 1976
Schachter and Neuhauser, 1981
Skillings et al., 1979
Taylor, 1976
Tunturi et al., 1979

SURGERY (NONSPECIFIC)

Abt, 1977
Barnes, 1977a, 1977b
Bunker, 1974
Bunker et al., 1977, 1978
Eddy, 1979
Gilbert et al., 1967
Green, 1977
Pauly, 1979

THERAPY
(NOT INCLUDED ELSEWHERE)

Armstrong and Armstrong, 1979
Aron and Daily, 1974
Bentkover and Drew, 1981
Charles et al., 1974
Collen, 1980
Culyer and Maynard, 1981
Fineberg and Pearlman, 1981
Griner, 1973
Linn et al., 1979
Pettinger, 1978
Rosenshein et al., 1980
Scheffler and Delaney, 1981
Schweitzer et al., 1979
Spratt, 1971
Stanaway, 1979
Thomson et al., 1978
Utian, 1977
Zapka and Averill, 1979

Appendix D

Selected Abstracts of Health Care CBA-CEAs

Three types of contributions to the literature on CBA-CEAs are included in the abstracts in this appendix: (1) many of the better-known articles on CBA-CEAs and methodology; (2) a few contributions to the general health care CBA-CEA literature which illustrate a variety of technical and methodological points; and (3) many of the case studies prepared or supported by the Office of Technology Assessment as part of its study of CBA-CEA applied to medical technologies. The OTA cases are found in U.S. Congress, Office of Technology Assessement, *The Implications of Cost-Effectiveness Analysis of Medical Technology; Background Paper no. 2: Case Studies of Medical Technologies*, published in 1981 and available from the Government Printing Office, Washington, D.C. This publication is identified in the abstracts as OTA (1981).

We followed no systematic rule in selecting the publications to be abstracted, although we did attempt to include most of the articles that were referred to frequently in the text. Certainly, neither inclusion nor exclusion should be construed as reflecting our judgment on the quality of a publication.

In general, we have evaluated the abstracted publications in the text (primarily in Chapter 4), not within the abstracts themselves.

Acton, J. 1975. *Measuring the Social Impact of Heart and Circulatory Disease Programs: Preliminary Framework and Estimates*. Report prepared for the National Heart and Lung Institute, National Institutes of Health. Santa Monica, Calif.: RAND Corp.

In this analysis the author demonstrates the application of alternative methodologies for valuing lifesaving by considering the case of heart and circulatory disease. He presents a strong argument that the willingness-to-pay approach is conceptually superior to the human capital approach because the former takes individual preferences into account. In practice, however, there is as yet no valid and reliable means of measuring willingness to pay. By contrast, the human capital approach is relatively straightforward mechanically, if flawed conceptually.

The author presents estimates of the major social impact associated with nine categories of heart and circulatory disease. These impacts include mortality, morbidity, disability, productivity losses, utilization of medical care services, and medical costs. The estimates show that heart and circulatory diseases impose a substantial burden on society, with their associated productivity losses and medical costs equaling 5 to 7 percent of the 1971 national income.

Comparison of estimates derived from the two different valuation techniques indicates that they produce qualitatively similar results, though the quantitative differences are not inconsequential. The conceptual weakness of the human capital approach leads the author to call for more research on the development of valuing techniques relying on expressions of individual preference.

Baker, C. and Way, L. 1978. Clinical Utility of CAT Body Scans. *Amer. J. Surg.* 136:37.

This CEA of computerized axial tomography (CAT) body scans employs an efficacy scale that ranges from one (given when the scan is deemed to have saved a patient's life) to eighteen (given when the scan is held to have led to a patient's death). In the course of the analysis, the sensitivity, specificity, and accuracy of CAT body scans are evaluated. The authors note that less expensive tests, primarily ultrasound, are bypassed or performed simultaneously with CAT scans. Analysis indicates that ultrasound and CAT scans are of about equal clinical value in any given situation, but ultrasound costs one-fourth as much as CAT scanning. The authors observe that clinicians, when employing CAT scanning, often seem to have no clear expectations that it can affect patient management. They also note that, for most conditions about which CAT body scans are informative, insufficient information is not the major factor limiting the success of therapy. Though this study, limited to hospitalized patients, would have missed any decreased admissions for diagnostic tests that may have resulted from the use of CAT body scanning, its authors believe that few savings can be expected from replacing other diagnostic procedures with CAT scans. They recommend that CAT body scans be ordered only if more information would truly affect patient management, more cost-effective diagnostic tests have failed, and the likelihood of disease is high.

The authors caution that their study was done as CAT technology was rapidly evolving. This evolution has obvious implications, including the likelihood that current use patterns (frequency and motivation) differ from what they will become if and when body scanning becomes standard practice. As such, the study fails to distinguish between cost-effectiveness today and in a steady state situation in the future. In addition, the study does not identify cost-effectiveness under optimal conditions. Despite these drawbacks, the study stands out as one of the very few that have attempted to identify and quantify patient management and health outcomes.

Banta, H. and Thacker, S 1979b. *Costs and Benefits of Electronic Fetal Monitoring: A Review of the Literature.*" DHEW Publication no. (PHS) 79-3245. Hyattsville, Md.: National Center for Health Services Research.

A relatively new technology, electronic fetal monitoring (EFM) is found in virtually all delivery rooms in the United States; it is used in the course of a large percentage of pregnancies. Despite its popularity, questions have arisen concerning its efficacy, safety, and cost. In this extensive review of the literature on EFM (nearly 300 references), the authors examine the understanding of the costs and benefits of the technology.

The paper opens with a history of EFM and of fetal monitoring generally. The authors identify unresolved medical issues concerning the data produced by monitoring, and they examine the impacts of EFM on therapy. For example, they estimate that half of the substantial increase in the cesarean section rate (from 4.5 percent of deliveries in 1965 to 12.1 percent in 1976) is attributable to EFM, and they question whether outcomes warrant this growth. All told, the authors conclude that the evidence of benefit from EFM is contradictory and generally limited to a small decrease in mortality among high-risk patients, especially babies with low weights at birth. The authors note the need for randomized, controlled studies of the technology.

The authors estimate that EFM adds over $400 million annually to the cost of childbirth, assuming that 50 percent of all deliveries are monitored electronically. In light of the questionable medical value of widespread use of EFM, the authors suggest that this may be an unduly high cost for society to bear in this era of constrained resources.

Barnes, B. 1977a. Cost-Benefit Analysis of Surgery: Current Accomplishments and Limitations. *Amer. J. Surg.* 133:438.

The general principles of CBA are presented, with a good program described as one in which the net discounted benefits exceed zero. The author says that CBA was first applied to health care in response to rapidly rising medical care expenditures. When conflict between individual and societal interests is discerned, the techniques of CBA must be applied with sensitivity to the individual and public interests involved. Limitations of CBA in health care include difficulties in accurately accounting for the numerous complex costs and benefits encountered, in identifying and valuing long-range effects, and in determining a discount rate when costs and benefits are deferred many years.

CBA is described as applicable only where effects are nearly equivalent, so that the analysis becomes, in effect, a cost comparison. Three examples of CBA as applied in health care are presented: cholecystectomy for silent gallstones, renal transplantation or chronic hemodialysis for end-stage renal disease, and intensive care unit support for different illnesses.

The author states that the accomplishments of CBA and related techniques in health are largely those of more comprehensive understanding of the advantages of a particular therapy or policy. In itself, CBA is seldom definitive, but, in conjunction with political and professional judgments, it can improve decision-making.

Bartlett, J. et al. 1978. Evaluating Cost-Effectiveness of Diagnostic Equipment: The Brain Scanner Case. *Brit. Med. J.* 2:815.

The bulk of this article is devoted to a comparison of the costs involved in five different options for implementing CAT scanning in a region of England. The net costs of CAT scanning are calculated as gross costs (for example, purchasing, installing, and staffing) minus savings from the decreased use of conventional neuroradiology and bed days presumed to result from the introduction of CAT. The article also includes a discussion of possible treatment improvements that, although unquantified and not included in the cost of calculations, may result from the use of CAT. There is little discussion of the cost-effectiveness of CAT scanning versus conventional neuroradiology, although the analysis of the five CAT implementation options seems based on the premises that CAT is more cost-effective in certain circumstances. The authors acknowledge the lack of precision and uncertainty involved in the savings calculations, but contend that some savings do result from the introduction of CAT and must be assessed in any analysis.

Bennett, W. 1976. Cost-Benefit Ratio of Pretransplant Bilateral Nephrectomy. *JAMA* 235:1703.

This paper is an example of how titles can be misleading. Despite the title, there is not a single cost-benefit ratio in the entire article. The author compares the posttransplant course of patients whose kidneys had been removed to that of patients who had had no pretransplant surgery. The latter group experienced fewer rejections and better survival.

Bentkover, J. and Drew, P. 1981. Cost-Effectiveness/Cost-Benefit of Medical Technologies: A Case Study of Orthopedic Joint Implants. U.S. Congress, Office of Technology Assessment, 1981 (OTA-BP-H-9(10)).

This study examines the feasibility and potential usefulness of undertaking CBA-CEA of orthopedic joint prostheses. Two specific issues are addressed: (1) whether it is feasible to evaluate carefully and completely the orthopedic joint implant technology within a CBA-CEA framework; and (2) whether such an evaluation could be useful in formulating public policy.

The authors present the state of the art of CBA-CEA as it pertains to this technology. They do not try to assess the technology. The study includes a description of the technology (joint implants) and alternative forms of treatment for arthritis. The authors point out an important difference between the alternatives (such as drugs) and joint implants: Most alternatives are only short-term measures, whereas joint implantation is a long-term measure.

Few data are available regarding the efficacy of joint implants. Data regarding the efficacy of hip replacements are better than the data for other joint implants or alternative measures. The authors speculate that hip replacement data may even be acceptable. Efficacy studies are in progress for some implants.

Potential direct benefits discussed include relief of pain, improved functional status of the joint, measures included in the sickness impact profile (such as social interactions, ambulation, sleep, leisure, and emotions), quality-adjusted life-years, and earnings. Potential indirect benefits include averted expenditures for the caring for, and treatment of, individuals handicapped with debilitated joints. The potential benefits are only enumerated; none is quantified or measured.

Most costs mentioned are not distinguished from charges, and avoidable costs are not specifically identified. Some indirect costs, such as loss of productivity when a patient is hospitalized, are identified. The authors point out that both indirect and direct costs of complications associated with joint implants must be included, as well as the costs of follow-up care and rehabilitation therapy. The authors note that all projected benefits and costs should be discounted, but they do not suggest any particular discount rate. They do suggest that variables with uncertain values be subjected to a sensitivity analysis. The authors briefly mention some potential public policy implications of conducting CBA-CEA of orthopedic joint implants, but their study does not contain specific results regarding the cost-effectiveness of implants.

Budetti, P. et al. 1981. Costs and Effectiveness of Neonatal Intensive Care. U.S. Congress, Office of Technology Assessment, 1981 (OTA-BP-H-9(10)).

This paper includes a review of the efficacy and effectiveness literature, as well as the cost and cost-effectiveness literature, on neonatal intensive care services. The authors note the rapid progress made in these services in the last fifteen years, emphasizing the range and sophistication of care that hospitals can now offer. Their study centers on an examination of costs, personnel, technologies, and procedures used and the efficacy and effectiveness of the intensive care services for seriously ill newborns.

Numerous problems are involved in analysis. First, definitions are tenuous. Neonatal services do not fit into the classifications used in many hospitals, and regulatory and reimbursement policies create incentives for hospitals to classify their neonatal units inappropriately. Providers, paying units, and regulators disagree on uniform definitions for levels of care.

The major focus of the study is on efficacy, effectiveness, and costs of neonatal intensive care. Outcomes are defined in terms of improved mortality and morbidity rates and mental and physical development of critically ill newborns. Costs are distinguished from charges. The study addresses the average cost per day of caring for the critically ill newborn and reimbursement policies and procedures.

The authors examine the incidence and severity of prematurity in the United States. They evaluate the social and biological aspects of prematurity, trends in infant mortality, the incidence of underweight infants in the last two decades, and the effect of neonatal intensive care units (NICUs) on mortality and morbidity of premature infants at various birth weights. They examine the use of NICUs through admission rates, estimated average length of stay, estimated total patient days, the number of hospitals with NICUs, and the number of intensive care beds.

The authors examine the costs of neonatal intensive care, warning that their data on use and cost are rough approximations. In general, costs are negatively correlated with low birth weight and prematurity. The average cost per day is $267, and the average stay is thirteen days. The average charge per day is about $395. The study looks at the existing system of reimbursement in five states and by five payers: commercial insurance, Blue Cross, Medicaid, self-pay, and private insurance.

NICUs have been shown to reduce mortality rates, and the authors believe that NICUs are cost-effective. More data are needed to determine their full impact. The authors also review other studies of the cost-effectiveness of neonatal intensive care.

They use a hybrid CBA-CEA developed by Marcia Kramer to measure the marginal costs of providing neonatal intensive care. They also compare methods of care in Great Britain and France with those in the United States.

The authors suggest that federal policies need to be changed to reflect changes that have occurred in neonatal care. In particular, guidelines that establish maximum numbers of beds per live births and minimum sizes of neonatal care units need to be revised; Medicaid and Social Security provisions for reimbursement of neonatal care costs need to be reexamined.

Bunker, J. et al., eds. 1977. *Costs, Risks, and Benefits of Surgery.* New York: Oxford Univ. Press.

This book includes case studies applying CBA-CEA to a variety of surgical procedures, including herniorrhaphy, cholecystectomy, hysterectomy, appendectomy, kidney transplantation, and coronary artery bypass. Several papers in the book discuss the application of CBA-CEA to surgery generally. The cases serve two functions: They provide guidance to both individual medical practitioners and health policymakers regarding specific issues of surgical treatment, and they illustrate the application and potential usefulness of several quantitative analytical techniques, including decision analysis, conditional probability, and CBA-CEA.

The book is structured to introduce the reader to these techniques and to the process of surgical innovation. Surgical cases are included in order to bring together method and substance.

Centerwall, B. and Criqui, M. 1978. Prevention of the Wernicke-Korsakoff Syndrome: A Cost-Benefit Analysis. *New Engl. J. Med.* 299:285.

The authors examine the costs and benefits of fortifying alcoholic beverages with thiamine in order to prevent Wernicke-Korsakoff syndrome, a serious thiamine-deficiency disorder found in alcoholics. The authors compare the cost of fortification—estimated between $3 million and $17 million per year—with the benefit—avoidance of the cost ($70 million per year) of long-term institutionalization for victims of the syndrome. The authors conclude that the benefits exceed the costs by a factor of from four to twenty-three.

The authors address several potential problems of fortification, but they find none that should hinder the effort. For example, thiamine is nontoxic (though there could be a possibility of generating toxic substances when it is combined in significant amounts with alcohol); in moderate amounts it does not seem to affect taste; and it is adequately soluble in alcoholic solutions. The authors find that their analysis strongly recommends a national program of thiamine fortification of alcoholic beverages.

An interesting feature of this study is that it could be viewed as a CEA, instead of a CBA, in which net cost is compared with a nonmonetary outcome such as number of cases of Wernicke-Korsakoff syndrome prevented. The costs of caring for victims of this disorder so greatly exceed the costs of preventing the disease that the net cost is negative—that is, the program produces positive net economic benefits at the same time that it serves a noneconomic health objective.

Cretin, S. 1977. Cost-Benefit Analysis of Treatment and Prevention of Myocardial Infarction. *Health Serv. Res.* 12:174.

This article, technically a CEA, compares the effects of three alternative methods for the treatment or prevention of myocardial infarction: (1) a coronary care unit, (2) a mobile coronary care unit, and (3) an intervention-prevention program aimed at reducing concentrations of cholesterol in the blood. Effects are measured in terms of the number of years of life added as a result of each alternative program. Costs are classified as direct and indirect. Costs and effects of each strategy are modeled on the basis of a cohort of ten-year-olds followed throughout their lives. In addition, the manner of implementation is varied. Costs and effects are calculated for each alternative method assuming (1) the method is newly introduced alone, and (2) it is newly introduced with the other alternatives already being used. "Cost-benefit" ratios are calculated as the dollar cost per added year of life for each alternative introduced alone. The author illustrates changes in the ratios that result from varying the discount rate (that is, she performs sensitivity analysis) from zero to 5 to 10 percent. She also discusses problems of selecting a discount rate for comparing alternative programs that incur costs and accrue benefits at widely separated times. The author finds the results of her analysis inconclusive. She notes that this and other modeling processes involve many simplifying assumptions and require that parameter values be estimated even when supporting data are scant.

Deane, R. and Ulene, A. 1977. Hysterectomy or Tubal Ligation for Sterilization: A Cost-Effectiveness Analysis. *Inquiry* 14:73.

The authors develop a ten-equation model of the costs and health consequences of two surgical sterilization procedures. The model considers both direct health effects and costs, including complications, and later indirect effects and costs (for example, cervical cancers developing in women who have had tubal ligations). The backbone of the model is a series of probability trees tracing the possible outcomes.
    The authors analyze the choice from both a societal and an individual point of view, using the human capital approach for the former and, for the latter, leaving determination of the dollar value of mortality to the individual patient.
    The analysis suggests that, for a discount rate of 5 to 15 percent, tubal ligation is preferred to hysterectomy for women of all ages, from both the societal and individual perspectives. The authors note that certain unmeasured costs of hysterectomy, such as its negative impact on marriages, would tend to support the finding. They estimate that the cost savings associated with tubal ligation would range from $200 to $400. As a result of their analysis, the authors suggest that patients, physicians, and society should prefer tubal ligations except in unusual cases (for example, patients with a family history of cervical or endometrial cancer, or a personal history of menstrual disorders).

Doherty, N. and Hicks, B. 1977. Cost-Effectiveness Analysis and Alternative Health Care Programs for the Elderly. *Health Serv. Res.* 12:190.

The authors discuss the methodology of CEA in general, contrast it with CBA, and illustrate it with an example involving alternative programs of health care for the elderly. They discuss the problems of measuring costs by market prices, which may "obscure the real opportunity costs of resource consumption." The authors note that many criteria of effectiveness can be specified only in terms of ordinal numbers denoting rank, and they warn against the temptation "to add the nonadditive and to compare the incomparable." In an analysis presented as an example, costs are classified as primary, secondary, and tertiary, denoting program costs, other health-related service costs, and personal living expenditures, respectively. The authors explain and illustrate the tabular display approach to presenting data, in which effectiveness criteria are presented in columns and alternative programs are presented as row headings. It is unlikely, the authors conclude, that one alternative will emerge as preferred on the basis of all relevant criteria. In their example, day care is preferred on the basis of effectiveness criteria, while home care is preferred on the basis of cost criteria.

Eddy, D. 1978. Rationale for the Cancer Screening Benefits Program Screening Policies: Implementation Plan, Part III. Paper read at the National Cancer Institute, Blue Cross Association, Chicago, Illinois.

This report describes the methods used to analyze the cost-effectiveness of alternative cancer screening policy options and the rationale for a recommended insurance benefits program. Five cancer sites—breast, colon, cervix, lung, and bladder—are selected for full analysis. The model translates screening-program effectiveness, and many variables that contribute to it, into quantitative terms and logical relationships. Probability formulas relating to the important variables are derived. The model, designed to be programmed on a computer, traces the expected fate of a patient under various program options. It will accept information about patient characteristics (age, relative risk, previous history, incidence rates, and so on) and will program options and present information on the costs and effectiveness of a specified program. Different discount rates can be used.

The author notes that creating a cancer screening program that is both medically effective and low in cost requires that many age, sex, and risk categories be used to define the optimal services and screening frequencies for various groups of individuals. Ideally, a program might include several screening protocols, each tailored to different categories. This is not possible, however, for a prepaid benefit program that will be purchased by a large, heterogeneous population. Thus, one objective is to design a benefit program in which services do not vary greatly. Marginal effectiveness, rather than absolute effectiveness, is considered the effectiveness criterion; on this basis, there is little difference in the cost-effective program between high-risk and average-risk groups. The benefit program designed includes the following provisions: (1) a standard screening program every four years for persons age twenty-five to forty-five; (2) a standard screening program every year for those over age forty-five; (3) an impregnated guaiac slide every year, beginning at age forty-five; (4) a Pap smear for women every four years, beginning at age twenty-five; (5) mammography for women covered by the high-option benefit every two years, beginning at age fifty; and (6) a proctosigmoidoscopy every five years, beginning at age fifty.

Eddy, D. 1980*b*. *Screening for Cancer: Theory, Analysis, and Design.* Englewood Cliffs, N.J.: Prentice-Hall.

The author presents the logic and mathematics that underlie work he did to assist the Blue Cross Association and the American Cancer Society in formulating their cancer screening policies and recommendations (Eddy 1978, 1980*a*). Using the case of breast cancer, the author takes the reader through the various steps involved in understanding the disease and the screening problem, developing the mathematical models needed to assess alternative screening strategies, programming the model on the computer for interactive decision-making, and running the model to assess the alternative strategies.

The author presents simulations illustrating the costs and effectiveness of a woman's following various screening programs. These are followed by extension of the model to the case of cancer of the colon. The book concludes with discussion of the screening recommendations that resulted from the author's work. (The preceding abstract provides additional detail on the modeling and its results.)

Eddy, D. 1981. Screening for Colon Cancer: A Technology Assessment. U.S. Congress, Office of Technology Assessment, 1981 (OTA-BP-H-9(3)).

This study focuses on the techniques that are available to screen for colon cancer—their development, evaluation, use, and cost-effectiveness.

The author examines the three basic techniques used in the detection of colon cancer: the digital exam, the sigmoidoscope, and the test for occult blood in the stool. For each method, the author notes, there is either some degree of uncertainty regarding the sensitivity and specificity of the tests, or some degree of risk to the patient involved.

The study points out that there have been few, if any, clinical studies of the digital exam. Its effectiveness is believed to have been proven through use and acceptable results at the patient-provider level. The effectiveness of sigmoidoscopes has been examined in a few clinical studies. The Hemoccult test has been through, and is going through, a number of large clinical trials to evaluate its efficacy. To date, the results are inconclusive.

The author discusses the problems that exist in trying to apply CEA to screening programs for colon cancer. He also examines a number of factors that affect CEA studies in the health care area in general. One is the need for, but absence of, information from formal, randomized clinical trials regarding the effect and value of screening techniques. The information that is available is usually from uncontrolled studies. Biases such as lead time, patient self-selection, and length of study, also present data problems.

The author discusses the special considerations that colon screening programs present to a CEA. These factors include patient characteristics and differences (in terms of effectiveness of screening programs), schedule (or history) and type of testing procedures used, varying accuracy of the different procedures, origins of the cancer (which require separate analysis), order and frequency of testing, and a host of other variables.

Once, or if, these data and methodological problems are solved, the author feels the central issue can be addressed: What is the value of screening for colon cancer? A screening program for a fifty-year-old average-risk woman is evaluated using eight different combinations and frequencies of screening tests. The relevant factors (costs, screening regimen, efficacy data, outcome information, and so on) are examined, using a sensitivity analysis to determine how the different variables affect the mortality rate and cost of the various screening programs. The result of the analysis is presented as a comparison between the decreasing probabilities of colon cancer's occurring with more frequent testing, improved life expectancy, increases in screening costs, and decreases in lost earnings as a result of the different levels of screening programs.

Fein, R. 1977. But, on the Other Hand: High Blood Pressure, Economics and Equity. *New Engl. J. Med.* 296:751.

This editorial accompanies and reacts to two articles explaining the methodology of CEA (Weinstein and Stason, 1977*b*) and applying it to the case of hypertension management (Stason and Weinstein, 1977). The author emphasizes the limitations of formal CEA; he fears that "[b]ecause the methods of cost-effectiveness analysis are elegant and powerful, they may be accepted without sufficient caution." In the case of health care CEA, this danger is particularly acute when the audience consists of health professionals unschooled in the techniques of CBA-CEA. The author's principal concern is that equity will be submerged in an ocean of quantitative analysis.

The author emphasizes that values underlie the presumably objective mathematics of CEA and that the arithmetic of CEA can imply a false precision. He worries that "a 'climate of opinion' is created: That which is measured is important and vice versa. The caring function is left to the soft-hearted idealists, and all of us are encouraged to become hard-headed realists."

Among the caveats that the author cites are the following: The discount rate may not accurately represent social values, yet in the calculus of CEA it affects valuation of social programs. Quality-adjusted life-years is a sound concept, but can it be made operational in a meaningful manner? And CEA ignores interpersonal utility comparisons, equating programs that have similar quantitative impacts but that affect different populations.

Fineberg, H. and Pearlman, L. 1981. Benefit and Cost Analysis of Medical Interventions: The Case of Cimetidine and Peptic Ulcer Disease. U.S. Congress, Office of Technology Assessment, 1981 (OTA-BP-H-9(11)).

The study has two major goals: One is to assess the available evidence regarding the benefits and costs of cimetidine in the treatment of peptic ulcer disease; the other is to develop a widely applicable cost-benefit model for evaluation of medical technology. The study combines these two objectives by applying the model to the evaluation of cimetidine and ulcer disease. The authors approach the analysis in three parts: (1) a development and discussion of a cost-benefit model that they feel can be applied to medical interventions in general; (2) an overview of peptic ulcer disease in the United States; and (3) a discussion of the development, diffusion, and use of cimetidine to treat, or manage, or both, peptic ulcer disease.

The foundation of their cost-benefit model is as follows: There are two principal classes of effects—clinical effects and health system effects—and the specific components of these effects depend on the population and intervention being examined. An evaluative model must apply to an identifiable patient population and specific health care interventions. A patient population may be defined in terms of a diagnostic category, clinical signs or symptoms, risk factors, or complications of disease. And clinical and health system effects interact to lead to an outcome (health status, resource costs, or both).

The authors examine studies dealing with the safety, efficacy, and effectiveness of cimetidine. Among the short-term clinical effects they assess are healing, pain relief, safety and adherence to the treatment plan, complications, recurrence, and recommendations for treating newly diagnosed, uncomplicated ulcers. The long-term clinical effects they examine are recurrence, safety, and complications.

The authors also examine the health system and outcome effects of cimetidine use. Among the variables evaluated are medication, diagnostic tests, physician visits, mortality, morbidity, and resource costs. Three areas—clinical effects, health system effects, and outcomes of cimetidine use—are the primary elements of the CBA they perform.

The authors discuss the following findings: Cimetidine promotes healing and provides faster and more complete pain relief for duodenal ulcers; it may be more effective than placebos for patients with gastric ulcers; when used for up to 2 months, cimetidine appears to be a relatively safe drug; most known side effects are minor or reversible; cimetidine plus moderate amounts of antacid cost no more than a therapeutically equivalent course of intense antacid therapy; and maintenance treatment with cimetidine for as long as a year significantly reduces the chance of ulcer recurrence (compared to a placebo) during the period of treatment. Cimetidine, according to a few studies, also appears to have contributed to a sharp decline in surgery for ulcer disease in 1978, as well as to have helped patients to lose significantly fewer days of work than patients given a placebo.

These findings and conclusions indicate that cimetidine provides a substantial benefit-cost ratio to the peptic ulcer patient and the health care system.

Geiser, E. and Menz, F. 1976. The Effectiveness of Public Dental Care Programs. *Med. Care* 14:189.

This CBA examines the costs and benefits of a public dental care program designed to maintain the integrity of the natural teeth in school-age children. Benefits are calculated by estimating the number of teeth saved in fifteen-year-olds as a result of the program, and then multiplying it by the cost of replacing a natural tooth with an artificial bridge. The current costs of saving a permanent tooth are used as a cost measure. Data from two actual public dental care programs are examined. The authors conclude that public dental care programs must be administered over a relatively long time (six to seven years) before net benefits begin to accrue on an annual basis. An even longer time (eleven to fourteen years) is required before the programs generate sufficient total benefits to cover total costs. The discounted present values of the program, using an 8 percent discount rate, were found to be particularly sensitive to changes in the cost of the care and the value of saving a tooth. Extensive sensitivity analysis is performed on the variables involved, making this article an excellent illustration of the use of sensitivity analysis in handling uncertainty.

Grosse, R. 1972b. Cost-Benefit Analysis of Health Services. *Ann. Amer. Acad. Polit. Soc. Sci.* 399:89.

This article presents an explanation of the rationale behind the use of CBA and CEA in the allocation of health resources and describes an application by HEW. Costs are described as foregone benefits: "The cost of saving a human life is not to be measured in dollars, but rather in terms of alternative lives to be saved or other social values sacrificed." The problem of incommensurability of benefits is discussed. HEW calculations of the cost per death averted and of productivity and medical treatment savings in various cancer control programs are presented and compared to other health programs (such as motor vehicle safety and arthritis). The article illustrates the changes in program priority that can occur when the criterion is changed from deaths averted to savings from avoided medical treatment and loss of productivity (measured as discounted lifetime earnings). The problem of uncertainty is discussed, and a matrix composed of relative payoffs and the probability of results is presented as one method of handling it. The final section of the article describes in detail the HEW maternal child health program analysis.

Hagard, S. and Carter, F. 1976a. Preventing the Birth of Infants With Down's Syndrome: A Cost-Benefit Analysis. *Brit. Med. J.* 1:753.

The costs and benefits of providing routine prenatal diagnosis, with termination of affected pregnancies, are examined. In the event of termination, two situations are considered: (1) Termination is followed by another pregnancy, assumed to be normal (replacement); and (2) termination is not followed by another pregnancy (no replacement). Since such prenatal testing could diagnose fetal myelocele, the costs and benefits involved in preventing this disease are also taken into consideration. For Down's syndrome between 1975 and 1994, the following numbers are estimated: (1) the number of births by five-year maternal age groups, (2) survival rates and the degree of handicap of survivors, (3) costs to society of caring for survivors, (4) characteristics, including the number of affected births prevented, of a prenatal diagnostic program, and (5) the costs of such a program. The benefit of preventing the birth of infants with Down's syndrome is calculated as the cost to the community of their care. In the case of replacement, this is the difference between the cost of caring for a handicapped person and the cost of caring for a normal person. In the case of no replacement, this is the cost of caring for a handicapped person. Results of the study indicate that the benefit-cost ratio of prenatal diagnosis is greater than 1 for women over forty years old, equal to 1 for women between thirty-five and forty, and less than 1 for women under thirty-five. The problems associated with different results for different age groups are discussed. A discount rate of 10 percent is used. The authors examine the changes in the results of the analysis that would occur if, after genetic counseling, only half of the women accepted amniocentesis and possible termination of pregnancy.

Hannan, E. and Graham, J. 1978. A Cost-Benefit Study of a Hypertension Screening and Treatment Program at the Work Setting. *Inquiry* 15:345.

This article explains the nature and application of a computer model designed to estimate the costs and benefits of hypertension screening and treatment programs in a variety of work settings. The purpose of the model is to assist specific businesses and other organizations in deciding whether they should establish such a program. Costs are defined as incremental costs for the personnel, supplies, equipment, and facilities needed to implement a detection and treatment program. Benefits include (1) savings resulting from decreases in hospitalization and physician fees for hypertension-related illnesses; (2) savings produced by decreases in hypertension-related disability or absenteeism; and (3) savings owing to decreases in hypertension-related mortality. Due to the complexity of assigning a meaningful value to the third category, the authors chose to predict only lives saved, leaving it to employers to value these implicitly.

The authors describe the steps required to assess costs and benefits for a specific company. Then they present the results of hypothetical runs of the computer model for eight types of companies, ranging in size from 400 to 51,000 employees. The runs suggest that indirect benefits (savings in absentee costs) roughly equal total costs, while direct benefits (savings in medical costs) equal only a little more than a quarter of costs. Together, direct and indirect benefits exceed total costs for all eight of the hypothetical companies. As noted above, however, the costs or benefits associated with the saving of lives are not included in the calculations.

The authors provide some sensitivity analysis, for example illustrating that the finding of positive net benefit is quite sensitive to the amount by which absenteeism is reduced. The effects of varying other variables are also discussed.

Harris, G. 1977. Introduction to Cost-Benefit Analysis Applied to New Health Technologies. Prepared by Arthur D. Little, Inc. Hyattsville, Md.: Health Resources Administration, Bureau of Health Planning and Resources Development.

This document describes the steps in CBA as the following: (1) articulation of the problem, (2) enumeration of alternatives to address the problem, (3) identification of their achievable effects, (4) measurement and valuation of the achievable effects, and (5) application of the economic decision criteria. Objectives are described as cost reduction, enhancing of benefits, or both. Costs and benefits are classified as direct, indirect, or intangible. The need to focus on incremental, rather than total, costs and benefits is explained. Discounting to present value and the problem of choosing a discount rate are discussed. Five criteria of preferredness are described: net present benefit, internal rate-of-return, benefit-cost ratio, payback period, and average rate of return. The advantages, disadvantages, and appropriate use of each criterion are presented. Threshold analysis, sensitivity analysis, and probability-risk analysis are described as methods of dealing with uncertainty. Common problems encountered in analysis, such as incomplete data, transitional costs, scope, and externalities, and the issue of equity and distribution are discussed.

Klarman, H. 1974a. Application of Cost-Benefit Analysis to the Health Services and the Special Case of Technologic Innovation. *Int. J. Health Serv.* 4:325.

In this methodology and review article, the author discusses the purposes and techniques of CBA-CEA, examines published health care CBA-CEAs, and considers the potential and limitations of using the techniques to assess health systems technology. The author illustrates the latter by use of two examples.

In his review of the literature, the author observes that relatively few complete health care CBA-CEAs have been carried out. He notes that many of the most prominent contributions to the field have themselves been incomplete as CBA-CEAs. Several important early studies assessed the costs of specific illnesses—and therefore the benefits of eradicating the illness—but none of these directly addressed the issue of how much specific programs could combat the respective diseases and their costs.

The paper concludes with a thoughtful treatment of the implications of trying to apply CBA-CEA to health systems technology. The author draws on a well-studied technology, automated multiphasic screening, and the case of services in hospitals.

Klarman, H. et al. 1968. Cost-Effectiveness Analysis Applied to the Treatment of Chronic Renal Disease. *Med. Care* 6:48.

The authors attempt to determine the best mix of center dialysis, home dialysis, and kidney transplantation in examining the costs and effects of treating chronic renal disease. A quality-of-life adjustment is made to account for the differences in lifestyle between patients on dialysis and those with effective transplants. (The freedom associated with the latter is valued at one-quarter of a year of life.) The calculations in the analysis are based on survivorship tables for transplant and dialysis cohorts of 1,000 persons each. The authors warn that, at the time of the analysis, there had not been enough experience with any of the three treatment modes to generate a life-expectancy table with great accuracy. The discount rate used is net of an anticipated inflation rate, resulting in a discount rate of 4 percent for transplant and center dialysis and 5 percent for home dialysis. The authors conclude that kidney transplantation is more cost-effective than the other two alternatives. Choice of the preferred treatment modality is independent of the quality-of-life adjustment because transplantation dominates even without the adjustment. No sensitivity analysis is presented for the discount rate, the anticipated inflation rate, or life expectancy.

Koplan, J. et al. 1979. Pertussis Vaccine—An Analysis of Benefits, Risks and Costs. *New Engl. J. Med.* 301:906.

The authors of this study use clinical and epidemiological data, combined with several analytical techniques (decision analysis, benefit-risk analysis, CBA, and sensitivity analysis), to compare the benefits, risks, and costs of routine childhood immunization against pertussis. They identify and quantify the principal relevant variables, assess their relative importance, determine for which of the variables better epidemiological data are needed, and perform the analyses comparing benefits, risks, and costs.

The paper presents a good example of how decision trees can be used to clarify the nature of a health care problem. The analysis leads to the following conclusions: (1) Without an immunization program, there would be a 71-fold increase in cases of the disease and almost a fourfold increase in deaths (2.0 to 7.6) per cohort of 1 million children. A vaccination program would lead to 0.1 case of encephalitis associated with pertussis and 5 cases of postvaccination encephalitis; without a program there would be only 2.3 cases of pertussis-associated encephalitis. Community vaccination would cost $721,000, compared with social costs of $1.866 million without a program; thus the program would reduce the costs associated with pertussis by 61 percent.

The authors conclude that community vaccination is desirable at all levels. They caution, however, that, in the worst possible situation, assuming the highest estimates of reaction rates, results are less clear-cut.

Korenbrot, C. et al. 1981. Elective Hysterectomy: Costs, Risks, and Benefits. U.S. Congress, Office of Technology Assessment, 1981 (OTA-BP-H-9(15)).

This study examines elective hysterectomy as it is used for sterilization and cancer prevention. The focus of the study is a review of the literature and the issues surrounding the costs, risks, and benefits of elective hysterectomy. The study does not attempt to establish the cost-effectiveness of hysterectomy. The authors examine the significant side effects of hysterectomy, such as change in medical utilization and psychological effects following surgery.

The authors review selected studies that evaluate the efficiency and cost-effectiveness of elective hysterectomies. Two studies contrast the direct costs of hysterectomy with the net lifetime costs of gynecological care. Future costs are discounted at rates varying from 3 to 6.5 percent. Another study examines the use of hysterectomy as a sterilization device versus the direct costs of tubal ligation plus the expense of future gynecological care that would have been averted by hysterectomy.

The effectiveness of hysterectomies in preventing pregnancy and cancer is not an issue, but the health risks of the procedure are. Efficacy and effectiveness of alternative means of accomplishing these objectives are assessed, but not in the cost-effectiveness studies reviewed. The cost-effectiveness studies reviewed do not attempt to identify, measure, or place a value on the side effects of surgery.

Costs are distinguished from charges, and issues of equity are discussed. Conclusions are drawn with respect to the cost-effectiveness of elective hysterectomies as they are used for the separate purposes that are examined.

Leroy, L. and Solkowitz, S. 1981. Costs and Effectiveness of Nurse Practitioners. U.S. Congress, Office of Technology Assessment, 1981 (OTA-BP-H-9 (16)).

This study reviews the literature on the cost-effectiveness of nurse practitioners who provide primary medical care services. Only limited data are available, and much of the information deals with other types of physician-extenders.

The authors note that nurse practitioners offer the potential for reducing the costs of health care and improving access to the health care system. Nurse practitioners can perform basic and routine medical care tasks, allowing physicians to focus their efforts on serious problems. Training costs and pay are less for nurse practitioners than for physicians, so costs should be lower for routine care if nurse practitioners are used. There are a number of problems associated with directly extrapolating to lower costs, however, and, depending on the system within which nurse practitioners operate, cost savings may or may not be realized.

A key question examined by this study deals with the nature of the services nurse practitioners perform and how they affect costs. In general, they provide both complementary and substitute services, although the nature of these services is difficult to document because data often indicate only "office visit."

Based on their literature review, the authors conclude that nurse practitioners appear to provide care that is of as high quality as that of physicians. There is some evidence that nurse practitioners, working in close conjunction with physicians, provide superior care when compared to solo practitioners. Productivity is more difficult to assess and depends on how nurse practitioners are used. There seems to be clear evidence that the use of nurse practitioners improves physicians' productivity, but it is not clear how this improved productivity affects costs. Supervisory time, duplicative work, and the fact that nurse practitioners spend more time per patient significantly affect the cost-effectiveness calculations.

The data needed to conduct a CEA of nurse practitioners include employment costs, training costs, and medical care costs. Unfortunately, each of these factors may be subject to changes as a result of alterations in another part of the system. The employment costs of nurse practitioners, for example, are a function (in part) of the demand for their services. Even more difficult to determine is price. Because they are most often hired by physicians or health institutions that have already established fee systems, any cost savings may be absorbed by the physicians or institutions and may not be reflected in the price of services delivered.

The paper cautions against the use of current data to determine new policy. Based on changes in the way nurse practitioners are used, costs could vary widely. This is a case in which a CEA may provide misleading policy advice, although the identification of variables required by the CEA may be very helpful.

LeSourd, D. et al. 1968. *Benefit-Cost Analysis of Kidney Disease Programs.* PHS Publication no. 1941. Washington, D.C.: Government Printing Office.

This analysis is one of a series of federally sponsored efforts to assess the costs and benefits of alternative approaches to the problem of kidney disease. The approaches include screening, prevention, and three treatment modalities (home dialysis, center dialysis, and transplantation). Employing a variety of assumptions (for example, risk population for the screening programs, size of treatment facilities), the authors conclude that early detection dramatically dominates the treatment approaches with respect to economic benefits and costs. Depending on the population screened, the former has benefit-cost ratios of 30:1 and greater. By contrast, the treatment alternatives produce benefit-cost ratios in the vicinity of 1:1. This ratio varies according to: the treatment method (transplantation producing the highest ratios); the scale of operation; the allocation of research costs; and high, low, and best-cost estimates in the two instances of dialysis. To estimate indirect benefits (that is, productivity losses avoided), the authors assume that 70 percent of the dialysis patients would be capable of resuming a normal earning capacity; the remaining 30 percent are assigned half the expected income of a comparable, but healthy, individual.

The qualitative findings of this analysis are supported by other studies undertaken at the same time.

Lubeck, D. and Bunker, J. 1981. The Artificial Heart: Costs, Risks, and Benefits. U.S. Congress, Office of Technology Assessment, 1981 (OTA-BP-H-9 (9)).

This study examines the many factors that have played a role in the development of the artificial heart: factors that are affected by, and in turn affect, three areas of public policy—R&D, reimbursement, and regulation.

The authors provide a backdrop of the history of the artificial heart development program. They also examine the safety and efficacy determinations arrived at through experiments and clinical trials. Current and potential technological developments in the artificial heart are described, and the numerous R&D needs that must be met before an artificial heart can be successfully used are explored.

The authors examine the economic aspects of the artificial heart from the patient's perspective and from a societal view, focusing on the costs of diagnosis, implantation, and postoperative care. These costs are compared to the costs associated with related procedures: cardiac pacemakers, aortocoronary bypass surgery, and heart transplants. The renal dialysis program is used to illustrate the possibility of the federal government's financing artificial heart procedures.

The authors also examine four areas of social cost: increased social expenditures, potential distributional inequities, effects of nuclear radiation if a nuclear energy source is used, and opportunity costs. They also examine the efficacy, potential benefits and costs, and likelihood of saving lives by cardiac disease prevention programs.

Quality of life is addressed for both the short- and long-term effects. The authors draw on the experiences of those who have had heart and kidney transplants to illustrate the types of impacts on the patient and the family that can occur. The potential effects include personal, marital, family, physical, medical, and psychological problems that can occur after a person undergoes major surgery.

On the benefits side, although the authors briefly discuss the technological spinoffs of the artificial heart program, their primary focus is on two areas: the potential for patients to return to an active life and the estimated years of life that may be gained. Morbidity, mortality, and added years of life are examined and estimated by a best case and worst case analysis if the artificial heart is implanted.

Luce, B. 1981. Allocating Costs and Benefits in Disease Prevention Programs: An Application to Cervical Cancer Screening. U.S. Congress, Office of Technology Assessment, 1981 (OTA-BP-H-9(7)).

This paper offers a CEA of cervical cancer screening for a given risk group from different perspectives. Screening for cervical cancer is used to demonstrate the cost-effectiveness of disease prevention programs. The disease process is modeled using a

Markov Chain technique to "age" a simulated population of thirty- to thirty-nine-year-old women for ten years (using disease transition probabilities reported in the literature). The cost-effectiveness of screening is then calculated at different intervals, ranging from annual screening to no screening for the ten-year period. The effects are evaluated for: different migration patterns, different risk groups, different modes of administering Pap tests, and joint production considerations. The author also tests the sensitivity of the results to various discount rates and to the range of error rates for Pap tests.

The results indicate that a private party always has a financial incentive to postpone screening, whereas society finds it more cost-effective to screen, but only at infrequent intervals. In addition, the cost-effectiveness of screening is markedly affected when a more efficient (less costly) delivery mode is simulated. Screening is significantly affected when joint production effects are considered. The cost-effectiveness of screening, however, is not very sensitive to small changes in the discount rate, initially set at 10 percent, nor to varying assumptions regarding error rates.

The author concludes that, if society wants the private sector to screen for cervical cancer at a socially determined optimal rate, then society must be willing to subsidize the cost of the program. The study also concludes that the cost-effectiveness of cervical cancer screening is much more affected by the cost assigned to screening than by different assumptions of the precise error and discount rates.

The cost-effectiveness of screening at each simulated interval is compared to no screening for a ten-year period. Efficacy information is addressed and different test error rates are used. The production of the Pap test is simulated, for cost purposes, at two levels: an expensive university hospital clinic using specialists, and an inexpensive health clinic using licensed nurses. Only lives and years of life saved are identified as benefits.

Costs are distinguished from charges, marginal costs are considered, and indirect costs are used.

Luft, H. 1976. Benefit-Cost Analysis and Public Policy Implementation: From Normative to Positive Analysis. *Pub. Pol.* 24:437.

The author argues that conventional CBA and CEA should be extended to include a predictive analysis of the implementation phase in order to determine whether and how a project will be done. The predictive analysis involves three steps: (1) a standard CBA to determine whether the project should be undertaken; (2) a CBA from the perspective of each decision-maker or interest group capable of influencing the success of the project, to determine the likelihood that the project will be undertaken; (3) a redesign of the project or the development of incentives to improve the likelihood of success for socially desirable projects.

In a case study of a surgicenter, it is noted that the resultant shifting of revenue from one set of providers to another, though only a pecuniary externality in standard cost-benefit analysis, has a substantial impact on the likelihood that a surgicenter will actually be implemented. The importance of identifying decision-makers and their respective power to influence the success of the project is discussed. The author points out that, in the second step of the analysis (the interest-group analysis), transfer payments, taxes, and pecuniary externalities should be explicitly considered so that the financial flows as perceived by the relevant interest groups are adequately represented. In addition, it may be appropriate to use substantially different discount rates for each interest group. The final step in the interest-group analysis is to estimate each group's utility function and its relative power to either promote or block implementation of the project.

Luft presents an application of predictive analysis to the use of a work evaluation unit for ascertaining functional work capacity following a myocardial infarction. The relevant interest groups in this analysis include the patient, family, physician, employer, insurer, and society. Luft estimates both the likely net effects on each interest group of using the work evaluation unit and each group's relative weight. The author concludes that this extended, positive form of cost-benefit analysis can improve the allocation of resources by helping to promote the implementation of desirable and feasible programs and "to prevent the adoption and implementation of proposals that appear promising in theory but are likely to be sabotaged in practice."

McNeil, B. 1979. Pitfalls in and Requirements for Evaluations of Diagnostic Technologies. DHEW Publication no. (PHS) 79-3254. Washington, D.C.: Government Printing Office.

Focusing on new diagnostic radiographic procedures, the author examines the basic but difficult issues that must be considered in evaluating diagnostic technologies. While one may generalize from the discussion, it is built around an early study comparing computerized tomography with radionuclide studies of patients suspected of having intracranial disease. The author raises and addresses each of the following questions: What data should be collected? What are the prerequisites for data collection involving imaging? By what criteria should evaluation be guided (improved diagnostic information; relevance for therapy planning; changes in short- and long-term health outcomes; impact on costs)? How should an evaluation of a diagnostic technology be conducted? What do diagnostic evaluations cost? Who should support them?

The author points out that the difficulties in evaluating therapeutic technologies are magnified in the case of diagnostic technologies, since the link between diagnosis and health outcome is exceedingly difficult to assess. She argues against the view that long-term patient health outcome is the only legitimate criterion for evaluating new technologies.

McNeil, B. et al. 1975a. Measures of Clinical Efficacy: Cost-Effectiveness Calculations in the Diagnosis and Treatment of Hypertensive Renovascular Disease. *New Engl. J. Med.* 293:216.

The authors measure the value, in terms of sensitivity and specificity, of intravenous pyelography and radiohippuran renography as diagnostic screening methods for hypertension caused by renovascular disease. Costs associated with both diagnosis and subsequent surgical treatment are also calculated. Financial costs of the diagnostic procedures are based on the Massachusetts relative value scale; hospital and operation costs are based on 1974 charges at Peter Bent Brigham

Hospital. Three aspects of cost-effectiveness in the management of renovascular hypertension are examined: (1) the financial costs of case-finding in relation to the sensitivity and specificity of both diagnostic procedures; (2) the total dollar cost of screening the American hypertensive population, making a definitive diagnosis, and performing corrective operations; and (3) the life and dollar cost of each surgical cure. The cost of case-finding is found to be approximately $2,000 per positive diagnosis when only one diagnostic examination is used for screening. This figure rises to $2,600 to $4,400 when both procedures are employed. The total costs of screening all patients with hypertension, performing arteriography on those with positive tests, and operating on all patients with renovascular disease amounts to $10 billion to $13 billion. The authors note that this estimate does not include the costs of initial identification of all hypertensive Americans. Thus, the authors estimate a cost of $15,000 to $20,000 per cure, and note that there are 15 deaths for every 100 surgical cures. The cost-effectiveness calculations are not sensitive to varying the assumptions regarding the prevalence of renovascular disease in hypertension patients from 10 to 5 percent.

Mushkin, S. 1979. *Biomedical Research: Costs and Benefits.* Cambridge, Mass.: Ballinger.

This book presents a comprehensive examination of the costs of illness in the United States for the period 1900-1975. The purpose of the book is to assess the impact of biomedical research on reducing morbidity and mortality, and thereby to compare the costs of research with its benefits. Indirect benefits are calculated using the human capital approach, valuing years of life saved and sickness avoided by their productive worth, measured by earnings.

The author provides an in-depth analysis of specific costs of illness and of the varied health impacts of biomedical advances, some of which are found to have saved costs while others apparently have increased costs. Overall, the author estimates that advances in biomedical science have kept national health expenditures below the level that would have been obtained without the advances.

In addition to the traditional measures of the cost of illness, the author strives to measure the costs of debility, the costs of pain, and the nonhealth-sector costs of illness. This difficult task is one that analysts generally have acknowledged as needed, but that few have attempted.

Neuhauser, D. 1977c. Elective Inguinal Herniorrhaphy versus Truss in the Elderly. In *Costs, Risks, and Benefits of Surgery,* ed. J. Bunker et al. New York: Oxford Univ. Press.

This CEA reviews available data in order to see what effect the choice of elective herniorrhaphy versus truss has on the life expectancy of a sixty-five-year-old person. The analysis includes a calculation of the average effects of having an immediate elective herniorrhaphy (with its low mortality, but the risk that the hernia will recur and require additional elective operations) or using a truss (with its attendant risk of obstruction, followed by an emergency operation with a high mortality rate). Using data obtained from the relevant literature, the author estimates: the mortality rates associated with elective and emergency surgery, the probability of recurrence of the hernia after an operation, the yearly probability of strangulation, and the life expectancy of the patient. Two sets of numbers are used in the analysis. The first set serves as a conservative test of the hypothesis that the truss prolongs life, because the values in this set are those that systematically place the benefit of the doubt in a direction favorable to the elective operation. The numbers in the second set are based on what seem to be the most reasonable and reliable data. (The author notes that there are insufficient data to consider a do-nothing alternative.)

The model takes the form of a decision tree, which is designed so that the payoffs equal the expected value of the average number of years of life lost. The results of the conservative test (used because it makes the strongest case for the elective operation, which is the standard of surgical practice uniformly proposed by current surgical literature) indicate that the elective operation has a higher loss of life associated with it for the sixty-five-year-old than does the truss. The test using the most reasonable estimates indicates that the elective operation has a mortality rate 5.5 times greater than the truss. This large relative difference, however, translates into an absolute difference of only 14.29 days. The author notes that, in view of this small absolute difference in mortality, the issue of quality of life becomes important. The article continues with a discussion of this type of adjustment, but no quality-of-life adjustments on the analysis data are attempted. The magnitude of the costs involved in the elective operation is noted, but a detailed analysis is not presented. On the basis of this study, the author observes that Medicare funds expended on elective herniorrhaphy serve, if anything, not to increase life expectancy, but rather to improve the quality of life. He asks, therefore, if these funds might better serve to improve the quality of life for the elderly in some other way (such as in reducing subway fares).

Neuhauser, D. and Lewicki, A. 1975. What Do We Gain From the Sixth Stool Guaiac? *New Engl. J. Med.* 293:226.

This article examines the costs and effects of the sixth sequential stool guaiac for screening asymptomatic colonic cancer. An analysis of the expenditures concludes that costs rise exponentially; the marginal cost of the sixth test may be 20,000 times the average cost. In addition, data indicate that there is little gain in the true positive rate from testing beyond the second guaiac examination. Thus, the cost per true positive becomes gigantic. The marginal cost is decreased with lower test sensitivity and increased with lower prevalence of colonic cancer. The authors conclude that defining a high-risk group, which would serve to lower marginal cost, is essential to justify such screening programs in a world of constrained resources.

Neutra, R. 1977. Indications for the Surgical Treatment of Suspected Acute Appendicitis: A Cost-Effectiveness Approach. In *Costs, Risks, and Benefits of Surgery*, ed. J. Bunker et al. New York: Oxford Univ. Press.

This article presents a quantitative approach to the costs and benefits associated with the interventionist and noninterventionist management of suspected appendicitis. The assessment considers lives, postoperative disability, and economic costs.

Since the author relied on the rather scanty data from the available literature and on many simplifying assumptions, however, he cautions that the analysis should not be viewed as definitive. The analysis addresses the question of when to operate, not alternative strategies such as a dietary prevention program or antibiotic therapy.

On the basis of two symptoms (location and severity of pain) and two signs (presence of right lower quadrant rebound tenderness and rectal tenderness), an appendicitis risk score is developed. Twenty-four symptom combinations are developed and the probability of appendicitis for each combination determined and ranked.

For example, the highest rank corresponds to the combination of right lower quadrant, severe pain with rebound, and rectal tenderness. Assumptions are presented regarding the distribution of cases and noncases of appendicitis along the risk scale, the prevalence of cases and noncases, and the net costs of the false negatives and false positives in terms of mortality, convalescence, and direct hospital costs. Two analyses are performed, one assuming that 100 percent of the appendicitis patients on whom surgery is not performed will perforate, the other assuming that 30 percent will perforate. The results indicate that a surgeon can ensure an acceptable mortality rate by taking an interventionist approach, but only at the cost of increasing convalescent days and hospital costs. Relaxing the indications for surgery to include patients who lack the most obvious symptoms saves lives, but at a diminishing rate. The few lives saved by operating on patients with minimal symptoms are purchased at great cost in convalescence and dollars associated with the removal of a large number of normal appendixes. The author suggests a solution to this dilemma—namely, increasing discrimination by using very complete diagnostic information and careful clinical interpretations. Increased discrimination can reduce the removal rate of normal appendixes without an increase (and possibly with a decrease) in the rate of perforation. The author estimates the possible savings in lives, convalescence, and money that may result from an increase in discrimination.

Pauker, S. and Kassirer, J. 1975. Therapeutic Decision-Making: A Cost-Benefit Analysis, *New Engl. J. Med.* 293:229.

A mathematical relationship is derived between the benefits and costs of a treatment of a given disease and the threshold of clinical suspicion of the disease. When the probability of a patient's illness exceeds this threshold, the better choice is to administer treatment; when the probability is below the threshold, the better choice is to withhold treatment. The benefit equals the net benefit of appropriate treatment and is calculated as the difference between the utility of administering treatment and the utility of withholding treatment from patients who could benefit from it. The cost is the net cost of unnecessary therapy and is calculated as the difference between the utility of avoiding treatment and the utility of administering treatment to those who do not have the disease. Using probabilities, the authors develop equations expressing the expected values of treatment and no treatment. The point of indifference is where the expected value of treatment equals the expected value of no treatment. The probability value at the point of indifference is the threshold. Using this concept in a clinical setting requires assessing the probability of the disease in a given patient and determining whether it is above or below the threshold. A unique threshold value must be calculated for each disease and its treatment in a given cohort of patients (defined as having common risk characteristics). Sensitivity analysis may be employed when significant uncertainty surrounds the probabilities and utilities involved in the calculations. In addition, if the clinical status of the patient or the circumstances of administration of the therapy differ notably from the typical case, benefits and costs must be adjusted appropriately.

Saxe, L. 1980. *The Implications of Cost-Effectiveness Analysis of Medical Technology; Background Paper no. 3: The Efficacy and Cost-Effectiveness of Psychotherapy* (OTA-BP-H-6). Washington, D.C.: Government Printing Office.

This case study describes a variety of methodological and substantive problems that arise in assessing the effects of mental health treatments. The report summarizes the existing literature and attempts to present the divergent perspectives within the research-policy community concerned with psychotherapy.

Part of the confusion about the effectiveness of psychotherapy has to do with reviewers' use of different definitions. The author uses a relatively broad definition of psychotherapy in order to best represent current therapy practice. The author also notes that psychotherapies are not distinguishable simply by their theoretical bases. In addition, patient variables (such as intelligence), therapist variables (such as empathy), and the nature of the treatment setting affect the nature of psychotherapy.

Although psychotherapy itself is complex and there is no clearly agreed-upon way of viewing it, the methods for assessing psychotherapy seem better established. The author describes the variety of experimental and quasi-experimental designs that have been used in assessing psychotherapy, along with an analysis of what types of information can be obtained by application of these techniques. The author also describes and analyzes various methodological strategies for measuring the outcomes of psychotherapeutic treatment and the ways in which the reliability and validity of measures are established. Unfortunately, research practice does not always meet these standards. Two explanations include the difficulties of withholding treatment and the problems of assessing effects over time. The author also considers the recent development of systematic procedures for synthesizing the findings of multiple investigations. The problems of such techniques, as well as their promise for detecting valid trends in the research literature, are analyzed.

The focus of the report's efficacy analysis is a discussion of six important earlier reviews of the psychotherapy literature. Despite some fundamental differences, the reviews all seem to support the finding that (under specified conditions) there is evidence as to psychotherapy's effectiveness. The author notes, however, that there is a great need for well-conducted research to evaluate psychotherapy for specific disorders under specified treatment conditions.

The author discusses the application of CBA-CEA to psychotherapy, which is much more recent, and hence less developed, than efficacy research. Nevertheless, a number of models are available for conducting such analyses. In general, the models are based on those used in other applications of CBA-CEA, and the problems engendered by their use are similar. A particular concern with such psychotherapy assessments is whether costs and benefits can be comprehensively measured. He notes, for example, that although the costs of psychotherapy treatments are relatively easy to measure, it is more difficult to determine and quantify what type of benefit has been achieved. Much of the CBA-CEA research to date has involved a comparison of psychotherapy treatments. Although such research indicates the potential use of CBA-CEA to improve the functioning of clinical settings where psychotherapy is given, its use for policymaking is less clear. He concludes that such work seems possible, however, and might be incorporated as part of large-scale efficacy assessments.

Scheffler, R. and Paringer, L. 1980. A Review of the Economic Evidence on Prevention. *Med. Care* 18:473.

The authors of this article review the economic evidence on preventive health care, classifying prevention activities as changes in life-style, public health measures, and screening programs. Changes in life-style include behavioral changes relating to automobile safety regulations and to the use of alcohol, tobacco, and other drugs. Public health measures include water fluoridation, immunization against communicable diseases, and food inspection. In the category of screening are found PKU screening of newborns, spina bifida cystica in fetuses, and hypertension.

The paper opens with a discussion of the techniques of CBA-CEA, their application to prevention, and the problems in implementing these approaches. Following their review of the literature, the authors conclude that a variety of preventive health care activities are cost-effective in the sense that they could produce resource savings. The authors observe that the measurable variables in CBA-CEAs may result in an understatement of net benefits since such nonpecuniary benefits as reduction of pain and suffering commonly are omitted from analysis.

Schoenbaum, S. et al. 1976a. Benefit-Cost Analysis of Rubella Vaccination Policy. *New Engl. J. Med.* 294:306.

The authors estimate the costs and benefits of various rubella vaccination strategies, each at 100 and 80 percent compliance. Benefits are the savings that result from the prevention of both acute rubella and congenital rubella. The direct costs of rubella (and hence the direct cost savings from prevention) are the costs of medical care, medication or special devices, and special education or rehabilitation. Indirect costs result from temporary disability during acute illness and complications, deaths from purpura or encephalitis, and permanent disability that results from congenital rubella syndrome. The costs of rubella vaccination are estimated on the basis of the cost of measles vaccination. Vaccination at ages ten to twelve appears preferable to vaccination at ages one to three for two reasons: (1) the gap between vaccinating and realizing benefits from prevention of congenital rubella is shorter the closer vaccination is to childbearing; and (2) the net benefits of preventing congenital rubella are greater than those associated with preventing acute rubella infection. The latter reason is demonstrated by employing conservative assumptions: Only the most obvious abnormalities associated with congenital rubella are included in the analysis, and the number of clinical cases of acute rubella is probably overestimated.

The results indicate that the economic benefits of a rubella vaccination program, assuming 100 percent compliance, are greater if offered once to girls at age twelve rather than to children of both sexes at age six or younger. If compliance is 80 percent instead, the least number of babies with congenital rubella will be born when vaccination is offered twice, once to children of both sexes at the age of two and again to girls at the age of twelve. Finally, the analysis indicates that, if the vaccine is to be offered to children at or before age two, it is more effective to use combined measles and rubella vaccine.

A discount rate of 6 percent is used throughout the analysis. It is assumed that complications of rubella vaccination in the age groups under consideration are negligible. The frequency of rubella infection is estimated on the basis of two serologic surveys.

Schoenbaum, S. et al. 1976*b*. The Swine-Influenza Decision. *New Engl. J. Med.* 295:759.

This CBA examines alternative strategies for a swine influenza vaccination program. The benefits of a vaccination program are described as the product of the direct and indirect costs that would be incurred in the event of an epidemic, the probability of an epidemic, and vaccine efficacy. The costs involved in the program include those associated with vaccine production and administration, resultant complications, and intangibles. Both private and public sector programs are examined. The Delphi method is used to obtain information regarding the probability of an epidemic, age-specific morbidity and mortality rates for both total and high-risk populations, vaccine efficacy and side effects, and vaccine acceptance rates. The net benefits for three strategies, which vary by age and risk of the target population, are calculated. The probability of an epidemic, vaccine efficacy, and vaccine acceptance rates are subjected to sensitivity analysis. The three strategies under consideration are found to be sensitive to acceptance rates. The results of the analysis indicate that expected net benefits are not maximized by the vaccination of everyone over the age of five. A policy of orienting the program toward the general adult population can be justified with low vaccine-administration costs, high vaccine efficacy, and high acceptance rates (59 percent), assuming further that the flu strain represents a potential pandemic. Otherwise, only high-risk group vaccination is warranted.

A major feature of this study—both in its design and achievement—is demonstration that a sound, useful analysis can be done in a matter of weeks.

Schweitzer, S. 1974. Cost Effectiveness of Early Detection of Disease. *Health Serv. Res.* 9:22.

The author presents a methodological framework for evaluating mass-screening diagnostic tests in the context of a CEA. The study illustrates the use of decision analysis in the evaluation of uncertain events. The author demonstrates how the decision rule rests on disease incidence, probabilities of test error, cost of the test and of treatment for cases identified, and the economic value (measured as expected lifetime earnings) of additional life for those cured. Extensions of the method would permit: (1) estimation of the incidence of the disease at which a test or a therapy would become cost-effective; (2) estimation of the break-even price of test and therapy, given disease incidence; and (3) determination of the optimal frequency of testing.

While the model is generalizable, and the principal intent of the paper is to present it as such, the author illustrates the approach by applying it to the case of Pap test screening for cervical cancer. This analysis shows that the test is socially cost-effective as a one-time screening device.

The author is careful to point out limitations of the method, observing that this form of analysis omits nonquantifiable costs and benefits, "such as a more complete value of human life and pain and suffering."

Schweitzer, S. and Scalzi, C. 1981. The Cost-Effectiveness of Bone Marrow Transplant Therapy and Its Policy Implications. U.S. Congress, Office of Technology Assessment, 1981 (OTA-BP-H-9(6)).

The study is a CEA of a highly technical and very costly emerging medical technology. The cost and effectiveness (lives and years of life saved) data the authors use are derived from the bone marrow transplant (BMT) program at the University of California at Los Angeles. Much of the effectiveness data have been previously published. Quality-of-life data were collected by a single observer, a BMT program nurse.

Patients with aplastic anemia and leukemia are studied. Since there were insufficient resources to allow all eligible patients into the program, the authors compare patients who received transplants to those judged eligible but not selected. The sample sizes are very small, and survival data are limited to three years as a result of the newness of the technology.

The authors compare bone marrow transplant procedures to conventional therapy, even though there is no indication that conventional treatment is efficacious. They consider the cost of transplant procedures to be the incremental—or avoidable—cost above that which would have been spent anyway.

Efficacy data are derived from the study of patients admitted to the program, extrapolated to normal life expectancy for successful transplants (defined as those patients still living after three years), and compared to the group of nonselected patients.

The authors identify a wide range of benefits and attempt to value and combine quality of life with projected increase in life. They use hospital charges for costs and calculate indirect costs. They discount future benefits (years of life saved) and assume all costs occur in the present. Sensitivity analysis is not used.

The results of the analysis are expressed as a cost-effectiveness ratio (cost per year of life saved). The authors do not qualify these results by discussing the confidence the reader can place in them, but they do provide an extensive discussion on the relevance this study has to public policy. Finally, the authors compare the cost-effectiveness ratios developed for bone marrow transplant procedures to the cost-effectiveness ratios for other lifesaving programs.

Showstack, J. and Schroeder, S. 1981. The Cost-Effectiveness of Upper Gastrointestinal Endoscopy. U.S. Congress, Office of Technology Assessment, 1981 (OTA-BP-H-9(8)).

This report examines the use of the fiberoptic endoscope to visualize the upper gastrointestinal (UGI) tract from the esophagus to the upper portion of the small intestine. The study covers the effectiveness and economic costs of this common form of endoscopy. Issues related to evaluating endoscopy's benefits and costs are discussed, though no formal comparison of costs and benefits is undertaken.

The report discusses the clinical effectiveness of UGI endoscopy, which is used to diagnose conditions of the UGI tract and to obtain specimens of tissue. Studies of the diagnostic value of the technique suggest that endoscopy significantly contributes to the amount of diagnostic information. Very often, however, the medical condition being diagnosed is such that the information gained does not improve morbidity or mortality for the patient.

The authors state that the more common dangers associated with endoscopy are perforation (esophagus or stomach), bleeding, cardiopulmonary effects, and infection. These complications are relatively rare, yet not insignificant given the large number of endoscopies performed nationally (at least 500,000 each year).

The authors distinguish between the cost of performing the procedure and the charges for it. Using data from California, they provide a median charge of $240, and, by extrapolation, a total national expenditure of $122 million. Using a hypothetical cost analysis, they then estimate that the average cost to a physician for performing a routine procedure ranges from $41 to $83.

The study addresses issues in evaluating benefits and costs of endoscopies. The authors point out the difficulties of adequately estimating the value of a diagnostic procedure such as endoscopy. They cite the ethical difficulties of conducting a clinical trial when conditions such as gastric cancer are involved. They also cite other difficulties, such as problems in extrapolating from the results of clinical trials in the event that such trials were conducted. The authors maintain that cost-effectiveness studies would be limited in their usefulness because of these difficulties in assessing benefits. Though theoretically possible, measurements of costs and benefits are unlikely because they cannot realistically be made sensitive enough to provide an accurate and useful assessment for decision-makers.

The authors also discuss the use of endoscopy and policy considerations, such as incentives leading to its use and the regulatory issues involved. Finally, the need for increased investigation of more narrowly defined indications for use of endoscopy is discussed.

Stange, P. and Sumner, A. 1978. Predicting Treatment Costs and Life Expectancy for End-Stage Renal Disease. *New Engl. J. Med.* 298:372.

The authors predict future medical care costs and life expectancy of patient cohorts in facility dialysis, home dialysis, and cadaveric transplantation over the next decade; they also estimate the cumulative effect on costs and life expectancy of 1,000-patient cohorts changing methods of treatment in each of the ten years. Three treatment transition options are evaluated: facility dialysis to home dialysis, facility dialysis to cadaveric transplantation, and home dialysis to cadaveric transplantation. They discount both costs and life expectancy at a rate of 7 percent. They obtain the 10-year survival and cost estimates through linear extrapolation of recent trends in data and predict the experience of the cadaveric-transplantation cohort for two survival-rate assumptions. The low assumption is based on rates reported in 1976, and the high assumption is an estimate of the average national survival rates over the next ten years. The results of the first phase of the analysis indicate that, over the next decade, each of the dialysis cohorts is predicted to have more added years of life than the transplantation group. Though the predicted number of years of life for both forms of dialysis is approximately equal over the ten-year period, treatment for the home-dialysis cohort will cost about $43 million less than that for the facility-dialysis cohort. Transplantation is less costly than either form of dialysis.

The second phase of the analysis indicates that undergoing home dialysis instead of facility dialysis (the first option) provides approximately the same life expectancy, but at 34 percent lower costs. The second option, moving from facility dialysis to transplantation, also results in a substantial reduction in costs, but there is an accompanying reduction in life expectancy as well. The third option, moving from home dialysis to transplantation, has results similar to those of the second option. The authors conclude that, while it is clear that there are potential savings to society from public policies that encourage able and willing patients to shift from facility to home dialysis, cost-effectiveness of the two dialysis-to-transplant options is ambiguous. Transplantation is less costly than dialysis over the ten-year period, but attention must also be paid to the impact of the shift in life expectancy. No cost-effectiveness ratios are presented. The authors caution that the intent of their analysis is not to promote any specific form of treatment, but to provide information such as the relative magnitude of the trade-offs between cost reduction and life expectancy in each of the treatment options.

Stason, W. and Fortess, E. 1981. Cardiac Radionuclide Imaging and Cost-Effectiveness. U.S. Congress, Office of Technology Assessment, 1981 (OTA-BP-H-9(13)).

The authors examine a range of issues in the recent growth of cardiac radionuclide imaging technology. The areas they address are the present and potential future characteristics of the technology; the market for and industry involvement in cardiac imaging innovations; the uses and users of these procedures; the clinical efficacy and risks associated with the techniques; the costs and charges of imaging technology use; and the cost-effectiveness of these procedures in different delivery situations.

The authors point out that much of the rapid diffusion and use of this technology are taking place without an understanding of the benefits and limitations of the various scanning techniques. To date, only a few patient populations have been evaluated out of a much broader spectrum of uses and techniques. Adding to the uncertainty are the rapid technological changes that are occurring and the poorly defined target population for cardiac scans.

Using the various suggested clinical indications and uses as a backdrop, the authors estimate that the potential target population for cardiac imaging could be 134 million people per year if all asymptomatic people age twenty and over were scanned, 70.8 million people per year if routine screening were limited to those forty and over, and 11.7 million people per year if scans were restricted to people with suspected or established coronary heart disease. The study looks at direct nonlabor costs (equipment, maintenance, radionuclides and so on), direct labor costs (personnel needs, training, support staff), and indirect costs (overhead) to estimate the costs of cardiac scanning services. The authors estimate the annual fixed costs of a model radionuclide laboratory to be $112,300 for the complete service, with the costs of the various individual procedures ranging from $72 to $258. Significant variations exist across the country regarding the charges for the various procedures. Nomenclature and billing procedures or listings are not comparable from hospital to hospital. As a result, it is extremely difficult to determine if there is a relative standard or range of charges for these techniques. The authors develop a set of suggested fee schedules for these procedures, ranging from $155 to $405 per scan.

The medical literature is examined to determine if there is a proper role for scanning techniques. The authors examine extant studies to determine what types of sample populations have been used, the reference or control groups used, the technical and medical standards against which radionuclide procedures were judged, and the clinical settings in which the studies were conducted. They also examine the risks associated with these procedures—both to health care professionals and patients—and assess the value of the diagnostic information that the scans provide to the diagnosis or understanding of the extent of the disease and its response to treatment.

The authors fit the many variables into a cost-effectiveness framework and conduct a limited analysis of cardiac imaging procedures. They conclude that "decision strategies based on threshold cutoff probabilities of a given disease(s) are cost effective compared to blanket testing . . . and the use of cardiac imaging appears to identify additional surgical candidates at reasonable cost when compared to exercise tolerance testing." The reasonableness of these additional costs will depend, to a large extent, on the incremental health benefits achieved by coronary artery surgery.

The authors identify many of the policy issues raised by this emerging technology. A few of the areas they discuss are issues of reimbursement, safety and efficacy determination, disposal of the radionuclide wastes, clinical standards and indications for use, allocation of resources, and responsibility for regulation and diffusion of these procedures throughout the medical community.

Stason, W. and Weinstein, M. 1977. Allocation of Resources to Manage Hypertension. *New Engl. J. Med.* 296:732.

The authors apply CEA to the management of essential hypertension in order to "determine how resources can be used most efficiently within programs to treat hypertension and to provide a yardstick for comparison with alternative health-related uses of the resources." Costs of treatment consist of the lifetime costs of hypertension treatment plus the costs of treating diseases that occur during the additional years of life minus the costs associated with avoided treatment of cardiovascular disease. Effectiveness is calculated in terms of increased years of life expectancy, adjusted for changes in the quality of life. The authors perform the analysis under three assumptions concerning the reduction of risk: full benefit, half benefit, and partial benefit varying with age.

The authors define one year of life with side effects to be the equivalent of 0.99 quality-adjusted life-years. They use a discount rate of 5 percent throughout the analysis and perform sensitivity analysis on several critical variables, including the discount rate, medical treatment costs, and the quality-of-life adjustment. In addition they examine the effects of incomplete adherence to the treatment regimen.

The results of the analysis indicate that in no case does treatment pay for itself. At best, only an average of 22 percent of gross treatment costs can be recovered from savings in the treatment of strokes and heart attacks. However, the analysis also indicates that, in terms of effectiveness, funds spent to improve adherence may be a better use of resources than efforts to screen a maximum number of subjects.

Steiner, K. and Smith, H. 1973. Application of Cost Benefit Analysis to a PKU Screening Program. *Inquiry* 10:34.

The authors compare and contrast the techniques of CBA and CEA, stating that, although equally sound decisions may be reached by either method, one of the two is usually better suited for a particular problem. The authors believe that CBA is the best approach for screening programs, and it is this technique that they subsequently use in evaluating a PKU screening program in Mississippi.

Direct costs associated with PKU are defined in this study as the actual expenditures for medical and other services attributable to the disease. Indirect costs are defined as a loss of economic productivity attributable to the disease. These costs serve to measure the benefits of a successful prevention program. The analysis is performed from both a retrospective and a prospective point of view. The retrospective approach measures the costs of the current population with PKU and estimates what the costs of screening, detecting, and treatment would have been. For this study, the direct costs associated with PKU are estimated using data from three mental institutions in Mississippi. Indirect costs are measured by loss of income, assuming that the PKU victim remains incapacitated for life. Detection costs are based on estimates of the incidence of PKU. The retrospective analysis indicates that the total costs of institutionalization and lost earnings associated with the current Mississippi population with PKU (twenty-five persons) amounts to $2,314,595. The costs of detecting and treating the twenty-five cases are estimated at $1,392,668, yielding a cost-benefit ratio of 1 to 1.66.

The prospective method compares the cost of screening all live births in a given year to treating those found to be suffering from PKU. In this study, calculations are based on the 1967 live births in Mississippi. Testing the 46,714 live births that year would have detected an average of 1.76 PKU cases. The costs associated with these cases are $135,062 if the minimum expected length of institutionalization (thirty years) is assumed, and $256,418 if institutionalization is assumed to cover the normal life expectancy of a one-year-old child born in 1967 (70.8 years). Program costs are estimated at $98,518, yielding cost-benefit ratios of 1 to 1.37 and 1 to 2.6, respectively. The authors state that, in all calculations, detection costs are high and the total illness costs (that is, possible benefit) are low in order to produce conservative results. A discount rate of 4 percent is applied to the lost earnings data, but not to direct or detection costs.

U.S. Congress, Office of Technology Assessment. 1979. *A Review of Selected Federal Vaccine and Immunization Policies.* Based on Case Studies of Pneumococcal Vaccine (OTA-H-96). Washington, D.C.: Government Printing Office.

This study includes an examination of the cost-effectiveness of applying a primary preventive technology—vaccination against pneumococcal pneumonia—to different age groups. Costs of medical care and effects of health associated with a preventive program are explored from the perspectives of society and of a third-party payer such as Medicare.

A CEA is used to calculate the expected change in health and in medical costs resulting from vaccination versus continuation of the present situation, in which pneumococcal pneumonia is treated if it occurs. In the analysis, costs are limited to expenditures and savings within the medical care sector, and changes in health status are expressed in years of healthy life. Thus, the cost-effectiveness ratio represents the net medical cost per year of healthy life that would be gained by a vaccinated person. The calculations are based on a single hypothetical vaccination program conducted in June 1978. The analysis uses a simulation model to estimate the costs and effects that would result from 1978 to 2050 for two populations, one vaccinated and the other unvaccinated. Costs and effects are discounted at 5 percent per year. Separate cost-effectiveness ratios are calculated for five different age groups: two to four years, five to twenty-four, twenty-five to forty-four, forty-five to sixty-four, and sixty-five and older. A sensitivity analysis is used to test the effect on the results of varying the values of several uncertain parameters over reasonable ranges.

Net effects on health are expressed in quality-adjusted life-years (QALY). Mortality rates for pneumonia as an underlying cause of death form the basis for estimating 1978 pneumonia mortality among the unvaccinated. Unpublished age-specific data are used to estimate the days of pneumonia morbidity among the unvaccinated.

Costs of medical care, expressed in dollars, include additional expenditures for vaccinations and for treatment of side effects; reduced expenditures for treating pneumococcal pneumonia that would be expected to occur without vaccination; and additional expenditures for other illness in the extended years of life gained by vaccinees who avoid death from pneumococcal pneumonia.

The study finds that, given the range of factors involved, vaccinations would entail positive medical expenditures for every age group and would be most cost-effective for those age sixty-five or over. The cost-effectiveness ratio is about $4,800 per QALY gained for all ages and $1,000 per QALY for ages sixty-five and over. The analysis finds that vaccination of 21.5 percent of the population age sixty-five and over would result in a net cost to society of about $23 million and would yield about 22,000 QALYs over the lifetimes of those vaccinated. The study also concludes that vaccination for all age groups in the population would have a net cost of about $150 million, for a gain of 31,000 QALYs.

The study also examines policy implications of these findings, including a possible change in the Medicare law to permit federal payment for pneumococcal vaccine for the elderly.

VanPelt, A. and Levy, H. 1974. Cost-Benefit Analysis of Newborn Screening for Metabolic Disorders. *New Engl. J. Med.* 291:1414.

This article examines the costs and benefits of a Massachusetts program designed to detect inborn errors of metabolism in newborn infants. The costs, based on a survey of all hospitals with obstetric and newborn units in Massachusetts, include those for routine specimen collection, laboratory analysis, the collection of additional specimens, confirmatory testing, and follow-up care and therapy. For fiscal year 1972–73, these costs amounted to $460,638. Benefits are calculated as the estimated savings from the prevention of mental retardation and other complications. For 1972–73, estimated total savings amounted to $825,300, yielding a net benefit of $364,662 or a benefit-cost ratio of nearly 1.8 to 1. Indirect costs of metabolic disorders (such as reduced economic productivity due to disability and premature mortality) that would be averted as a result of a screening program are not included in the calculation of benefits. Presumably, the inclusion of the present value of such benefits, when considered along with a similar future stream of the other costs and benefits (also discounted to present value), would result in even higher net benefits.

Wagner, J. 1981a. The Feasibility of Economic Evaluation of Diagnostic Procedures: The Case of CT Scanning. U.S. Congress, Office of Technology Assessment, 1981 (OTA-BP-H-9(2)).

This study examines the appropriate methodology of CBA-CEA for diagnostic procedures. Following the development of a framework for analysis, the author reviews the literature on the cost-effectiveness of CT scanning, critically evaluating it in terms of the evaluation model.

The author describes a theoretically ideal evaluative model, in which the analysis compares alternative diagnostic pathways, each of which begins with the presentations of signs and symptoms and ends with outcome. The purpose of the evaluation is not to examine the technology per se, but to evaluate its use. The author describes the need for an appropriate means of identifying homogeneous patient groups, specifying diagnostic pathways, measuring diagnostic accuracy, measuring diagnostic and therapeutic costs, and specifying outcomes of the diagnostic and therapeutic process.

In a review of the literature on the economic impact of CT scanning, only one study that attempted to specify diagnostic pathways is identified. Most of the other studies examine the impact CT has on diagnostic costs or the cost of case-finding.

Efficacy information is addressed both for diagnostic studies in general and for CT scanners in particular. Comments regarding the potential benefits associated with negative findings are also included.

Costs are distinguished from charges; marginal, or avoidable, costs are recommended; the difficulty of capturing true costs is discussed extensively. Indirect costs are not considered.

Despite major limitations in applying principles of economic evaluation to diagnostic procedures, such evaluations are feasible. For CT scanning, some specific uses appear to be cost-effective when sufficient demand exists to operate a scanner at full capacity.

Warner, K. 1979*b*. The Economic Implications of Preventive Health Care. *Soc. Sci. Med.* 13C:227.

The author examines understanding of the costs and benefits of disease prevention efforts. He reviews the relevant literature within the following classification of preventive health care activities: whether the activity is personal or environmental; whether it involves primary or secondary prevention (that is, respectively, reducing later development of disease by reducing health hazards or identifying disease in a presymptomatic stage in order to achieve cure or to minimize ill effects); whether it requires active or passive involvement on the part of the recipient; and whether it is produced by an individual professional or a community.

The review of the literature supports the conventional wisdom that primary prevention activities are frequently cost-effective, particularly when the recipient's role is relatively passive and when the prevention measure is a public good delivered to an entire community (for example, fluoridation of water).

Given successes with traditional public health preventive measures, the author suggests that "future prevention opportunities may lie in nontraditional activities which violate 'rules' of effective health care delivery or communication of prevention information. For example, the broadcast media may prove to be a cost-effective vehicle for health education, despite the impersonal character of the media and the required 'activation' of the viewer-listener."

The paper concludes by placing the cost-effectiveness of prevention in the context of the political debate on health care cost containment.

Weinstein, M. 1979. Economic Evaluation of Medical Procedures and Technologies: Progress, Problems, and Prospects. DHEW Publication no. (PHS) 79-3254. Washington, D.C.: Government Printing Office.

This paper presents the state of the art of CBA and CEA of medical procedures. CBA-CEAs are defined and distinguished from each other. The author advocates the use of multiattribute accounting in conjunction with CBA and CEA, in which unquantifiable concerns, such as equity and ethical issues, are considered along with the traditional, measurable impacts. Basic methodological principles are reviewed, including estimation of event rates, sensitivity analysis, choosing a discount rate, measurement of costs, and measurement of benefits. The controversy surrounding the assignment of monetary value of lifesaving and health improvement in CBA is discussed.

Selected applications, classified as treatment, secondary prevention, screening, and immunization, are reviewed. The author states that diagnostic procedures other than screening have not received much attention, in part because of methodological obstacles. He predicts that technology evaluation will be the area in which the next major advances in CBA and CEA will develop. He discusses current methodological problems, classified as valuation of multiattributed outcomes, evaluation of diagnostic tests, evaluation of multifaceted technologies, and uncertainty concerning efficacy, costs, and ultimate uses of evolving technology.

The paper concludes with a generally optimistic assessment of the prospects of CBA and CEA in medical care and of overcoming current methodological problems. The author recommends a multidisciplinary approach to analysis, including the expertise of physicians, engineers, and economists. He notes that the value of formal economic analysis lies not so much in the actual results, but rather in the ability of such analysis to highlight uncertainty and the most important value trade-offs involved in alternative policies.

Weinstein, M. and Pearlman, L. 1981. Cost-Effectiveness of Automated Multichannel Chemistry Analyzers. U.S. Congress, Office of Technology Assessment, 1981 (OTA-BP-H-9(4)).

The authors illustrate the possible techniques for evaluating the cost-effectiveness of automated, multichannel chemistry analyzers. They also examine and discuss limitations caused by deficient data, areas for future research, and influences of clinical practice on the evaluation of such analyzers.

The history of multichannel clinical chemistry technology is reviewed, and the authors present an analytical framework for evaluating the cost-effectiveness of the multichannel analyzer. They review the available data on costs and examine the evidence on the cost-effectiveness of using cardiac enzymes and isoenzymes in the diagnosis of myocardial infarction.

The authors discuss several important issues related to the clinical efficacy and cost-effectiveness of clinical laboratory chemical tests. A prominent example is the potential influences on physicians' test-ordering behavior that may be induced by the availability of multichannel analyzers.

Various types of automated, multichannel chemistry analyzers could be compared to one another under specified circumstances. The authors also compare the cost-effectiveness of using multichannel analyzers to obtain laboratory values with not obtaining that laboratory value at all. Further, they advocate comparing the efficiency of using the analyzers under varying work loads (that is, the number of tests performed per unit of time).

Information on efficacy is not plentiful, but studies designed to produce efficacy data are under way. The authors also discuss the variability of benefits resulting from use of multichannel analyzers. Potential benefits are described from a societal perspective; they include potential reduced costs from reduced incidence of unnecessary hospitalization.

Costs are distinguished from charges, and several direct costs are identified. Fixed, variable, and induced costs are all addressed. The authors state that indirect costs have not been adequately studied and may not be extensively affected by the analyzers. Discounting should be included in analyses, as should sensitivity analysis.

Results are not derived from this case study; however, many different ways the CEA could be conducted are discussed. Each approach would yield results with a different meaning; hence several caveats would be needed for each approach and set of results.

The authors discuss the potential public policy implications of this analysis; it could affect reimbursement policies regarding laboratory tests, the use of automated analyzers by hospitals and physicians, and the design of equipment by manufacturers. No conclusions regarding the cost-effectiveness of automated, multichannel chemistry analyzers can be drawn from this study: It was not designed to be an actual assessment, it was intended to illustrate how a CEA of automated analyzers could be performed.

Weinstein, M. and Stason, W. 1977*b*. Foundations of Cost-Effectiveness Analysis for Health and Medical Practices. *New Engl. J. Med.* 296:716.

This article presents principles of CEA as they are applied to the allocation of health care resources. The authors caution that, in conducting an analysis, the objectives of the actual decision-maker may be more relevant than the societal point of view. Whenever possible, measures of effectiveness should be expressed in outcome-oriented terms, such as length of life and quality of life. Trade-offs between present and future health benefits and costs, and hence the use of discounting, are discussed. Net health care costs are expressed as the sum of costs associated with treatment, side effects, and increased longevity, minus the savings from decreased morbidity. Net health effectiveness is expressed as the expected number of quality-adjusted life-years gained. It is calculated by adjusting the expected number of years of life for improvements in the quality of life caused by alleviation or prevention of morbidity and side effects of treatment. Sensitivity analysis is described and its use is recommended whenever uncertainty is involved in the estimation of key variables (for example, discount rates, clinical efficacy, and prevalence). The article ends with a discussion of the value and application of CEA in health care and concludes that its principal value is that it forces one to be explicit about the beliefs and values that underlie allocation decisions.

Weisbrod, B. 1971. Costs and Benefits of Medical Research: A Case Study of Poliomyelitis. *J. Polit. Econ.* 79:527.

In this CBA of poliomyelitis research, benefits are calculated as savings from avoided premature mortality, morbidity, and treatment and rehabilitation costs. The analysis requires an estimation of the time stream of research expenditures directed toward poliomyelitis, the time streams of a number of forms of benefits resulting from (or predicted to result from) the application of the knowledge generated by the research, and the cost of applying that knowledge.

Using this information, the author calculates internal rates of return on research expenditure. Savings per case prevented, application costs, the time horizon, and research expenditures are all subjected to sensitivity analysis. The internal rates of return are found to be sensitive to application costs, varying from 4 to 14 percent. In approximating the present value of expenditures and benefits, the author uses a discount rate of 10 percent. No sensitivity analysis is performed on this variable. The difficulties encountered in trying to associate specific medical research expenditures with a particular disease are discussed. These include the fact that basic research is often not directed at a specific disease and even disease-specific research frequently yields knowledge relevant to the prevention or treatment of other diseases. The data used here are estimates of awards for poliomyelitis research from 1930 to 1956. The author stresses the need to include the costs involved in the application of new medical knowledge, as well as the costs of generating it, when attempting to comprehensively analyze a medical research program.

The article concludes with a discussion of the impact on private market allocative efficiency when a collective consumption good (such as medical research) requires for its application a procedure (such as vaccination) that is provided individually and from which nonpayers may be excluded. The author also discusses the effects of externalities on the provision of medical research and its application for contagious diseases.

Witte, J. et al. 1975. The Benefits From 10 Years of Measles Immunization in the United States. *Pub. Health Rep.* 90:205.

The authors estimate the costs the nation would have sustained between 1963 and 1972 without measles immunization (that is, the benefits of measles immunization) and the actual costs of measles during that period in terms of illness and associated resources consumed. The research costs of developing and testing the measles vaccine are not included because of the difficulty in identifying them and in determining the share applicable to the United States in the period under consideration.

The benefits associated with the measles immunization program considered in this analysis include savings in costs of physician services and long-term institutional care for those who would have become retarded, and avoidance of production losses due to morbidity and premature mortality. Program costs are those incurred in vaccine production, distribution, administration, and promotion. The analysis concludes that the net benefits achieved through immunization in the United States totaled $1.3 billion for that period. A discount rate of 4 percent is used. The authors assume that the national immunization effort had no significant effect on the demand for medical care or on the size and composition of the labor force.

Bibliography

Items preceded by an asterisk were referred to in the text but were not classified as part of the CBA-CEA bibliography. See Appendix A for an explanation of the classification procedure.

Abel-Smith, B. 1973. Cost-Effectiveness and Cost-Benefit in Cholera Control. *WHO Chron.* 27:407.

Abrams, H. and McNeil, B. 1978. Computed Tomography: Cost and Efficacy Implications. *Amer. J. Roentgenol..* 131:81.

Abt, C. 1977. The Issue of Social Costs in Cost-Benefit Analysis of Surgery. In *Costs, Risks, and Benefits of Surgery,* ed. J. Bunker et al., New York: Oxford Univ. Press.

Acton, J. 1973. *Evaluating Public Programs to Save Lives: The Case of Heart Attacks.* Santa Monica, Calif.: RAND Corp.

————. 1975. *Measuring the Social Impact of Heart and Circulatory Disease Programs: Preliminary Framework and Estimates.* Report prepared for the National Heart and Lung Institute, National Institutes of Health. Santa Monica, Calif.: RAND Corp.

*————. 1976. Measuring the Monetary Value of Lifesaving Programs. *Law Contemp. Prob.* 40:47.

Adelstein, S. and McNeil, B. 1978. A New Diagnostic Test for Pulmonary Embolism: How Good and How Costly. *New Engl. J. Med.* 299:305.

Aikawa, J. 1974. Proceedings: The Cost-Effectiveness of the C.U. Computerized Clinical Laboratory System. *Biomed. Sci. Instr.* 10:89.

Akehurst, R. and Holterman, S. 1978. Application of Cost-Benefit Analysis to Programmes for the Prevention of Mental Handicap. In *Major Mental Handicap: Methods and Costs of Prevention,* Ciba Foundation Symposium 59. New York: Elsevier, Excerpta Medica.

Albert, D. 1978. Decision Theory in Medicine: A Review and Critique. *Milbank Mem. Fund Q.* 56:362.

Albritton, R. 1978. Cost-Benefits of Measles Eradication: Effects of a Federal Intervention. *Pol. Anal.* 4:1.

Allanson, J. 1978. School Nursing Services: Some Current Justifications and Cost-Benefit Implications. *J. Sch. Health* 48:603.

Alter, J. et al. 1979. Cost-Effectiveness: Allied Medical Personnel. *Ohio State Med. J.* 75:279.

Altman, S. and Blendon, R., eds. 1979. *Medical Technology: The Culprit Behind Health Care Costs?* Proceedings of the Sun Valley Forum on National Health,

DHEW Publication no. (PHS) 79–3216. Washington, D. C.: Government Printing Office.

Alvord, D. 1977. Innovation in Speech Therapy: A Cost-Effective Program. *Except. Child.* 43:520.

Ambrosch, F. et al. 1979. Cost-Benefit Analysis of BCG-Vaccination in Austria. *Devel. Biol. Stand.* 43:121.

Ament, A. 1980. Observations on the Application of Cost Benefit Analysis in Health Care. *Ned. T. Genusk.* 124:1423.

American Dietetic Association. 1979. *Costs and Benefits of Nutritional Care— Phase 1.* Chicago: American Dietetic Association.

*American Medical Association. 1978. *Report of the National Commission on the Cost of Medical Care.* Chicago: American Medical Association.

Angle, C. et al. 1977. The Myelodysplasia and Hydrocephalics Program in Nebraska: A 15-Year Review of Costs and Benefits. *Nebr. Med. J.* 62:391.

Armstrong, B. and Armstrong, R. 1979. Tympanostomy Tubes: Their Use, Abuse, and Cost-Benefit Ratio. *Laryngoscope* 89:443.

*Arnstein, S. 1977. Technology Assessment: Opportunities and Obstacles. *IEEE Trans. Syst. Man Cyb.* SMC-7:571.

Aron, W. and Daily, D. 1974. Short- and Long-Term Therapeutic Communities: A Follow-Up and Cost-Effectiveness Comparison. *Int. J. Addict.* 9:619.

Arthur D. Little, Inc. 1976. Automated Electrocardiography in the United States. HRA 23075–0212. Hyattsville, Md.: Health Resources Administration.

Ashmole, R. et al. 1973. Cost Effectiveness of Current Awareness Sources in the Pharmaceutical Industry. *Proc. Roy. Soc. Med.* 66:459.

Atherley, G. et al. 1976. An Approach to the Financial Evaluation of Occupational Health. *J. Soc. Occup. Med.* 26:21.

Averill, R. et al. 1977. A Cost-Benefit Analysis of Continued Stay Certification. *Med. Care* 15:158.

Axnick, N. et al. 1969. Benefits Due to Immunization Against Measles. *Pub. Health Rep.* 84:673.

Backhaut, B. 1973. Refining Cost Benefit Estimates of Methadone Programs. *Natl. Conf. Meth. Treat. Proc.* 2:1227.

Bagdonoff, M. 1972. Cost Allocation and the Evaluation of New Procedures. *Arch. Intern. Med.* 130:295.

Bahr, A. 1978. Efficacy of Computed Tomography of the Head in Changing Patient Care and Health Costs: A Retrospective Study. *Amer. J. Roentgenol.* 131:45.

Bailar, J. 1976. Screening for Early Breast Cancer: Pros and Cons. *Cancer* 39:2783.

Baker, C. and Way, L. 1978. Clinical Utility of CAT Body Scans. *Amer. J. Surg.* 136:37.

Balatskii, O. 1976. An Approach to the Determination of the Economic Effectiveness of Investment in Public Health. *Matekon.* 12:84.

Banerjie, A. 1972. Cost-Benefit Analysis of Health Measures at Local Level: A Plan for a Pilot Project. *Indian J. Pub. Health* 16:141.

Banta, H. and McNeil, B. 1978a. Cost and Benefits of ECT Therapy for Depression. Paper read at the conference on ECT: Efficacy and Impact, New Orleans, Louisiana.

————. 1978b. Evaluation of the CT Scanner and Other Diagnostic Technologies. *Health Care Man. Rev.* 3:7.

Banta, H. and Sanes, J. 1978. Assessing the Social Impacts of Medical Technologies. *J. Comm. Health* 3:245.

Banta, H. and Thacker, S. 1979a. Assessing the Costs and Benefits of Electronic Fetal Monitoring. *Obstet. Gyn. Surv.* 34:627.

————. 1979b. *Costs and Benefits of Electronic Fetal Monitoring: A Review of the Literature.* DHEW Publication no. (PHS) 79-3245. Hyattsville, Md.: National Center for Health Services Research.

Barach, A. 1975. The Indiscriminate Use of IPPB. *JAMA* 231:1141.

Baram, M. 1979. Regulation of Health, Safety, and Environmental Quality, and the Use of Cost-Benefit Analysis. Paper read at the Administrative Conference of the United States, Washington, D.C.

Barnes, B. 1977a. Cost-Benefit Analysis of Surgery: Current Accomplishments and Limitations. *Amer J. Surg.* 133:438.

————. 1977b. An Overview of the Treatment of End-Stage Renal Disease and a Consideration of Some of the Consequences. In *Costs, Risks, and Benefits of Surgery,* ed. J. Bunker et al. New York: Oxford Univ. Press.

Barnes, B. et al. 1977. Evaluation of Surgical Therapy by Cost-Benefit Analysis. *Surgery* 82:21.

Barrett, T. et al. 1977. Making Evaluation Systems Cost-Effective. *Hosp. Comm. Psychol.* 3:173.

Bartlett, J. et al. 1978. Evaluating Cost-Effectiveness of Diagnostic Equipment: The Brain Scanner Case. *Brit. Med. J.* 2:815.

Bay, K. et al. 1976. The Worth of a Screening Program: An Application of a Statistical Decision Model for the Benefit Evaluation of Screening Projects. *Amer. J. Pub. Health* 66:145.

Bendixen, H. 1977. The Cost of Intensive Care. In *Cost, Risks, and Benefits of Surgery,* ed. J. Bunker et al. New York: Oxford Univ. Press.

Bennett, M. and Winchester, J. 1977. *Heart and Circulatory Problems in New Mexico: A Benefit-Cost Perspective.* Albuquerque: Univ. of New Mexico Medical Center.

Bennett, M. et al. 1978. Balancing Quality and Cost in Health Care: An Example of Culturing for Streptococcus Bacteria. Paper read at the annual meeting of the American Public Health Association, Los Angeles, California.

Bennett, W. 1976. Cost-Benefit Ratio of Pretransplant Bilateral Nephrectomy. *JAMA* 235:1703.

Bentkover, J. and Drew, P. 1981. Cost-Effectiveness/ Cost-Benefit of Medical Technologies: A Case Study of Orthopedic Joint Implants (OTA-BP-H-9 (14)). In *The Implications of Cost-Effectiveness Analysis of Medical Technology: Background Paper no. 2: Case Studies of Medical Technologies.* Washington, D. C.: Government Printing Office.

*Bergner, M. et al. 1976a. The Sickness Impact Profile: Conceptual Formulation and Methodology for the Development of a Health Status Measure. *Int. J. Health Serv.* 6:393.

Bergner, M. et al. 1976b. The Sickness Impact Profile: Validation of a Health Status Measure. *Med. Care* 14:57.

Berman, E. 1971. Cost-Benefit Analysis of Selected Preventive Dentistry Programs. Unpublished paper. McLean, Va.: Mitre Corp.

Bernard, J. 1979. Cost-Benefit Analysis and Mental Retardation Center Funding. *Ment. Retard.* 17:156.

Berry, R., Jr. 1974. Cost and Efficiency in the Production of Hospital Services. *Milbank Mem. Fund Q.* 52:291.

Bertera, E. and Bertera, R. 1981. The Cost-Effectiveness of Telephone vs. Clinic

Counseling for Hypertensive Patients: A Pilot Study. *Amer. J. Pub. Health* 71:626.

Bertera, R. et al. 1979. Cost-Effectiveness Evaluation of a Home Visiting Triage Program for Family Planning in Turkey. *Amer. J. Pub. Health* 69:950.

Berwick, D. et al. 1976. Screening for Cholesterol: Costs and Benefits. In *Genetic Counseling*, ed. H. Lubs and F. Delacuz. New York: Raven Press.

Binner, P. et al. 1976. Workload Levels, Program Costs, and Program Benefits: An Output Value Analysis. *Admin. Ment. Health* 3:156.

Bishop, S. 1979. Cost-Effectiveness: Pharmacy Systems. *Ohio State Med. J.* 75: 287.

Blair, H. 1978. Capsule of the Cost-Effective Health Care Conference. *J. Med. Assoc. Ga.* 67:891.

Bloom, B. and Peterson, O. 1973. End Results, Costs and Productivity of Coronary-Care Units. *New Engl. J. Med.* 288:72.

Blount, J. 1973. Gonorrhea Epidemiology: Insuring The Best Return for Resources Expended. *J. Reprod. Med.* 11:125.

Blumstein, A. and Cassidy, R. 1973. Benefit-Cost Analysis of Family Planning. *Socio-Econ. Plan. Sci.* 7:151.

Boddy, F. 1971. Cost-Effectiveness, Cost-Benefit Analysis and the Use of Audio-visual Resources. *Scot. Med. J.* 16:117.

Boden, L. 1979. Cost-Benefit Analysis: Caveat Emptor. *Amer. J. Pub. Health* 69:1210.

Boggs, D. 1973. Applying the Techniques of Cost Effectiveness to the Delivery of Dental Services. *J. Pub. Health Dent.* 33:222.

Boissoneau, R. 1975. Point of View: Cost Effectiveness in the Health Care System. *J. Amer. Diet. Assoc.* 66:504.

Bond, M. et al. 1968. An Occupational Health Program: Costs vs. Benefits. *Arch. Environ. Health* 17:408.

Bredin, H. and Prout, G., Jr. 1976. One-Stage Radical Cystectomy for Bladder Carcinoma: Operative Mortality, Cost-Benefit Analysis. *Trans. Amer. Assoc. Genitourin. Surg.* 68:47.

Bredin, H., et al. 1977. One-Stage Radical Cystectomy for Bladder Carcinoma: Operative Mortality, Cost-Benefit Analysis. *J. Urol.* 117:447.

Brian, E. et al. 1976. Cost-Benefit Analysis of Installation of a Spectra System at Santa Monica Hospital. Unpublished paper. Los Angeles: Univer. of Southern California.

Briggs, D. et al. 1979. Cost-Effectiveness: Occupational Medicine. *Ohio State Med. J.* 75:305.

Brodsky, L. and Scherzer, N. 1976. An Analysis of Alternative Gonorrhea Control Programs in New York City—March, 1971. In *Analysis of Urban Health Problems*, ed. I. Leveson and J. Weiss. New York: Spectrum.

*Brook, R. et al. 1979. Overview of Adult Health Status Measures Fielded in RAND's Health Insurance Study. *Med. Care* 17 (suppl.):7.

Brooks, R. 1969. Cost-Benefit Analysis of Patients Treated at a Rheumatism Center. *Ann. Rheum. Dis.* 28:655.

Brown, J. 1979. Reducing the Cost of Medical Care: Prevention as a Cost Effective Measure. *Tex. J. Med.* 75:73.

Brown, S. 1975. *A Case Study of Medical Efficacy: Tonsillectomy.* Washington, D.C.: National Academy of Sciences, Institute of Medicine.

Bryant, N. et al. 1974. Comparison of Care and Cost Outcomes for Stroke Patients With and Without Home Care. *Stroke* 5:54.

Bryers, E. and Hawthorne, J. 1978. Screening for Mild Hypertension: Costs and Benefits. *J. Epidem. Comm. Health* 32:117.

Budetti, P. et al. 1981. Costs and Effectiveness of Neonatal Intensive Care (OTA-BP-H-9 (10)). In *The Implications of Cost-Effectiveness Analysis of Medical Technology; Background Paper no. 2: Case Studies of Medical Technologies.* Washington, D.C.: Government Printing Office.

Bunker, J. 1974. Risks and Benefits of Surgery. In *Benefits and Risks in Medical Care: A Symposium Held by the Office of Health Economics,* ed. D. Taylor. Lutan, England: White Crescent Press.

Bunker, J. et al. 1978. Surgical Innovation and Its Evaluation. *Science* 200:937.

Bunker, J. et al., eds. 1977. *Costs, Risks and Benefits of Surgery.* New York: Oxford Univ. Press.

Burt, B., ed. 1978. The Relative Efficiency of Methods of Caries Prevention in Dental Public Health. Unpublished proceedings. Ann Arbor.

Burt, B. and Warner, K. Forthcoming. Prevention of Oral Disease: Its Potential for Containing the Costs of Dental Care. In *Controlling the Cost of Dental Care,* ed. L. Meskin and R. Kudrle. Minneapolis: Univ. of Minnesota Press.

Burt, M. 1974. Policy Analysis: Introduction and Applications to Health Programs. Unpublished paper. Washington, D.C.: Information Resources Press.

Burton, G. et al. 1975. Respiratory Care Warrants Studies for Cost-Effectiveness. *Hospitals* 49:64.

Bush, J. et al. 1973. Cost-Effectiveness Using a Health Status Index: Analysis of the New York State PKU Screening Program. In *Health Status Indexes: Proceedings of a Conference,* ed. R. Berg. Chicago: Hospital Research and Educational Trust.

Buxton, M. and West, R. 1975. Cost-Benefit Analysis of Long-Term Haemodialysis for Chronic Renal Failure. *Brit. Med. J.* 2:376.

Carlson, D. 1977. Cost-Effectiveness of Laboratory Improvement Programs: The Viewpoint From the Private Sector. *Health Lab. Sci.* 14:199.

Carr, A. 1978. Cost-Effective Nursing. *Nurs. Times* 74:906.

Carrera, G. et al. 1977. Computed Tomography of the Brain in Patients With Headache or Temporal Lobe Epilepsy: Findings and Cost-Effectiveness. *J. Comput. Assist. Tomogr.* 1:200.

Catford, J. and Fowkes, F. 1979. Economic Benefits of Day Care Abortion. *Comm. Med.* 1:115.

Centerwall, B. 1979. Prevention of the Wernicke-Korsakoff Syndrome: An Updated Cost-Benefit Analysis. *New Engl. J. Med.* 300:320.

Centerwall, B. and Criqui, M. 1978. The Prevention of Wenicke-Korsakoff Syndrome: A Cost-Benefit Analysis. *New Engl. J. Med.* 299:285.

Chadwick, J. et al. 1970. Cost and Operational Analysis of Autotmated Multiphasic Health Testing. HSM 110-69-411, PB 193880. Menlo Park, Calif.: Stanford Research Institute.

Chamberlain, J. 1978. Human Benefits and Costs of a National Screening Program for Neural-Tube Defects. *Lancet* 8103(2):1293.

Chapalain, M. 1978. Perinatality: French Cost-Benefit Studies and Decision on Handicap and Prevention. In *Major Mental Handicap: Methods and Costs of Prevention.* Ciba Foundation Symposium 59. New York: Elsevier, Excerpta Medica.

Chapman, C. 1976. Nursing—A Cost-Benefit Analysis. *Roy. Soc. Health J.* 96:208.

Charles, E., Jr. et al. 1974. Spinal Cord Injury: A Cost Benefit Analysis of Alternative Treatment Models. *Paraplegia* 12:222.

Charles, E. J. et al. 1978. Economics of the Coronary Artery Bypass. Paper read at the Health Economics Research Organization, American Economic Association Annual Meeting, Chicago, Illinois.

Chawla, M. and Steinhardt, B. 1975. Episode of Care Accounting Methodology for a Cost-Effectiveness Approach to Quality Assurance in a HMO. Unpublished paper. PHS-HSM-110-73-402. Bethesda, Md.: Public Health Service.

Chen, M. et al. 1976. Maximizing Health System Output With Politcal and Administrative Constraints Using Mathematical Programming. *Inquiry* 13:215.

Christie, D. 1977. Screening for Breast Cancer: The Role of Mammography. *Med. J. Aust.* 2:398.

Chung, Y. et al. 1980. A Cost-Benefit Analysis of Fieldwork Education in Occupational Therapy. *Inquiry* 17:216.

Civetta, J. 1973. The Inverse Relationship Between Cost and Survival. *J. Surg. Res.* 14:265.

Clayman, C. 1980. Mass Screening: Is It Cost-Effective? *JAMA* 243:2067.

Cochrane, A. 1972. *Effectiveness and Efficiency: Random Reflections on Health Services.* London: Burgess & Son, Nuffield Provincial Hospitals Trust.

Cohen, J. 1973. On Determining the Cost of Radiation Exposure to Populations for Purposes of Cost-Benefit Analysis. *Health Phys.* 25:527.

Cohen, J. et al. 1971. Benefit-Cost Analysis for Mental Retardation Programs, Theoretical Considerations and a Model for Application. Unpublished paper. Ann Arbor: University of Michigan, Institute for the Study of Mental Retardation and Related Disabilities.

Cohn, E. 1972. Assessment of Malaria Eradication Costs and Benefits. *Amer. J. Trop. Med. Hyg.* 21:663.

————. 1973. Assessing the Costs and Benefits of Anti-Malaria Programs: The Indian Experience. *Amer. J. Pub. Health* 63:1086.

Cohodes, D. n.d. *Listening to Babies: Benefit-Cost Analysis and Its Application to Fetal Monitoring.* Cambridge, Mass.: Urban Systems Research and Engineering.

Cole, P. 1976. Elective Hysterectomy: Pro and Con. *New Engl. J. Med.* 295:264.

Collen, M. 1980. Biofeedback (A Technology Assessment of a New Treatment Modality). Unpublished paper. Medical Methods Research, The Permante Medical Group.

Collen, M. et al. 1969. Cost Analysis of a Multiphasic Screening Program. *New Engl. J. Med.* 280:1043.

Collen, M. et al. 1970. Dollar Cost Per Positive Test for Automated Multiphasic Screening. *New Engl. J. Med.* 283:459.

Collen M. et al. 1973. Multiphasic Checkup Evaluation Study: Preliminary Cost Benefit Analysis for Middle Aged Men. *Prevent. Med.* 2:236.

Collen, M. et al. 1977. Cost Analysis of Alternative Health Examination Modes. *Arch. Intern. Med.* 137:73.

Collis, P. et al. 1973. Adenovirus Vaccines in Military Recruit Populations: A Cost-Benefit Analysis. *J. Infect. Dis.* 128:745.

Committee for the Study of Inborn Errors of Metabolism. 1975. An Economic Perspective on Evaluating Screening Programs. In *Genetic Screening: Programs, Principles, and Research.* Washington, D.C.: National Research Council.

*Committee on Principles of Decision Making for Regulating Chemicals in the Environment, Commission on Natural Resources. 1975. *Decision Making for Regulating Chemicals in the Environment.* Washington, D.C.: National Academy of Sciences.

Conley, R. 1975a. *The Economics of Vocational Rehabilitation.* Baltimore: Johns Hopkins Univ. Press.

————. 1975b. Issues in Benefit-Cost Analyses of the Vocational Rehabilitation Program. *Amer. Rehab.* 1:19.

————. 1976. Mental Retardation: An Economist's Approach. *Ment. Retard.* 14:20.

Conley, R. and Milunsky, A. 1975. The Economics of Prenatal Genetic Diagnosis. In *The Prevention of Genetic Disease and Mental Retardation,* ed. A. Milunsky. Philadelphia: Saunders.

*Cooper, B. and Rice, D. 1976. The Economic Cost of Illness Revisited. *Soc. Sec. Bull.* 39:21.

Cost-Effective Health Care. 1976. *Nurs. Times* 72:119.

Cost-Effectiveness of Health Services. 1968. *New Engl. J. Med.* 278:1069.

Cost-Effectiveness Studies. 1978. *Brit. Med. J.* 2:848.

Costs and Benefits. 1974. *Lancet* 2:7889.

Costs and Benefits of Hysterectomy. 1976. *New Engl. J. Med.* 295:1085.

Coyne, J. 1980. Multihospital System Types: Comparing Costs and Occupancy. *Hosp. Prog.* 61:50.

Crabtree, M. 1978. Application of Cost-Benefit Analysis to Clinical Nursing Practice: A Comparison of Individual and Group Preoperative Teaching. *J. Nurs. Admin.* 8:11.

Creese, A. et al. 1977. Hospital or Home Care for the Severely Disabled: A Cost Comparison. *Brit. J. Prevent. Soc. Med.* 31:116.

Cretin, S. 1977. Cost-Benefit Analysis of Treatment and Prevention of Myocardial Infarction. *Health Serv. Res.* 12:174.

Criley, J. et al. 1975. Mobile Emergency Care Units: Implementation and Justification. *Adv. Cardiol.* 15:9.

Cromwell, J. and Gertman, P. 1977. The Early Detection of Cancer: Some Economic Issues. Paper read at a conference of the American Society of Preventive Oncology, New York.

*Cromwell, J. et al. 1975. *Incentives and Decisions Underlying Hospitals' Adoption and Utilization of Major Capital Equipment.* DHEW contract no. HSM 110-73-513. Cambridge, Mass.: ABT Associates.

Crystal, R. and Brewster, A. 1966. Cost-Benefit and Cost-Effectiveness Analyses in Health Field: An Introduction. *Inquiry* 3:3.

Culyer, A. and Maynard, A. 1981. Cost-Effectiveness of Duodenal Ulcer Treatment. *Soc. Sci. Med.* 15C:3.

Cuzacq, G. and Glass, R. 1972. The Projected Financial Savings in Dental Restorative Treatment: The Result of Consuming Fluoridated Water. *J. Pub. Health Dent.* 32:52.

Dales, L. et al. 1979. Evaluating Periodic Multiphasic Health Checkups: A Controlled Trial. *J. Chron. Dis.* 32:385.

Davies, G. 1973a. Fluoride in the Prevention of Dental Caries: A Tentative Cost-Benefit Analysis; Part 1: The Effect of Fluoridation on Dental Caries and Dental Treatment. *Brit. Dent. J.* 135:79.

————. 1973b. Fluoride in the Prevention of Dental Caries: A Tentative Cost-Benefit Analysis; Part 2: Cost-Benefits of Fluoridation. *Brit. Dent. J.* 135:131.

_____. 1973c. Fluoride in the Prevention of Dental Caries: A Tentative Cost-Benefit Analysis; Part 3: School Fluoridation. *Brit. Dent. J.* 135:173.

_____. 1973d. Fluoride in the Prevention of Dental Caries: A Tentative Cost-Benefit Analysis; Part 4: Fluoridation Tablets. *Brit. Dent. J.* 135:233.

_____. 1973e. Fluoride in the Prevention of Dental Caries: A Tentative Cost-Benefit Analysis; Part 5: The Cost-Effectiveness of Professionally-Administered Topical Applications of Fluoride Solutions. *Brit. Dent. J.* 135:293.

_____. 1973f. Fluoride in the Prevention of Dental Caries: A Tentative Cost-Benefit Analysis; Part 6: The Cost-Benefits of Professionally-Administered Topical Applications of Fluoride Solutions. *Brit. Dent. J.* 135:333.

Dawson, P. et al. 1976. Cost-Effectiveness of Screening Children in Housing Projects. *Amer. J. Pub. Health* 66:1192.

Dawson, P. et al. 1979. Cost Effectiveness of Screening Children in Health Centers. *Pub. Health Rep.* 94:362.

Deane, R. and Ulene, A. 1977. Hysterectomy or Tubal Ligation for Sterilization: A Cost-Effectiveness Analysis. *Inquiry* 14:73.

Deinard, A. et al. 1977. Screening of a High-Risk Ambulatory Female Population for Urinary Tract Infection: A Cost-Effectiveness Study. *Minn. Med.* 60:123.

delBueno, D. et al. 1980. How Cost-Effective is Your Staff Development Program? *J. Nurs. Admin.* 10:31.

Desimone, A. 1974-75. Individualizing Rehab Plans for Cost-Effective Gains. *Soc. Rehab. Rec.* 2:24.

Dhillon, W. and Bennett, A. 1975. A Cost-Performance Analysis of Alternative Manpower Technology Combinations for Delivering Primary Health Care. Unpublished paper. McLean, Va.: Mitre Corp.

Dickhaus, E. 1974. Economic Evaluation of Missouri Automated Radiology System, MARS: A Case Study. Dissertation, William Woods College, Fulton, Missouri.

Dickinson., L. 1972. Evaluation of the Effectiveness of Cytologic Screening for Cervical Cancer: Cost-Benefit Analysis. *Mayo Clin. Proc.* 47:550.

Dittman, D. and Smith, K. 1979. Consideration of Benefits and Costs: A Conceptual Framework for the Health Planner. *Health Care Man. Rev.* 4:45.

Doberneck, R. 1980. Breast Biopsy: A Study of Cost-Effectiveness. *Amer. Surg.* 192:152.

Dodge, W. 1977. Cost Effectiveness of Renal Disease Screening. *Amer. J. Dis. Child.* 131:1274.

Doherty, N. and Hicks, B. 1977. Cost-Effectiveness Analysis and Alternative Health Care Programs for the Elderly. *Health Serv. Res.* 12:190.

Doherty, N., and Powell, E. 1974. Effects of Age and Years of Exposure on the Economic Benefits of Fluoridation. *J. Dent. Res.* 53:912.

Doherty, N. et al. 1975. The Use of Cost-Effectiveness Analysis in Geriatric Day Care. *Gerontologist* 15:412.

*Donabedian, A. 1969. Evaluating the Quality of Medical Care. In *Program Evaluation in the Health Fields*, ed. H. Schulberg, et al. New York: Behavioral Publications.

Donabedian, A. et al. 1977. The Numerology of Utilization Control Revisited: When To Recertify. *Inquiry* 14:96.

Donner, E. 1977. Cost-Benefit Evaluation of Alternative Hospital Structures. In *Systems Science in Health Care*, ed. A. Coblenta and J. Walter. London: Taylor and Francis.

Doyle, L. et al. 1978. Attacking the Cost Crisis. *Int. Med. J.* 153:298.

Dunlop, D. 1975. Benefit-Cost Analysis: A Review of Its Applicability in Policy Analysis for Delivering Health Services. *Soc. Sci. Med.* 9:133.

Dyckman, Z. 1973. A Cost-Benefit Analysis of Federal Support for Medical Education. Paper read at an Engineering Foundation Conference, South Berwick, Maine, August 19–24.

*Eastaugh, S. 1981. *Medical Economics and Health Finance*, Boston, Mass.: Auburn House.

Eddy, D. 1978. Rationale for the Cancer Screening Benefits Program Screening Policies: Implementation Plan, Part III. Paper read at the National Cancer Institute, Blue Cross Association, Chicago, Illinois.

—————. 1979. Measuring the Effectiveness of Therapeutic Surgical Procedures: A Master Plan. In *Medical Technology Research Priorities*, ed. J. Wagner. Washington, D.C.: Urban Institute.

—————. 1980a. The ACS Report on the Cancer-Related Health Checkup: Recommendations and Rationale. Report to the American Cancer Society, New York, New York.

—————. 1980b. *Screening for Cancer: Theory, Analysis, and Design.* Englewood Cliffs, N.J.: Prentice-Hall.

—————. 1981. Screening for Colon Cancer: A Technology Assessment (OTA-BP-H-9(3)). In *The Implications of Cost-Effectiveness Analysis of Medical Technology; Background Paper no. 2: Case Studies of Medical Technologies.* Washington, D.C.: Government Printing Office.

Eden, H. and Eden, M., eds. 1981. *Microcomputers in Patient Care.* Park Ridge, N.J.: Noyes Medical Publications.

*Egdahl, R. and Gertman, P. 1978. *Technology and the Quality of Health Care.* Germantown, Md.: Aspen.

Ekblom, M. et al. 1978. Costs and Benefits of Measles Vaccination in Finland. *Scand. J. Soc. Med.* 6:111.

Elo, O. n.d. Health and Economic Consequences of Rubella. *Acta Univ. Tamp.* 60:27.

Emlet, H., Jr. 1969. Definition of Cost Analysis, Cost-Effectiveness Analysis, and Cost-Benefit Analysis in Medicine. Unpublished paper. Falls Church, Va.: Analytic Services, Inc.

Emlet, H., J. et al. 1968. Use of Cost-Benefit Analysis in Solutions to National Health Problems. Unpublished paper. Falls Church, Va.: Analytic Services, Inc.

Emlet, H., Jr. et al. 1973. Estimated Health Benefits and Cost of Post-Onset Care for Stroke. Unpublished paper. Arlington, Va.: Analytic Services, Inc.

*Enthoven, A. 1978. Consumer-Choice Health Plan. *New Engl. J. Med.* 298:650 and 709.

Evans, W. 1977. *Cost-Effectiveness Studies.* National Health Watch, Inc.

Evens, R. and Jost, R. 1976. Economic Analysis of Computed Tomography Unit. *Amer. J. Roentgenol.* 127:191.

—————. 1977. The Cranial Efficacy and Cost Analysis of Cranial Computed Tomography and the Radionuclide Brain Scan. *Sem. Nucl. Med.* 2:129.

—————. 1978. Economic Analysis of Body Computed Tomography Units Including Data on Utilization. *Radiology* 127:151.

Evens, R. et al. 1977a. The Clinical Efficacy and Cost Analysis of Cranial Computed Tomography and the Radionuclide Brain Scan. *Sem. Nucl. Med.* 7:129.

Evens, R. et al. 1977b. Utilization, Reliability, and Cost Effectiveness of Cranial Computed Tomography in Evaluating Pseudotumor Cerebri. *Amer. J. Roentgenol.* 129:263.

Evens, R. et al. 1979a. Utilization of Body Computed Tomography Units: In Installations With Greater Than One-and-a-Half Years' Experience. *Radiology* 131:695.

Evens, R. et al. 1979b. Utilization of Head Computed Tomography Units: In Installations With Greater Than Two-and-a-Half Years' Experience. *Radiology* 131:691.

Fabricius, J. 1978. A Cost Benefit Analysis of Different Types of Pacemakers. *Scand. J. Thor. Cardiov. Surg.* 22(suppl.): 35.

*Fanshel, S. and Bush, J. 1970. A Health Status Index and Its Application to Health-Services Outcomes. *Oper. Res.* 18:1021.

Farber, M. and Finkelstein, S. 1978. A Cost Benefit Analysis of a Mandatory Premarital Rubella-Antibody Screening Program. *New Engl. J. Med.* 300:856.

Fast, J. 1978. Feasibility Study for the Evaluation of Methodologies for Cost-Benefit Analysis of Restoration Services in Rehabilitation. Unpublished paper. Falls Church, Va.

Feigenson, J. 1979. Stroke Rehabilitation: Effectiveness, Benefits, and Cost, Some Practical Considerations. *Stroke* 10:1.

Feigenson, J. et al. 1978. A Comparison of Outcome and Cost for Stroke Patients in Academic and Community Hospital Centers. *JAMA* 240:1878.

Fein, R. 1958. *Economics of Mental Illness.* New York: Basic Books.

_____. 1976. On Measuring Economic Benefits of Health Programs. In *Ethics and Health Policy,* ed. R. Veach and R. Branson. Cambridge, Mass.: Ballinger.

_____. 1977. But, On the Other Hand: High Blood Pressure, Economics and Equity. *New Engl. J. Med.* 296:751.

Feingold, A. 1975. Cost Effectiveness of Screening for Tuberculosis in a General Medical Clinic. *Pub. Health Rep.* 90:544.

Felch, W. 1976. The Routine Physical and Examination—Opiate of the Masses. Is it Worth the Cost? An Overview of the Problem. *J. Tenn. Med. Assoc.* 69:177.

Feldstein, M. 1966. Measuring the Costs and Benefits of Health Services. Copenhagen: World Health Organization.

*_____. 1971a. A New Approach to National Health Insurance. *Pub. Interest* 23:93.

*_____. 1971b. *The Rising Cost of Hospital Care.* Washington, D.C.: Information Resources Press.

Feldstein, P. 1974. Financing Hypertension: The Costs and Benefits of Government Intervention. Unpublished paper. The Hypertension Coordinating and Planning Corporation of Southwestern Michigan.

*_____. 1977. *Health Associations and the Demand for Legislation: The Political Economy of Health.* Cambridge, Mass.: Ballinger.

*_____. 1979. *Health Care Economics.* New York: Wiley.

Fenwick, A. 1972. The Costs and a Cost-Benefit Analysis of an S. Mansoni Control Programme on an Irrigated Sugar Estate in Northern Tanzania. *Bull. WHO* 47:573.

Ferguson, R. 1975. Cost and Yield of the Hypertensive Evaluation: Experience of a Community-Based Referral Clinic. *Ann. Intern. Med.* 82:761.

Fernandez, P. 1972. Costs and Benefits of Rehabilitation of Heroin Addicts. Dissertation, Claremont Men's College, Claremont, California.

Field, H. and Jong, A. 1971. Cost Effectiveness of Bussing Pupils to a Dental Clinic. *HSMHA Health Rep.* 86:222.

Fielding, J. 1979. Preventive Medicine and the Bottom Line. *J. Med.* 21:79.

Fineberg, H. 1978. Life, Death . . . and Dollars. *Sciences* 18:30.

*_____. 1979. Clinical Chemistries: The High Cost of Low-Cost Diagnostic Tests. In *Medical Technology: The Culprit Behind Health Care Costs?* ed. S. Altman and R. Blendon. DHEW Publication no. (PHS) 79-3216. Washington, D.C.: Government Printing Office.

Fineberg, H. and Pearlman, L. 1981. Benefit and Cost Analysis of Medical Interventions: The Case of Cimetidine and Peptic Ulcer Disease (OTA-BP-H-9(11)). In *The Implications of Cost-Effectiveness Analysis of Medical Technology; Background Paper no. 2: Case Studies of Medical Technologies.* Washington, D.C.: Government Printing Office.

Finkler, S. 1979. Cost-Effectiveness of Regionalization: the Heart Surgery Example. *Inquiry* 16:264.

Fitzpatrick, G. et al. 1977. Cost-Effectiveness of Cholecystectomy for Silent Gallstones. In *Costs, Risks, and Benefits of Surgery,* ed. J. Bunker et al. New York: Oxford Univ. Press.

Fitzpatrick, P. 1974. Cost-Effectiveness in Cancer. *Canad. Med. Assoc. J.* 111:652.

Flagle, C. 1976. Some Approaches to Cost-Benefit Analysis and Evaluation in Cardiovascular Disease. *Cardiov. Res. Cent. Bull.* 15:29.

Fofar, J. 1979. Effectiveness and Cost in the Pediatric Service. *Scot. Med. J.* 24:233.

Foley, H. et al. 1973. The Cost-Effectiveness of a Mental Center: An Experiment. Paper read at an Engineering Foundation Conference, South Berwick, Me., August 19-24.

Foltz, A. and Kelsey, J. 1978. The Annual Pap Test: A Dubious Policy Success. *Milbank Mem. Fund Q.* 56:426.

Foote, A. et al. 1977. Controlling Hypertension: A Cost-Effective Model. *Prevent. Med.* 6:319.

Forst, B. 1971. The Grisly Analytics of Death, Disability and Disbursements. Paper read at the 40th National Meeting of the Operations Research Society of America, Anaheim, Ca., October.

_____. 1973. An Analysis of Alternative Periodic Health Examination Strategies. In *Benefit-Cost and Policy Analysis—1972,* ed. W. Niskanen et al. Chicago: Aldine.

Francis, G. et al. 1976. The Economic Benefits of Early Diagnosis and Training for Handicapped Children. *Amer. Correct. Ther. J.* 30:47.

Fraser, R. 1971. Canadian Hospital Costs and Efficacy. Unpublished paper. Ottawa: Information Canada.

*Freeland, M. et al. 1980. Projections of National Health Expenditures, 1980, 1985, and 1990. *Health Care Finan. Rev.* 1(3):1.

Freeman, R. et al. 1976. Economic Cost of Pulmonary Emphysema: Implications for Policy on Smoking and Health. *Inquiry* 13:15.

Freireich, E. 1980. Can We Afford to Treat Acute Leukemia? *New Engl. J. Med.* 302:1084.

*Friedman, M. 1962. *Capitalism and Freedom.* Chicago: Univ. of Chicago Press.

*Fuchs, V. 1974. *Who Shall Live? Health, Economics, and Social Choice.* New York: Basic Books.

*_____. 1976. The Earnings of Allied Health Personnel—Are Health Workers Underpaid? *Explor. Econ. Res.* 3:408.

*_____. 1978. The Supply of Surgeons and the Demand for Operations. *J. Hum. Res.* 13(suppl.):35.

_____. 1980. What is CBA/CEA and Why Are They Doing This to Us? *New Engl. J. Med.* 303:937.

Fudenberg, H. 1972. The Dollar Benefits of Biomedical Research: A Cost Analysis. *J. Lab. Clin. Med.* 70:353.

Fulchiero, A. et al. 1978. Can PSROs Be Cost Effective? *New Engl. J. Med.* 299:574.

Galliher, H. 1976. Cost-Effective Planned Lifetime Schedule of Pap Smears: Estimated Maximal Potentials. Unpublished paper. Ann Arbor: University of Michigan, Department of Industrial and Operations Engineering.

Garrison, L. 1978. Studies in the Economics of Surgery. Ph.D. dissertation, Stanford University, Palo Alto, California.

Geiser, E. and Menz, F. 1976. The Effectiveness of Public Dental Care Programs. *Med. Care* 14:189.

Gelfand, D. et al. 1978. Costs of Gastrointestinal Examinations: A Comparative Study. *Gastroint. Radiol.* 3:135.

Geller, N. and Yockmowitz, M. 1975. Regional Planning of Maternity Services. *Health Serv. Res.* 10:63.

Gellman, D. 1974. Cost-Benefit in Health Care: We Need To Know Much More. *Canad. Med. Assoc. J.* 111:998.

Gelman, C. 1970. Health Economics. The Cost of Illness, Cost-Benefit and Cost-Effectiveness Analysis of Screening Programs: Cost Analysis. In *Multiphasic Health Testing—Screening Systems State of the Art.* New York: American Health Foundation.

Gempel, P. et al. 1977. *Comparative Cost Analysis: Computed Tomography vs. Alternative Diagnostic Procedures, 1977–1980.* Cambridge, Mass.: Arthur D. Little.

Giauque, W. 1972. Prevention and Treatment of Streptococcal Sore Throat and Rheumatic Fever—A Decision Theoretic Approach. Dissertation, Harvard University, Cambridge, Massachusetts.

Gibson, W. 1980. The Cost of Not Doing Medical Research. *JAMA* 244:1817.

Gilbert, J. et al. 1967. Progress in Surgery and Anesthesia: An Evaluation of Therapy. In *Cost–Effectiveness Analysis: New Approaches in Decisionmaking,* ed. J. Goldman. Washington, D.C.: Praeger.

Gill, R. 1974. Emergency Ambulance Service (A) and (B). In *Cases in Urban Management,* ed. J. Russell. Cambridge, Mass.: MIT Press.

Gillum, R. et al. 1978. Screening for Hypertension: A Rational Approach. *J. Comm. Health* 4:67.

Ginsberg, A. and Offsend, F. 1968. An Application of Decision Theory to a Medical Diagnosis-Treatment Problem. *IEEE Trans. Sys. Sci. Cyb.* 4:355.

Ginsberg, G. et al. 1977. Costs and Benefits of Behavioral Psychotherapy: A Pilot Study of Neurotics Treated by Nurse-Therapists. *Psychol. Med.* 7:685.

Glasgow, J. 1970. Cost-Benefit and Cost-Effectiveness Analyses in the Health Field. Paper read at the National Regional Medical Programs Conference and Workshop on Evaluation, University of Chicago Center for Continuing Education, Chicago, Illinois, September 28–30.

Glass, N. 1973. Cost-Benefit Analysis and Health Services. *Health Trends* 5:51.

———. 1975. Economic Aspects of the Prevention of Down's Syndrome. In *Systems Aspects of Health Planning.* ed. N. Bailey and M. Thompson, Amsterdam: Elsevier–North Holland Publishing Co.

Glass, N. and Russell, I. 1974. Proceedings: Cost-Benefit Analysis in the Health Service—A Case Study of Elective Herniorrhaphy. *Brit. J. Prevent. Soc. Med.* 28:68.

Glass, N. et al. 1977. Cost-Benefit Analysis and the Evaluation of Psychiatric Services. *Psychol. Med.* 7:701.

Godfrey, A. 1980. The Cost of School Dental Care—Some Thoughts on Economic Analysis. *Aust. Dent. J.* 25:20.

Goldhaber, S. et al. 1974. Effects of the Fiberoptic Laparoscope and Colonoscope on Morbidity and Cost. *Ann. Surg.* 179:160.

Goldschmidt, P. 1976. A Cost-Effectiveness Model for Evaluating Health Care Programs: Application to Drug Abuse Treatment. *Inquiry* 13:29.

Gorry, G. et al. 1977. Cost-Effectiveness of Cardiopulmonary Resuscitation Training Programs. *Health Serv. Res.* 12:30.

Grab, B. and Cvjetanovic, B. 1971. Simple Method for Rough Determination of the Cost-Benefit Balance Point of Immunization Programmes. *Bull. WHO* 45:536.

*Grabowski, H. 1976. *Drug Regulation and Innovation: Empirical Evidence and Policy Options*. Washington, D.C.: American Enterprise Institute.

Gragono, A. 1977. Temporal Units for Expressing Cost Effectiveness. *New Engl. J. Med.* 297:284.

Grainger, R. 1973. Cost-Benefit Analysis: Application to Dental Services. *J. Canad. Dent. Assoc.* 39:693.

*Gramlich, E. 1981. *Benefit-Cost Analysis of Government Programs*. Englewood Cliffs, N.J.: Prentice-Hall.

Grande, P. et al. 1980. Optimal Diagnosis in Acute Myocardial Infarction. A Cost-Effectiveness Study. *Circulation* 61:723.

Gravelle, H. 1976. The Economic Evaluation of Screening for Breast Cancer: A Tentative Methodology.

Green, J. 1977. Cost-Benefit Analysis of Surgery: Some Additional Caveats and Interpretations. In *Costs, Risks, and Benefits of Surgery*, ed. J. Bunker et al. New York: Oxford Univ. Press.

*_____. 1978. Physician-Induced Demand for Medical Care. *J. Hum. Res.* 13(suppl.):21.

Green, L. 1974. Toward Cost-Benefit Evaluations of Health Education: Some Concepts, Methods, and Examples. *Health Educ. Monogr.* 2(suppl.):34.

_____. 1976. The Potential of Health Education Includes Cost Effectiveness. *Hospitals* 50:57.

Green, V. 1970. Cost-Effectiveness and Hospital Environmental Sanitation. *Canad. Hosp.* 47:34.

Greenwood, C. et al. 1979. Selecting a Cost-Effective Screening Measure for the Assessment of Preschool Social Withdrawal. *J. Appl. Behav. Anal.* 12:639.

Griffith, J. and Chernow, R. 1977. Cost-Effective Acute Care Facilities Planning in Michigan. *Inquiry* 14:229.

Griner, P. 1973. Treatment of Acute Pulmonary Edema: Conventional or Intensive Care? *Ann. Intern. Med.* 182:1102.

_____. 1976. Cost Versus Effectiveness of Laboratory Studies. *J. Tenn. Med. Assoc.* 69:179.

Grosse, R. 1970. Problems of Resource Allocation in Health. In *Public Expenditures and Policy Analysis*, ed. R. Haveman and J. Margolis. Chicago: Markham.

_____. 1971. Cost-Benefit Analysis in Disease Control Programs. In *Cost-Benefit Analysis*, ed. M. Kendall. New York: American Elsevier.

_____. 1972a. Analysis in Health Planning. In *Analysis of Public Systems*, ed. A. Drake, et al. Cambridge, Mass.: MIT Press.

_____. 1972b. Cost-Benefit Analysis of Health Services. *Ann. Amer. Acad. Polit. Soc. Sci.* 399:89.

*Grossman, R. 1981. A Review of Physician Cost Containment Strategies and Implications for the Future. Unpublished paper. Univerity of Michigan, Ann Arbor.

Guillette, W. et al. 1978. Day Hospitalization as a Cost Effective Alternative to Inpatient Care: A Pilot Study. *Hosp. Comm. Psychol.* 29:525.

Gumbhir, A. and Brown, W. 1975. Cost-Benefit Analysis of Unit Dose Drug Distribution Systems: A Conceptual Approach. *Hosp. Topics* 53:35.

Gunn, A. 1978. Cost Effectiveness? It's Time to Blow the Whistle. *Crit. Care Med.* 6:352.

Haber, Z. and Leatherwood, E., Jr. 1969. A Dental Program for Head Start Children in New York City: A Retrospective Study of Utilization and Costs. *Med. Care* 7:281.

Hagard, S. and Carter, F. 1976a. Preventing the Birth of Infants With Down's Syndrome: A Cost-Benefit Analysis. *Brit. Med. J.* 1:753.

Hagard, S. et al. 1976b. Screening for Spina Bifida Cystica: A Cost-Benefit Analysis. *Brit. J. Prevent. Soc. Med.* 30:40.

Hallstrom, A. et al. 1981. Modeling the Effectiveness and Cost-Effectiveness of an Emergency Service System. *Soc. Sci. Med.* 15C:13.

Hamilton, J. 1968. A Method for Estimating the Cost, Growth Rate, and Efficiency of Radioisotope Laboratories. *Amer. J. Med. Technol.* 34:473.

Hannan, E. and Graham, J. 1978. A Cost-Benefit Study of a Hypertension Screening and Treatment Program at the Work Setting. *Inquiry* 15:345.

Hannan, T. 1975. *The Economics of Methadone Maintenance.* Lexington, Mass.: Lexington Books.

————. 1976. The Benefits and Costs of Methadone Maintenance. *Pub. Pol.* 24:197.

Harder, E. 1977. Searching for Cost-Effective Measures That Also Improve Care. *Hospitals* 51:155.

Harris, G. 1977. Introduction to Cost-Benefit Analysis Applied to New Health Technologies. Prepared by Arthur D. Little, Inc. Hyattsville, Md.: Health Resources Administration, Bureau of Health Planning and Resources Development.

*Hartunian, N. et al. 1981. *The Incidence and Costs of Cancer, Motor Vehicle Injuries, Coronary Heart Disease, and Stroke: A Comparative Analysis.* Lexington, Mass.: Lexington Books.

Havia, T. and Schuller, H. 1978. The Re-Use of Previously Implanted Pacemakers. *Scand. J. Thor. Cardiov. Surg.* 22(suppl.):33.

*Havighurst, C. 1979. Private Cost Containment. *New Engl. J. Med.* 300:1298.

Hawkins, B. 1978. Cost-Benefit Analysis as a Tool To Evaluate Capital Acquisitions. *Hospitals* 52:60.

Hazell, J. et al. 1972. Intermediate Benefit Analysis—Spencer's Dilemma and School Health Services. *Amer. J. Pub. Health* 62:560.

Heagarty, M. et al. 1970. Some Comparative Costs in Comprehensive Versus Fragmented Pediatric Care. *Pediatrics* 46:596.

Hefner, D. 1979. *A Study to Determine the Cost-Effectiveness of a Restrictive Formulary: The Louisiana Experience.* Washington, D.C.: National Pharmaceutical Council.

Hellinger, F. 1980. Cost-Benefit Analysis of Health Care: Past Applications and Future Prospects. *Inquiry* 17:204.

Henry, F. 1980. Cost Effectiveness. *Ohio State Med. J.* 76:342.

Hertzman, M. et al. 1977. Cost-Benefit Analysis and Alcoholism. *J. Stud. Alcohol.* 38:1371.

Hessel, S. 1977. Perspectives on Benefit-Cost Analysis in Medical Care. *Amer. J. Roentgenol.* 129:753.

Hiatt, H. 1975. Protecting the Medical Commons: Who Is Responsible? *New Engl. J. Med.* 293:235.

———. 1977. Lessons of the Coronary-Bypass Debate. *New Engl. J. Med.* 297:1462.

Hilbert, S. 1977. Prevention. *Amer. J. Pub. Health* 67:35.

*Hodgson, T. and Meiners, M. 1979. *Guidelines for Public Health Service Cost of Illness Studies.* Hyattsville, Md.: National Center for Health Services Research.

Hoffman, K. et al. 1975. The "Cost-Effectiveness" of Sim One. *J. Med. Educ.* 50:1127.

Hohn, A. et al. 1980. Proficiency and Cost-Effectiveness in Pediatric Hospitals. *Amer. Heart J.* 99:403.

Holahan, J. 1970. The Economics of Drug Addiction and Control in Washington, D.C.: A Model for Estimation of Costs and Benefits of Rehabilitation. Unpublished paper. Washington, D.C.: District of Columbia Department of Corrections.

———. 1973. Measuring Benefits From Alternative Heroin Policies. *Nat. Conf. Meth. Treat. Proc.* 2:1219.

Holler, A. 1976. Risks Versus Benefits in Breast Cancer Diagnosis. *CA-A Cancer J. Clin.* 26:63.

Holmin, T. et al. 1980. Selective or Routine Intraoperative Cholangiography: A Cost-Effectiveness Analysis. *World J. Surg.* 4:315.

Holtman, A. 1965. Alcoholism and the Economic Value of a Man. *Rev. Soc. Ecol.* 23:143.

Hookey, P. 1979. Cost-Benefit Evaluation in Primary Health Care. *Health Soc. Work* 4:151.

Horowitz, H. et al. 1979. Methods of Assessing the Cost-Effectiveness of Caries Preventive Agents and Procedures. *Int. Dent. J.* 29:106.

*Hu, T. and Sandifer, F. 1981. Synthesis of Cost-of-Illness Methodology. National Center for Health Services Research, PHS Contract no. 233-79-3010. Unpublished paper. Washington, D.C.: Georgetown University, Public Service Laboratory.

Hu, T. et al. 1978. Cost-Effectiveness Study of Drug Prevention Programs. Unpublished paper. Pennsylvania State University, Institute for Policy and Research and Evaluation.

*Hudson, J. and Braslow, J. 1979. Cost Containment Education Efforts in United States Medical Schools. *J. Med. Educ.* 54:835.

Huggins, D. 1980. An Approach to Cost-Effectiveness. *Ohio State Med. J.* 76:10.

*Hughes, E. et al. 1978. *Hospital Cost Containment Programs: A Policy Analysis.* Cambridge, Mass.: Ballinger.

Hughes, J. 1974. A Method To Determine the Cost Effectiveness of Occupational Health Programs. *J. Occup. Med.* 16:156.

Hughes, J. 1974. A Method To determine the Cost Effectiveness of Occupational Health Programs. *J. Occup. Med.* 16:156.

Hur, D. et al. 1979. Is ECG Monitoring in the Operating Room Cost Effective? *Biotelem. Patient Monit.* 6:200.

Hurtado, A. et al. 1972. The Utilization and Cost of Home Care Facility Services in a Comprehensive, Prepaid Group Practice Program. *Med. Care* 10:8.

Huston, M. 1979. Cost-Effectiveness: School Health Programs. *Ohio State Med. J.* 75:308.

Ingalls, J. et al. 1978. Attacking the Cost Crisis. *Int. Med. J.* 153:125.

Inman, R. 1978. On the Benefits and Costs of Genetic Screening. *Amer. J. Hum. Genet.* 30:219.

Jackson, M. et al. 1978. Elective Hysterectomy: A Cost-Benefit Analysis. *Inquiry* 15:275.

Jackson, S. and Ward, D. 1976. Prevention of Institutionalization: A Cost-Effectiveness Model of Community Based Alternatives. Paper read at the Annual Meeting of the American Public Health Association, Miami Beach, Florida, October 17-21.

*Jacobs, P. 1980. *The Economics of Health and Medical Care: An Introduction.* Baltimore: University Park Press.

Jaffe, F. et al. 1977. Short-Term Benefits and Costs of U.S. Family Planning Programs, 1970-1975. *Fam. Plan. Perspect.* 9:77.

Janke, T. 1980. Cost Accounting: The Vital Link to Cost Effectiveness. *J. Amer. Diet. Assoc.* 77:167.

Jeffers, J. and Johnson, J. 1973. A Cost-Benefit Analysis of Heroin Abuse Control Programs. Bureau of Business and Economic Research working paper. University of Iowa, Iowa City.

Joehnk, M. and McGrail, G. 1977. Benefit-Cost Ratios for Family Practice Residency Centers. *Man. Account.* 58:41.

Joglekar, P. 1980. Cost-Benefit Studies of Health Care Programs: Choosing Methods for Desired Results. Paper read at the Joint National Meeting of the Operations Research Society of America, Washington, D.C., May.

Johns, M. et al. 1976. *Benefit-Cost Analysis of Alcoholism Treatment Centers.* Rockville, Md.: National Institute on Alcohol Abuse and Alcoholism.

Jonas, A. 1976. Cost-Effectiveness of Developing Animal Models. In *Animal Models of Thrombosis and Hemorrhagic Diseases.* Bethesda, Md.: National Institutes of Health.

*Jones-Lee, M. 1976. *The Value of Life: An Economic Analysis.* Chicago: Univ. of Chicago Press.

Jong, A. and Gluck, G. 1974. Factors Influencing the Cost-Effectiveness of Community Health Center Dental Programs in the USA. *Comm. Dent. Oral Epidemiol.* 2:263.

Kagan, A. and Skinner, D. 1978. Detection of Metastatic Disease in the Urologic Patient: An Opinion on Cost Versus Benefit. *J. Urol.* 120:140.

Kane, R. 1978. Societal Values and Modern Medicine: How Do We Measure Costs and Benefits? *J. Comm. Health* 4:97.

Kane, R. et al. 1974. Can Nursing-Home Care Be Cost-Effective? *J. Amer. Geriat. Soc.* 22:265.

Kane, R. et al. 1976. Is Good Nursing-Home Care Feasible? *JAMA* 235:516.

*Kaplan, R. et al. 1976. Health Status: Types of Validity for an Index of Well-Being. *Health Serv. Res.* 11:478.

*Kaplan, R. et al. 1978. The Reliability, Stability, and Generalizability of a Health Status Index. In *Proceedings of the American Statistical Association, Social Statistics Section, Part II.* Washington, D.C.: American Statistical Association.

*Kaplan, R. et al. 1979. Health Status Index: Category Rating Versus Magnitude Estimation for Measuring Levels of Well-Being. *Med. Care* 17: 501.

Kaser, M. 1974. Choice of Technique. In *The Economics of Health and Medical Care,* ed. M. Perlman. New York: Wiley.

*Keeler, E. et al. 1976. *The Demand for Supplementary Health Insurance, or Do Deductibles Matter?* Publication no. R-1958-HEW. Santa Monica, Calif.: RAND Corp.

Keith, L. et al. 1975. Gonorrhea Detection in a Family Planning Clinic: A Cost-Benefit Analysis of 2,000 Triplicate Cultures. *Amer. J. Obstet. Gyn.* 121:399.

Kirby, W. 1971. Cost-Benefit Analysis in a Large Health Care System. In *Cost-Benefit Analysis*, ed. M. Kendall. New York: American Elsevier.

Klarman, H. 1965*a*. *The Economics of Health.* New York: Columbia Univ. Press.

———. 1965*b*. The Socioeconomic Impact of Heart Disease. In *The Second National Conference on Cardiovascular Disease, the Heart and Circulation.* Washington, D.C.: Federation of American Societies for Experimental Biology.

———. 1967. Present Status of Cost-Benefit Analysis in the Health Field. *Amer. J. Pub. Health* 57:1948.

———. 1974*a*. Application of Cost-Benefit Analysis to the Health Services and the Special Case of Technologic Innovation. *Int. J. Health Serv.* 4:325.

———. 1974*b*. Application of Cost-Benefit Analysis to Health Systems Technology. *J. Occup. Med.* 16:172.

———. 1979. Observations on Health Care Technology: Measurement, Analysis, and Policy. In *Medical Technology: The Culprit Behind Health Care Costs?* ed. S. Altman and R. Blendon. DHEW Publication no. (PHS) 79-3216. Washington, D.C.: Government Printing Office.

Klarman, H., and Guzick, D. 1976. Economics of Influenza. In *Influenza: Virus, Vaccines, and Strategy*, ed. P. Selby. New York: Academic Press.

Klarman, H., et al. 1968. Cost Effectiveness Analysis Applied to the Treatment of Chronic Renal Disease. *Med. Care* 6:48.

Knapper, D. and Dungy, C. 1978. Cost-Benefits of Using Practitioners in a School-Based CHDP Program. Paper read at the annual meeting of the American Public Health Association, Los Angeles, California, October 19.

Knaus, W. and Davis, D. 1978. Utilization and Cost-Effectiveness of Cranial Computed Tomography at a University Hospital. *J. Comput. Assist. Tomogr.* 2:209.

Knaus, W. et al. 1981. CT for Headache: Cost-Benefit for Subarachnoid Hemorrhage. *Amer. J. Neuroradiol.* 1:567.

Knobel, R. and Longest, B. 1974. Problems Associated With the Cost-Benefit Analysis Technique in Voluntary Hospitals. *Hosp. Admin.* 19:42.

Knox, E. 1976. Ages and Frequencies for Cervical Cancer Screening. *Brit. J. Cancer* 34:444.

Kodlin, D. 1972. A Note on the Cost-Benefit Problem in Screening for Breast Cancer. *Method. Info. Med.* 11:242.

Koplan, J. et al. 1979. Pertussis Vaccine—An Analysis of Benefits, Risks and Costs. *New Engl. J. Med.* 301:906.

Korenbrot, C. et al. 1981. Elective Hysterectomy: Costs, Risks, and Benefits (OTA-BP-H-9(15)). In *The Implications of Cost-Effectiveness Analysis of Medical Technology; Background Paper no. 2: Case Studies of Medical Technologies.* Washington, D.C.: Government Printing Office.

Kramer, M. 1976. Ethical Issues in Neonatal Intensive Care: An Economic Perspective. In *Ethics of Newborn Intensive Care*, ed. A. Joneson and M. Garland. Berkeley: Institute of Governmental Studies.

Krause, B. et al. 1977. Is Coronary Artery Surgery So Expensive? *New Zeal. Med. J.* 86:570.

Kridel, R. and Winston, D., eds. 1978. *Cost-Effective Medical Care.* Chicago: Resident Physicians Section, American Medical Association.

Kriedel, T. 1980. Cost-Benefit Analysis of Epilepsy Clinics. *Soc. Sci. Med.* 14C:35.

Kristein, M. 1977*a*. Cost Effectiveness of Various Smoking Cessation Methods. Unpublished paper. New York: American Health Foundation.

———. 1977*b*. Economic Issues in Prevention. *Prevent. Med.* 6:252.

_____. 1978. Economics of Secondary Prevention: Screening for Disease—An Example From Colorectal Cancer. Paper read at the American Society of Preventive Oncology, Washington, D.C., March 9.

_____. 1979. Cost-Effectiveness Analysis for HSA Planning. Paper read at the annual meeting of the American Public Health Association, New York, New York, November 7.

_____. n.d. *The Economics of Screening for Colo-Rectal Cancer.* New York: American Health Foundation.

Kristein, M., and Arnold, C. 1978. Mammographic Screening for Breast Cancer—An Economic Analysis. Paper read at the annual meeting of the American Public Health Association, Los Angeles, California, October 17.

_____. 1980. A Mini Cost-Effectiveness Analysis of Mammography as a Procedure for the Mass Screening of Asymptomatic Populations. Paper read at the Annual Western Economic Association, San Diego, California, June 17.

Kristein, M., and Jonas, S. 1980. A Cost-Effectiveness Manual for HSA Planning. Paper prepared for the National Center for Health Services Research, Hyattsville, Maryland.

Kristein, M. et al. 1977. Health Economics and Preventive Care. *Science* 195:457.

Kuschner, J. 1976. A Benefit-Cost Analysis of Nurse Practitioner Training. *Canad. J. Pub. Health* 67:405.

Laguna, J. et al. 1977. Impact of Computerized Tomography in Medical Practice: Cost-Effectiveness Considerations. *Ariz. Med.* 34:344.

Lasdon, G. et al. 1977. Evaluating Cost-Effectiveness Using Episodes of Care. *Med. Care* 15:260.

Lashof, J. 1977. Do Benefits Exceed Costs of Alternatives to Institutional Care? *Geriatrics* 32:33.

Lave, J. and Lave, L. 1977. Measuring the Effectiveness of Prevention: I. *Milbank Mem. Fund. Q.* 55:273.

La Violette, S. 1979. Dollar Benefits, Costs Break Even. *Mod. Health Care* 9:46.

Lavor, J. et al. 1976. Home Health Cost Effectiveness: What Are We Measuring? *Med. Care* 14:866.

Layde, P. et al. 1979. Maternal Serum Alpha-Fetoprotein Screening: A Cost-Benefit Analysis. *Amer. J. Pub. Health* 69:566.

Ledley, R. et al. 1978. Medical Technology and Cost Containment: Two Applications of Operations Research. *Science* 202:979.

Leitch, I. 1968. Value for Money in Health and Welfare: A Local Study of the Home Help Service. *Roy. Soc. Health J.* 88:159.

Leroy, L. and Solkowitz, S. 1981. Costs and Effectiveness of Nurse Practitioners (OTA-BP-H-9(16)). In *The Implications of Cost-Effectiveness Analysis of Medical Technology; Background Paper no. 2: Case Studies of Medical Technologies.* Washington, D.C.: Government Printing Office.

Leslie, A. 1976. A Benefit-Cost Analysis of New York City Heroin Addiction Problems and Programs—1971. In *Analysis of Urban Health Problems,* ed. I. Levinson and J. Weiss. New York: Spectrum.

LeSourd, D. et al. 1968. *Benefit-Cost Analysis of Kidney Disease Programs.* PHS Publication no. 1941. Washington, D.C.: Government Printing Office.

Leveson, I. 1973. Cost-Benefit Analysis and Program Target Populations: The Narcotics Addiction Treatment Case. *Amer. J. Econ. Sociol.* 32:129.

Leveson, I. and Weiss, J. 1976. *Analysis of Urban Health Problems.* New York: Spectrum.

Levin, A. 1968. Cost-Effectiveness in Maternal and Child Health: Implications for Program Planning and Evaluation. *New Engl. J. Med.* 278:1041.

Lewis, D. et al. 1972. Initial Dental Care Time, Cost and Treatment Requirements Under Changing Exposure to Fluoride During Tooth Development. *J. Canad. Dent. Assoc.* 38:140.

Linn, B. et al. 1979. Do Dollars Spent Relate to Outcomes in Burn Care? *Med. Care* 17:835.

Litsios, S. 1976. Developing a Cost and Outcome Evaluation System. *Int. J. Health Serv.* 6:345.

Loewy, E. 1980. Cost Should Not be a Factor in Medical Care. *New Engl. J. Med.* 302:697.

Longest, B. 1978. An Empirical Analysis of the Quality-Cost Relationship. *Hosp. Health. Serv. Admin.* 23:20.

Lubeck, D. and Bunker, J. 1981. The Artificial Heart: Costs, Risks, and Benefits (OTA-BP-H-9(9)). In *The Implications of Cost-Effectiveness Analysis of Medical Technology; Background Paper no. 2: Case Studies of Medical Technologies*, Washington, D.C.: Government Printing Office.

Lucas, S. 1979. Cost Effectiveness: Radiologic Services. *Ohio State Med. J.* 75:290.

Luce, B. 1979. Allocating Costs and Benefits in Disease Prevention–Health Promotion Programs. Paper read at the annual meeting of the American Public Health Association, New York, New York, November.

_____. 1981. Allocating Costs and Benefits in Disease Prevention Programs: An Application to Cervical Cancer Screening (OTA-BP-H-9(7)). In *The Implications of Cost-Effectiveness Analysis of Medical Technology; Background Paper no. 2: Case Studies of Medical Technologies*. Washington, D.C.: Government Printing Office.

Luft, H. 1976. Benefit-Cost Analysis and Public Policy Implementation: From Normative to Positive Analysis. *Pub. Pol.* 24:437.

*_____. 1978. How Do Health Maintenance Organizations Achieve Their "Savings"—Rhetoric and Evidence. *New Engl. J. Med.* 298:1336.

*_____. 1980. Assessing the Evidence on HMO Performance. *Milbank Mem. Fund Q.* 58:501.

McCaffee, K. 1969. The Cost of Mental Health Care Under Changing Treatment Conditions. In *Program Evaluation in the Health Fields*, ed. H. Schulberg et al. New York: Behavioral Publications.

McCarthy, N. 1979. Benefit-Cost and Cost-Effectiveness Analysis: Theory and Application. *Devel. Biol. Stand.* 43:403.

McCombie, F. 1979. Cost-Effectiveness Considerations in Planning a Preventive Dental Programme for British Columbia. *Int. Dent. J.* 29:125.

McGhan, W. et al. 1978. Cost-Benefit and Cost-Effectiveness: Methodologies for Evaluating Innovative Pharmaceutical Services. *Amer. J. Hosp. Pharm.* 35:133.

McGlothlin, W. et al. 1972. Alternative Approaches of Opiate Addiction Control: Costs, Benefits and Potential. Bureau of Narcotics and Dangerous Drugs Report SC10-TR-7, Washington, D.C.: Government Printing Office.

McGregor, M. and Pelletier, G. 1978. Planning of Specialized Health Facilities: Size vs. Cost and Effectiveness in Heart Surgery. *New Engl. J. Med.* 299:179.

Macklin, F. 1976. Mainstreaming: The Cost Issue. *Amer. Ann. Deaf.* 121:364.

McNeil, B. 1976. A Summary of Cost-Effectiveness Calculations in the Diagnosis and Treatment of Hypertensive Renovascular Disease. *Bull. N.Y. Acad. Med.* 52:680.

————. 1978. Rationale for the Use of Bone Scans in Selected Metastatic and Primary Bone Tumors. *Sem. Nucl. Med.* 8:299.

————. 1979. Pitfalls in and Requirements for Evaluations of Diagnostic Technologies. In *Medical Technology*, ed. J. Wagner. DHEW Publication no. (PHS) 79-3254. Washington, D.C.: Government Printing Office.

McNeil, B. and Adelstein, S. 1975. The Value of Case Finding in Hypertensive Renovascular Disease. *New Engl. J. Med.* 293:221.

————. 1976. Determining the Value of Diagnostic and Screening Tests. *J. Nucl. Med.* 117:439.

McNeil, B. et al. 1975*a*. Measures of Clinical Efficacy: Cost-Effectiveness Calculations in the Diagnosis and Treatment of Hypertensive Renovascular Disease. *New Engl. J. Med.* 293:216.

McNeil, B. et al. 1975*b*. Primer on Certain Elements of Medical Decision Making. *New Engl. J. Med.* 293:211.

McNeil, B. et al. 1976. Measures of Clinical Efficacy: III—The Value of the Lung Scan in the Evaluation of Young Patients With Pleuritic Chest Pain. *J. Nucl. Med.* 17:163.

*Maloney, T. and Rogers, D. 1979. Medical Technology—A Different View of the Contentious Debate over Costs. *New Engl. J. Med.* 301:1413.

Mandel, M. 1975. Cost Analysis of Regionalized Versus Decentralized Abortion Programs. *Med. Care* 13:137.

Mani, M. et al. 1976. The Economics of Peritoneal Dialysis: A Cost-Efficiency Study. *Nephron* 17:130.

Marram, G. 1976. The Comparative Costs of Operating a Team and Primary Nursing Unit. *J. Nurs. Admin.* 6:21.

Marram, G. et al. 1975. Comparison of the Cost-Effectiveness of Team and Primary Nursing Care Modalities. Unpublished paper. Boston: New England Deaconess Hospital, Nursing Office.

Marshall, A. 1965. Cost-Benefit Analysis in Health. Unpublished paper. Santa Monica, Calif.: RAND Corp.

Martin, G. and Newman, I. 1973. The Costs and Effects of a Student Health-Aide Program. *J. Amer. Coll. Health Assoc.* 21:237.

Martin, J. 1978. Research Priorities. *Dimen. Health Serv.* 55:8.

Martin, S. et al. 1974. Inputs Into Coronary Care During 30 Years: A Cost-Effectiveness Study. *Ann. Intern. Med.* 81:289.

Marty, A. et al. 1977. The Variation in Hospital Charges: A Problem in Determining Cost-Benefit for Cardiac Surgery. *Ann. Thor. Surg.* 24:409.

*Marvin, K. and Rouse, A. 1970. The Status of PPB in Federal Agencies: A Comparative Perspective. In *Public Expenditures and Policy Analysis*, ed. R. Haveman and J. Margolis. Chicago: Markham.

Mather, H. 1979. Cost-Effective Patient Care. *J. Roy. Coll. Physicians* 13:93.

Mather, H. et al. 1971. Acute Myocardial Infarction: Home and Hospital Treatment. *Brit. Med. J.* 3:334.

Matlack, D. 1974. Cost-Effectiveness of Spinal Cord Injury Center Treatment. *Paraplegia* 12:222.

Maturi, V. 1976. An Automated Cost-Effective HMO. *Pub. Health Rep.* 91:188.

May, P. 1970*a*. Cost-Effectiveness of Mental Health Care: Sex as a Parameter of Cost in the Treatment of Schizophrenia. *Amer. J. Pub. Health* 60:2269.

————. 1970*b*. Cost-Efficiency of Mental Health Delivery System: A Review of the Literature on Hospital Care. *Amer. J. Pub. Health* 60:2060.

_____. 1971*a*. Cost-Efficiency of Mental Health Care: Treatment Method as a Parameter of Cost in the Treatment of Schizophrenia. *Amer. J. Pub. Health* 61:127.

_____. 1971*b*. Cost-Efficiency of Treatments for the Schizophrenic Patient. *Amer. J. Psychiat.* 127:1382.

Maynard, A. 1977. Avarice, Inefficiency and Inequality: An International Health Care Tale. *Int. J. Health Serv.* 7:179.

Menz, F. 1971. Economics of Disease Prevention: Infectious Kidney Disease. *Inquiry* 8:3.

Merck, Sharp and Dohme. n.d. *Vaccine Cost-Benefit Analysis Program.* West Point, Pa.: Merck, Sharp, and Dohme.

*Mervin, K. and Rouse, A. 1970. The Status of PPB in Federal Agencies: A Comparative Perspective. In *Public Expenditures and Policy Analysis*, ed. R. Haveman and J. Margolis. Chicago: Markham.

Michels, R. et al. 1976. Mental Health Services for Students: Cost Benefit and Value. *J. Amer. Coll. Health Assoc.* 24:208.

Mikkelsen, M. et al. 1976. Cost-Benefit Analysis of Prevention of Down's Syndrome. In *Prenatal Diagnosis*, ed. A. Baue. Paris: Institut National de la Sante et de la Recherche Medicale.

Miller, M. 1976. The Cost-Effectiveness of Medical Device Standards. *Med. Instr.* 10:28.

Minnesota Medical Association. 1979. New Directions for Health Care. Report and Recommendations of the Minnesota Medical Association Commission on Health Care Costs. *Minn. Med.* 62(suppl. 2):1.

Moore, G. et al. 1975. Comparison of Television and Telephone for Remote Medical Consultation. *New Engl. J. Med.* 92:729.

Moore, R. and Hoover, A. 1974. NIOSH Interest in the Cost Effectiveness of Occupational Health Programs. *J. Occup. Med.* 16:154.

Morrow, J. et al. 1976. U.S. Health Manpower Policy: Will the Benefits Justify the Costs? *J. Med. Educ.* 51:791.

Moskowitz, M. and Fox, S. 1979. Cost Analysis of Aggressive Breast Cancer Screening. *Radiology* 130:253.

Moskowitz, M. et al. 1976. Breast Cancer Screening: Benefit and Risk for the First Annual Screening. *Radiology* 120:431.

Moulding, T. 1971. Chemoprophylaxis of Tuberculosis: When Is the Benefit Worth the Risk and Cost? *Ann. Intern. Med.* 74:761.

Mulford, H. 1979. Treating Alcoholism Versus Accelerating the Natural Recovery Process: A Cost-Benefit Comparison. *J. Stud. Alcohol.* 40:505.

Muller, A. 1980. Evaluation of the Costs and Benefits of Motorcycle Helmet Laws. *Amer. J. Pub. Health* 70:586.

Muller, C. et al. 1977. Cost Factors in Urban Telemedicine. *Med. Care* 15:251.

Murphy, J. et al. 1976. A Cost-Benefit Analysis of Community Versus Institutional Living. *Hosp. Comm. Psychol.* 27:165.

Mushkin, S. 1962. Health as an Investment. *J. Pol. Econ.* 70:129.

_____. 1977*a*. Evaluation of Health Policies and Actions. *Soc. Sci. Med.* 11:491.

_____. 1977*b*. Knowledge and Choices in Health: Cost-Benefit Analysis in Health Policy. Unpublished paper. Washington, D.C.: Georgetown University, Public Services Laboratory.

_____. 1979. *Biomedical Research: Costs and Benefits.* Cambridge, Mass.: Ballinger.

Mushkin, S. and Cotton, J. 1967. The Cost of Mental Health Care Under Changing Treatment Methods: One Criterion Out of Many. *Int. J. Psychol.* 4:162.

Muskin, S. and Weisbrod, B. 1963. Investment in Health—Lifetime Health Expenditures on the 1960 Work Force. *KYKLOS* 16:583.

Muskin, S. et al. 1977. Returns to Biomedical Research 1900–1975: An Initial Assessment of Impacts on Health Expenditures. Unpublished paper. Washington, D.C.: Georgetown University, Public Services Laboratory.

Mushkin, S. et al. 1978. Cost of Disease and Illness in the United States in the Year 2000. *Pub. Health Rep.* 93:493.

Mustard, R. 1977. Major Cardiac Surgery: Are the Benefits Worth the Cost? *Ann. Thor. Surg.* 24:400.

Nason, F. and Delbanco, T. 1976. Soft Services—A Major Cost-Effective Component of Primary Medical Care. *Soc. Work Health Care* 1:297.

*National Academy of Sciences. 1979. *Medical Technology and the Health Care System.* Washington, D.C.: National Academy of Sciences.

National Institute of Mental Health. 1975. Development and Test of a Cost-Effectiveness Methodology for Community Mental Health Centers. Unpublished paper. Rockville, Md.: National Institute of Mental Health.

Nelson, W. 1978. An Economic Evaluation of a Genetic Screening Program for Tay-Sachs Disease. *Amer. J. Hum. Genet.* 30:160.

Nelson, W. et al. 1976. Cost-Benefit Analysis of Fluoridation in Houston, Texas. *J. Pub. Health Dent.* 36:88.

Nelson, W. et al. 1978. A Comment on the Benefits and Costs of Genetic Screening. *Amer. J. Hum. Genet.* 30:663.

Neuhauser, D. 1977a. Cost-Effective Clinical Decision-Making. *Pediatrics* 60:756.

————. 1977b. Cost-Effective Clinical Decision-Making: Implications for the Delivery of Health Services. In *Costs, Risks, and Benefits of Surgery*, ed. J. Bunker et al. New York: Oxford Univ. Press.

————. 1977c. Elective Inguinal Herniorrhaphy versus Truss in the Elderly. In *Costs, Risks, and Benefits of Surgery*, ed. J. Bunker et al. New York: Oxford Univ. Press.

Neuhauser, D. and Halperin, W. 1973. *Cost-Effective Clinical Decision-Making, Parts I and II.* Ford Foundation Series on the Delivery of Urban Health Services. Boston: Harvard University.

Neuhauser, D. and Lewicki, A. 1975. What Do We Gain From the Sixth Stool Guaiac? *New Engl. J. Med.* 293:226.

————. 1976. National Health Insurance and the Sixth Stool Guaiac. *Pol. Anal.* 2:175.

Neutra, R. 1977. Indications for the Surgical Treatment of Suspected Acute Appendicitis: A Cost-Effectiveness Approach. In *Costs, Risks, and Benefits of Surgery*, ed. J. Bunker et al. New York: Oxford Univ. Press.

Newhouse, J. 1971. Allocation of Public Sector Resources in Medical Care: An Economist Looks at Health Planning. *Econ. Bus. Bull.* 23:8.

*————. 1978. *The Economics of Medical Care: A Policy Perspective.* Reading, Mass.: Addison-Wesley.

Norcross, K. 1977. Society and the Doctor. *Amer. Heart J.* 94:261.

Nordgerg, O. et al., eds. 1975. *Action for Children.* Uppsala, Sweden: Dag Hammarskjold Foundation.

Norling, R. 1975. Cost and Effectiveness Models for Hospital Programs. Ann Arbor: University Microfilms International.

Nowlan, D. 1980. Costs and Benefits. *Irish Med. J.* 73:146.

Nyiendo, J. et al. 1979. Cost-Effective Clinical Microbiology. *Amer. J. Med. Technol.* 45:393.

O'Boyle, E. 1980. Cost-Effective Clinical Decision Making. *Pediatrics* 62:371.

Olavi, E. n.d. Health and Economic Consequences of Rubella. *Acta Univ. Tamp.*, Series A.

Oldenburg, T. 1980. Cost Effectiveness and Human Welfare. *J. Amer. Dent. Assoc.* 100:10.

On Cost-Benefit and Cost-Effectiveness Analysis. 1976. *NIHAE Bull.* 9:166.

Osteria, T. 1973. A Cost-Effectiveness Analysis of Family Planning Programs in the Philippines. *Stud. Fam. Plan.* 4:191.

Packer, A. 1968. Applying Cost-Effectiveness Concepts to the Community Health System. *Oper. Res.* 16:227.

Pantell, R. 1977. Cost-Effectiveness of Pharyngitis Management and Prevention of Rheumatic Fever. *Ann. Intern. Med.* 86:497.

Panzetta, A. 1973. Cost-Benefit Studies in Psychiatry. *Compr. Psychiat.* 14.

Parker, B. 1978. Quantitative Decision Techniques for the Health-Public Sector Policy-Maker: An Analysis and Classification of Resources. *J. Health Pol. Policy Law* 3:388.

Patiala, H. et al. 1976. Cost-Benefit Analysis of Synovectomy of the Knee. *Scand. J. Rheumatol.* 5:227.

Pauker, S. 1976. Coronary Artery Surgery: The Use of Decision Analysis. *Ann. Intern. Med.* 85:8.

Pauker, S. and Kassirer, J. 1975. Therapeutic Decision-Making: A Cost-Benefit Analysis. *New Engl. J. Med.* 293:229.

*Pauly, M. 1968. The Economics of Moral Hazard: Comment. *Amer. Econ. Rev..* 58:531.

_____. 1979. What Is Unnecessary Surgery? *Milbank Mem. Fund Q.* 57:95.

*Peltzman, S. 1974. *Regulation of Pharmaceutical Innovation: The 1962 Amendments*. Washington, D.C.: American Enterprise Institute.

Penner, D. 1978. Cost Effectiveness of the Autopsy in Maintaining and Improving the Standard of Patient Care. *Amer. J. Clin. Pathol.* 69:250.

Pettingiee, B. 1978. Cost Effectiveness of Hospital Treatment. *Dimen. Health Serv.* 55:19.

Pfahl, S. 1979. Cost-Effective Health Care: The Balance of Cost and Quality. *Ohio State Med. J.* 75:262.

Phelps, C. 1976. Benefit-Cost Assessment for Quality Assurance Program. Unpublished paper. Santa Monica, Calif.: RAND Corp.

Phillips, C. and Wolfe, J. 1977. *Clinical Practice and Economics*. London: Pitman.

Phillips, R. and Hughes, J. 1974. Cost-Benefit Analysis of the Occupational Health Program: A Generic Model. *J. Occup. Med.* 16:158.

Piachaud, D. and Weddell, J. 1972. The Economics of Treating Varicose Veins. *Int. J. Epidem.* 1:287.

Pliskin, J. 1974. The Management of Patients With End-Stage Renal Failure: A Decision Theoretic Approach. Dissertation, Harvard University, Cambridge, Massachusetts.

Pliskin, J. and Beck, C., Jr. 1976. A Health Index for Patient Selection: A Value Function Approach With Applications to Chronic Renal Failure Patients. *Man. Sci.* 22:1009.

Pliskin, N. and Taylor, A. 1977. General Principles: Cost-Benefit and Decision

Analysis. In *Costs, Risks, and Benefits of Surgery*, ed. J. Bunker et al. New York: Oxford Univ. Press.

Pole, J. 1968. Economic Aspects of Screening for Disease. In *Screening in Medical Care*, ed. T. McKeown. London: Oxford Univ. Press.

──────. 1971a. The Cost-Effectiveness of Screening. *Proc. Roy. Soc. Med.* 64: 1256.

──────. 1971b. Mass Radiography: A Cost-Benefit Approach. In *Problems and Progress in Medical Care: Essays in Current Research*, ed. G. McLachlan. New York: Oxford Univ. Press.

──────. 1972. The Economics of Mass Radiography. In *The Economics of Medical Care*, ed. M. Hauser. London: Allen and Unwin.

*Policy Analysis, Inc. Forthcoming. *Evaluation of Cost-of-Illness Ascertainment Methodology*. PHS Contract no. 233-79-2048. Brookline, Mass.: Policy Analysis, Inc.

Pomrinse, S. et al. 1972. Cost-Benefit Analysis of Computer. *Hospitals* 46:76.

Ponnighaus, J. 1980. The Cost-Benefit of Measles Immunization: A Study From Southern Zambia. *J. Trop. Med. Hyg.* 83:141.

Popkin, B. et al. 1980. Benefit-Cost Analysis in the Nutrition Area: A Project in the Philippines. *Soc. Sci. Med.* 14C:207.

Porro de Somenzi, C. 1979. Analysis of Cost-Benefits of Vaccination Against Measles. *Ann. Sclavo.* 21(suppl.):373.

Potchen, E. et al. 1977. Value Measurement of Nuclear Medicine Procedures. In *Financial Operation and Management Concepts in Nuclear Medicine*, ed. J. Bennington et al. Baltimore: University Park.

Prescott, P. 1979. Cost-Effectiveness: Tool or Trap? *Nurs. Outlook* 27:722.

Preston, T. 1977. *Coronary Artery Surgery: A Critical Review*. New York: Raven Press.

*Quade, E. 1975. *Analysis for Public Decisions*, New York: American Elsevier.

Quilligan, E. and Paul, R. 1975. Fetal Monitoring: Is It Worth It? *Obstet. Gyn.* 45:96.

Rabello, Y. and Paul, R. 1976. Fetal Monitoring: What Does It Cost? What Is the Benefit? *JOGN Nurs.* 5:715.

Radtke, H. 1974. Benefits and Costs of a Physician to a Community. *Amer. J. Agr. Econ.* 56:586.

Ramaiah, T. 1976. Cost-Effectiveness Analysis of the Intensified Campaign Against Smallpox in India. *Nat. Inst. Health Admin. Educ. (India) Bull.* 9:169.

Raskin, M. 1975. Quality Assurance and Cost Effectiveness for Prepaid Care. *N. Y. State Dent. J.* 41:464.

Rathbone-McCuan, E. et al. 1975. *Cost-Effectiveness Evaluation of the Levindale Adult Day Treatment Center*. Baltimore: Levindale Geriatric Research Center.

*Redisch, M. 1974. Hospital Inflationary Mechanisms. Paper read at the meeting of the Western Economic Association, Las Vegas, Nevada, June 10–12.

Rees, P. et al. 1978. Medical Care in a Tropical National Reference and Teaching Hospital: Outline Study of Cost-Effectiveness. *Brit. Med. J.* 2:102.

Reid, M. and Morris, J. 1979. Perinatal Care and Cost Effectiveness: Changes in Health Expenditures and Birth Outcome Following the Establishment of a Nurse-Midwife Program. *Med. Care* 17:491.

Reiff, T. 1978. It Can Happen Here. *JAMA* 239:2761.

*Reinhardt, U. 1975. *Physician Productivity and the Demand for Health Manpower*. Cambridge, Mass.: Ballinger.

*Reiss, J. 1980. A Conceptual Model of the Case-Based Payment Scheme for New Jersey Hospitals. *Health Serv. Res.* 15:161.

Reiss, J. et al. 1980. Issues in the Cost and Regulation of New Medical Technologies and Procedures: Heart Transplants as a Case Study. Paper read at the Harvard-MIT Conference on Critical Issues in Medical Technology—Innovation, Diffusion, Utilization, and Cost, Boston, Massachusetts, April 13–16.

Retka, R. 1977. Cost Accountability in Drug Abuse Prevention. Rockville, Md.: National Institute on Drug Abuse.

*Rettig, R. 1976. The Policy Debate on Patient Care Financing for Victims of End-Stage Renal Disease. *Law Contemp. Prob.* 40:196.

*_____. 1979. End-Stage Renal Disease and the "Cost" of Medical Technology. In *Medical Technology: The Culprit Behind Health Care Costs?* ed. S. Altman and R. Blendon. DHEW Publication no. (PHS) 79–3216. Washington, D.C.: Government Printing Office.

_____. 1981. Formal Analysis, Policy Formulation, and End-Stage Renal Disease (OTA-BP-H-9(1)). In *The Implications of Cost-Effectiveness Analysis of Medical Technology; Background Paper no. 2: Case Studies of Medical Technologies.* Washington, D.C.: Government Printing Office.

Reynell, P. and Reynell, M. 1972. The Cost-Benefit of a Coronary Care Unit. *Brit. Heart J.* 34:897.

*Rice, D. 1966. Estimating the Cost of Illness. Unpublished paper. Washington, D.C.: U.S., Department of Health Education, and Welfare, Public Health Service, Health Economics Series no. 6.

Rich, G. et al. 1976. Cost-Effectiveness of Two Methods of Screening for Asymptomatic Bacteriuria. *Brit. J. Prevent. Soc. Med.* 30:54.

Rios, J. et al. 1978. The Quest for Optimal Electrocardiography: Task Force V—Cost-Effectiveness of the Electrocardiogram. *Amer. J. Cardiol.* 41:175.

*Rivlin, A. 1971. *Systematic Thinking for Social Action.* Washington, D.C.: Brookings Institution.

Roberts, J. 1974. Economic Evaluation of Health Care: A Survey. *Brit. J. Prevent. Soc. Med.* 28:210.

Roberts, S. et al. 1980. Cost-Effective Care of End-Stage Renal Disease: A Billion Dollar Question. *Ann. Intern. Med.* 92:243.

Robinson, D. 1971. Cost and Effectiveness of a Program To Prevent Rheumatic Fever. *Health Serv. Ment. Health Admin. Health Rep.* 86:385.

Robinson, W. 1979. The Cost Per Unit of Family Planning Services. *J. Biosoc. Sci.* 11:93.

Rogers, P. et al. 1981. Is Health Promotion Cost Effective? *Prevent. Med.* 10:324.

Romm, J. et al. 1978. Survey and Evaluation of the Physician Extender Reimbursement Study: Cost Effectiveness. Paper read at the annual meeting of the American Public Health Association, Los Angeles, California, October 18.

Rosenshein, M. et al. 1980. The Cost Effectiveness of Therapeutic and Prophylactic Leukocyte Transfusion. *New Engl. J. Med.* 302:1058.

Rosenthal, G. 1979. Anticipating the Costs and Benefits of New Technology: A Typology for Policy. In *Medical Technology: The Culprit Behind Health Care Costs?* ed. S. Altman and R. Blendon. DHEW Publication no. (PHS) 79-3216. Washington, D.C.: Government Printing Office.

Ross, D. et al. 1980. Comprehensive Clinical Electrophysiologic Studies in the Investigation of Documented or Suspected Tachycardias. Time, Staff, Problems and Costs. *Circulation* 61:1010.

Round-table Discussion: Maximizing the Clinical Usefulness and Cost-Effectiveness of EEG and EMG. 1979. *Clin. Electroenceph.* 10:5.

Rowe, D. and Bisbee, J. 1978. Preventive Health Care in the HMO: Cost-Benefit Issues. *J. Amer. Coll. Health Assoc.* 26:298.

Ruchlin, H. and Levey, S. 1972. Nursing Home Cost Analysis: A Case Study. *Inquiry* 9:3.

Rundell, O. et al. 1979. Benefit-Cost Methodology in the Evaluation of Therapeutic Services to Alcoholism. *Alcoholism* 3:324.

*Russell, L. 1976. Making Rational Decisions About Medical Technology. Paper read at a meeting of the American Medical Association's National Commission on the Cost of Medical Care, Chicago, Illinois, November 23.

*_____. 1977. How Much Does Medical Technology Cost? Paper read at the Annual Health Conference of the New York Academy of Medicine, New York, New York, April 29.

Russell, R. et al. 1976. Unstable Angina Pectoris: National Cooperative Study Group to Compare Medical and Surgical Therapy. *Amer. J. Cardiol.* 37:896.

*Salkever, D. and Bice, T. 1979. *Hospital Certificate-of-Need Controls: Impact on Investment, Costs, and Use.* Washington, D.C.: American Enterprise Institute.

Salvatierra, O. et al. 1979. Analysis of Cost and Outcomes of Renal Transplantation at One Center: Its Implications. *JAMA* 241:1469.

Sarna, S. et al. 1979. Optimization Procedures in Turn Zygosity Diagnosis by Genetic Markers. A Cost-Effectiveness Analysis. *Acta Genet. Med. (Roma)* 28:139.

Saslaw, M. et al. 1965. Cost of Rheumatic Fever and Its Prevention. *Amer. J. Pub. Health* 55:429.

Saunders, J. 1970. Results and Costs of a Computer-Assisted Immunization Scheme. *Brit. J. Prevent. Soc. Med.* 24:187.

Savas, B. 1969. Simulation and Cost-Effectiveness Analysis of New York's Emergency Ambulance Service. *Man. Sci.* 15:B608.

Saxe, L. 1980. *The Implications of Cost-Effectiveness Analysis of Medical Technology; Background Paper no. 3: The Efficacy and Cost-Effectiveness of Psychotherapy* (OTA-BP-H-6). Washington, D.C.: Government Printing Office.

Scanlon, J. 1976. Proceedings: Cost Savings-Benefit Analysis of Drug Abuse Treatment. *Amer. J. Drug Alcohol Abuse* 3:95.

Schachter, K. and Neuhauser, D. 1981. Surgery for Breast Caner. In *The Implications of Cost-Effectiveness Analysis of Medical Technology; Background Paper no. 2: Case Studies of Medical Technologies.* Washington, D.C.: Government Printing Office.

Schaefer, M. 1975. Demand Versus Need for Medical Services in a General Cost-Benefit Setting. *Amer. J. Pub. Health* 65:293.

Scheffler, R. 1973. A Methodological Framework for Cost-Benefit Analysis in Health. Paper read at an Engineering Foundation Conference, South Berwick, Me. August 19–24.

Scheffler, R. and Delaney, M. 1981. Assessing Selected Respiratory Therapy Modalities: Trends and Relative Costs in the Washington, D.C., Area. In *The Implications of Cost-Effectiveness Analysis of Medical Technology; Background Paper no. 2: Case Studies of Medical Technologies.* Washington, D.C.: Government Printing Office.

Scheffler, R. and Paringer, L. 1980. A Review of the Economic Evidence on Prevention. *Med. Care* 18:473.

Scheffler, R. and Rovin, S. 1981. Periodontal Disease: Assessing the Effectiveness and Costs of the Keyes Technique (OTA-BP-H-9(5)). In *The Implications of Cost-Effectiveness Analysis of Medical Technology Background Paper no. 2: Case Studies of Medical Technologies.* Washington, D.C.: Government Printing Office.

Schelling, T. 1968. The Life You Save May Be Your Own. In *Problems in Public Expenditure Analysis,* ed. S. Chase, Jr. Washington, D.C.: Brookings Institution.

Schippers, H. and Kalff, M. 1976. Cost Comparison: Hemodialysis and Renal Transplantation. *Tissue Antigens* 7:86.

Schoenbaum, S. et al. 1976*a*. Benefit-Cost Analysis of Rubella Vaccination Policy. *New Engl. J. Med.* 294:306.

Schoenbaum, S. et al. 1976*b*. The Swine-Influenza Decision. *New Engl. J. Med.* 295:759.

Schramm, C. 1977. Measuring the Return on Program Costs: Evaluation of a Multi-Employer Alcoholism Treatment Program. *Amer. J. Pub. Health* 67:50.

*Schroeder, S. et al. 1973. Use of Laboratory Tests and Pharmaceuticals: Variation Among Physicians and Effect of Cost Audit on Subsequent Use. *JAMA* 225:969.

Schultz, G. 1970. The Logic of Health Care Facility Planning. *Socioecon. Plan. Sci.* 4:383.

Schultz, P. and McGlone, F. 1977. Primary Health Care Provided to the Elderly by a Nurse Practitioner-Physician Team: Analysis of Cost-Effectiveness. *J. Amer. Geriat. Soc.* 25:443.

*Schultze, C. 1968. *The Politics and Economics of Public Spending.* Washington, D.C.: Brookings Institution.

Schwartz, W. and Joskow, P. 1978. Medical Efficacy Versus Economic Efficiency: A Conflict in Values. *New Engl. J. Med.* 299:1462.

Schweitzer, S. 1974. Cost-Effectiveness of Early Detection of Disease. *Health Serv. Res.* 9:22.

Schweitzer, S. and Luce, B. 1979. *A Cost Effective Approach to Cervical Cancer Detection.* DHEW Publication no. 79-32371. Hyattsville, Md.: National Center for Health Services Research.

Schweitzer, S. and Scalzi, C. 1981. The Cost-Effectiveness of Bone Marrow Transplant Therapy and Its Policy Implications (OTA-BP-H-9(6)). In *The Implications of Cost-Effectiveness Analysis of Medical Technology; Background Paper no. 2: Case Studies of Medical Technologies.* Washington, D.C.: Government Printing Office.

Schweitzer, S. et al. 1979. Social Cost Versus Effectiveness of Bone Marrow Transplant Therapy. *UCLA Cancer Cent. Bull.* 6:3.

*Scitovsky, A. and McCall, N. 1976. *Changes in the Costs of Treatment of Selected Illnesses: 1951–1964–1971.* DHEW Publication no. (HRA) 77-3161. Hyattsville, Md.: National Center for Health Services Research.

Scriver, C. 1974. PKU and Beyond: When Do Costs Exceed Benefits? *Pediatrics* 54:616.

Seidman, H. 1977. Screening for Breast Cancer in Younger Women: Life Expectancy Gains and Losses: An Analysis According to Risk Indication Groups. *CA-A Cancer J. Clin.* 72:69.

Sencer, D. and Axnick, N. 1975. Utilization of Cost-Benefit Analysis in Planning Prevention Programs. *Acta Med. Scand.* 576:123.

Shapiro, S. 1977. Measuring the Effectiveness of Prevention: II. *Milbank Mem. Fund Q.* 55:291.

Sharfstein, S. et al. 1976. Community Care: Costs and Benefits for a Chronic Patient. *Hosp. Comm. Psychol.* 27:170.

Shattuck, L. 1850. *Report of a General Plan for the Promotion of Public Personal Health*. Boston: Dutton and Wentworth.

Sheehan, D. and Atkinson, J. 1974. Comparative Costs of State Hospital and Community-Based Inpatient Care in Texas: Who Benefits Most? *Hosp. Comm. Psychol.* 25:242.

Shepard, D. 1977. The Economics of Prevention: The Method of Cost-Effectiveness Analysis. Unpublished paper. Boston: Massachusetts Department of Public Health, Office of State Health Planning.

————. 1978. Cost Benefit Analysis in Health: A Selected Annotated Bibliography. Unpublished paper. Boston: Massachusetts Department of Public Health, Office of State Health Planning.

Shepard, D. and Thompson, M. 1979. First Principles of Cost-Effectiveness Analysis. *Pub. Health Rep.* 94:535.

Shepard, D. et al. 1978. Cost-Effectiveness of Interventions to Improve Compliance With Anti-Hypertensive Therapy. Paper read at the National Conference on High Blood Pressure Control, Washington, D.C., April 4–6.

Showstack, J. and Schroeder, S. 1981. The Costs and Effectiveness of Upper Gastrointestinal Endoscopy (OTA-BP-H-9(8)). In *The Implications of Cost-Effectiveness Analysis of Medical Technology; Background Paper no. 2: Case Studies of Medical Technologies*. Washington, D.C.: Government Printing Office.

Siebert, C. and Azidi, M. 1975. Benefit Cost Analysis in Health Care. *Biosci. Comm.* 1:193.

Silver, E. 1972. The Torrance et al. Cost-Effectiveness-Ranking Algorithm. *Health Serv. Res.* 7:322.

Simmons, H. 1976. The Routine Physical Exam: Is It Worth the Cost? *J. Tenn. Med. Assoc.* 69:183.

Sirotnik, K. et al. 1975. A Cost-Benefit Analysis for a Multimodality Heroin Treatment Project. *Int. J. Addict.* 10:443.

Siu, T. 1976. Cost Effectiveness of Early Detection. *Health Serv. Res.* 11:302.

Skillings, J. et al. 1979. Cost-Effectiveness of Operative Cholangiography. *Amer. J. Surg.* 127:26.

Smith, C. 1977. Cost-Benefit Ratio of Exfoliative Cytology of the Cervix. *Amer. J. Obstet. Gyn.* 129:476.

Smith, H. 1973. Application of Cost-Effectiveness Analysis to Patient Record Systems. *J. Amer. Pharm. Assoc.* 13:13.

Smith, W. 1968. Cost-Effectiveness and Cost-Benefit Analysis for Public Health Programs. *Pub. Health Rep.* 83:899.

Solomon, J. 1979. The Cost-Benefit Ratio in Psychoanalysis. *Amer. J. Psychiat.* 136:1482.

Sonenblum, S. et al. 1974. *Program Budgeting for Urban Health and Welfare Service With Special Reference to Los Angeles*. New York: Praeger.

Sonnenburg, A. et al. 1979. Cost-Benefit Calculation of Esophogo-Gastro-Duodenoscopy. *Z. Gastroent.* 17:773.

*Sorkin, A. 1975. *Health Econ.* Lexington, Mass.: Heath.

Spark, R. 1976. The Case Against Regular Physicals. *N.Y. Times Magazine*, July 25.

Spears, M. 1976. Concepts of Cost Effectiveness: Accountability for Nutrition, Productivity. *J. Amer. Diet. Assoc.* 68:341.

Spector, R. et al. 1975. Medical Care by Nurses in an Internal Medicine Clinic. Analysis of Quality and Its Cost. *JAMA* 232:1234.

Speight, A. 1975. Cost-Effectiveness and Drug Therapy. *Trop. Doct.* 5:89.

Spencer, D. and Axnick, N. 1973. Cost Benefit Analysis. *Sympos. Ser. Immunobiol. Stand.* 22:37.

Spitzer, W. et al. 1976*a*. Nurse Practitioners in Primary Care: Assessment of Their Deployment with the Utilization and Financial Index. *Canad. Med. Assoc. J.* 114:1103.

Spitzer, W. et al. 1976*b*. Nurse Practitioners in Primary Care: Development of the Utilization and Financial Index to Measure Effects of Their Deployment. *Canad. Med. Assoc. J.* 114:1099.

Spratt, J., Jr. 1971. Cost Effectiveness in the Post-Treatment Follow-Up of Cancer Patients. *J. Surg. Oncol.* 3:393.

―――――. 1978. Cancer: Do Early Diagnosis and Treatment Really Help? How Do We Relate Costs to Benefit in Cancer Control? *Oral Surg.* 45:220.

Stahl, J. n.d. Present State of Cost Benefit Analysis in Medical Evaluation. Lund, Sweden: Department of Economics, Lund University.

Stanaway, L. 1979. Assessment of the Cost-Effectiveness of Chemotherapy for Skin and Urinary Tract Infections Using in Vitro Sensitivity Testing. *New Zeal. Med. J.* 90:201.

Stanford Research Institute. 1978. *Feasibility and Cost-Effectiveness of Alternative Long-Term Care Settings.* Menlo Park, Calif.: Stanford Research Institute International.

Stange, P. and Sumner, A. 1978. Predicting Treatment Costs and Life Expectancy for End-Stage Renal Disease. *New Engl. J. Med.* 298:372.

Starr, J. 1975. Better Answer Alternatives to Institutional Care. Paper read at the 25th Annual Meeting of the National Council on Aging, Washington, D.C., September 30.

*Starr, P. 1976. The Undelivered Health System. *Pub. Interest* no. 42:66.

Stason, W. and Fortess, E. 1981. Cardiac Radionuclide Imaging and Cost Effectiveness (OTA-BP-H-9(13)). In *The Implications of Cost-Effectiveness Analysis of Medical Technology; Background Paper no. 2: Case Studies of Medical Technologies.* Washington, D.C.: Government Printing Office.

Stason, W. and Weinstein, M. 1977. Allocation of Resources To Manage Hypertension. *New Engl. J. Med.* 296:732.

Steiner, K. and Smith, H. 1973. Application of Cost Benefit Analysis to a PKU Screening Program. *Inquiry* 10:34.

*Steiner, P. 1974. Public Expenditure Budgeting. In *The Economics of Public Finance*, ed. A. Blinder et al. Washington, D.C.: Brookings Institution.

Stephen, K. et al. 1978. Caries Reduction and Cost-Benefit After 3 Years of Sucking Fluoride Tablets Daily at School: A Double-Blind Trial. *Brit. Dent. J.* 144:202.

Stewart C. 1971. Allocation of Resources to Health. *J. Hum. Res.* 6:104.

Stewart, J. et al. 1973. The Costs of Domiciliary Maintenance Haemodialysis: A Comparison With Alternative Renal Replacement Regimens. *Med. J. Aust.* 1:156.

Stilwell, J. 1976. Benefits and Costs of the Schools' BCG Vaccination Programme. *Brit. Med. J.* 1:1002.

Stokes, J. and Carmichael, D. 1975. A Cost-Benefit Analysis of Model Hypertension Control. Bethesda, Md.: National Heart and Lung Institute.

*Stokey, E. and Zeckhauser, R. 1978. *A Primer for Policy Analysis.* New York: Norton.

Strong, C. 1977. Surgically Correctable Causes of Hypertension. *Mayo Clin. Proc.* 52:585.

Sugar, J. 1978. An Ounce of Prevention Is Worth It: Benefits and Costs of Family

Planning. Paper read at the annual meeting of the American Public Health Association, Los Angeles, California, October 18.

Sullivan, W. and Thuesen, G. 1971. Cost Sensitivity Analysis for Radiology Department Planning. *Health Serv. Res.* 6:337.

Sussna, B. and Heinemann, H. 1972. The Education of Health Manpower in a Two-Year College: An Evaluation Model. *Socio-Econ. Plan. Serv.* 6:21.

Swartz, R. and Desharnius, S. 1977. Computed Tomography: The Cost-Benefit Dilemma. *Radiology* 125:251.

*Sweeney, G. 1980. The Market for Physicians' Services: Theoretical Implications and an Empirical Test of the Target Income Hypothesis. Paper read at the annual meeting of the American Economic Association, Denver, Colorado, September 5.

Swint, J. and Nelson, W. 1975. Cost-Benefit Analysis in Health Planning. Unpublished paper. Houston: Univ. of Texas.

Swint, J. et al. 1977a. The Application of Economic Analysis to Evaluation of Alcoholism Rehabilitation Programs. *Inquiry* 14:63.

Swint, J. et al. 1977b. Prospective Evaluation of Alcoholism Rehabilitation Efforts: The Role of Cost-Benefit and Cost-Effectiveness Analyses. *J. Stud. Alcohol.* 38:1386.

Swint, J. et al. 1978. The Economic Returns to Employment-Based Alcoholism Programs: A Methodology. *J. Stud. Alcohol.* 39:1633.

Swint, J. et al. 1979. The Economic Returns to Community and Hospital Screening Programs for a Genetic Disease. *Prevent. Med.* 8:463.

Taking Action to Contain Health Care Costs. 1980. *Pers. J.* August–September.

Taylor, D. 1974. *Benefits and Risks in Medical Care.* London: Office of Health Economics.

————. 1976. The Costs of Arthritis and the Benefits of Joint Replacement Surgery. *Proc. Roy. Soc. Lond.* 192:145.

Taylor, F. 1977. Cost and Benefits of Rare Earth Screens. *Brit. J. Radiol.* 50:294.

Taylor, V. 1970. How Much Is Good Health Worth? *Pol. Sci.* 1:49.

Teeling-Smith, G. 1972. A Cost-Benefit Approach to Medical Care. In *The Economics of Medical Care,* ed. M. Hauser et al. London: Allen & Unwin.

————. 1975. The Economics of Screening. In *Screening in General Practice,* ed. C. Hart. Edinburgh: Churchill Livingstone.

————. 1976. Cost-Benefit Paralysis. *Nurs. Times* 72:88.

Terrill, J., Jr. 1972. Cost-Benefit Estimates for the Major Sources of Radiation Exposure. *Amer. J. Pub. Health* 62:1008.

Terris, M. 1980. Preventive Services and Medical Care: the Costs and Benefits of Basic Change. *Bull. N.Y. Acad. Med.* 56:108.

Thomson, J. 1977. Cost-Effectiveness of an EMI Brain Scanner. A Review of a 2-Year Experience. *Health Trends* 9:16.

————. 1978. Epidemiology and Health Services Administration: Future Relationships in Practice and Education. *Milbank Mem. Fund Q.* 56:253.

Thomson, K. et al. 1978. Scope of Interventional Radiology 1977. *Appl. Radiol.* 7:73.

Thorbury, J. et al. 1977. Cost-Benefit Analysis, Medical Decision Making and the Individual Radiologist. *Curr. Prob. Diag. Radiol.* 7:1.

Thrall, R. 1976. Benefit-Cost Estimation, Alternatives, Requirements, Advantages and Disadvantages. In *Workshops From the Centennial Conference on Laryngeal Cancer,* ed. P. Alberti and D. Bryce, New York: Appleton-Century-Crofts.

Thrall, R. and Cardus, D. 1974. Benefit-Cost and Cost-Effectiveness Analysis in Rehabilitation Research Programs. *Method. Info. Med.* 13:147.

Tolpin, H. 1980. The Necessity of a Cost-Benefit Approach: Economics of Health Care. *J. Amer. Diet. Assoc.* 76:217.

Tompkins, R. et al. 1977*a*. An Analysis of the Cost Effectiveness of Pharyngitis Management and Acute Rheumatic Fever Prevention. *Ann. Intern. Med.* 86:481.

Tompkins, R. et al. 1977*b*. The Effectiveness and Costs of Acute Respiratory Illness Medical Care by Physicians and Algorithm-Assisted Physicians' Assistants. *Med. Care* 15:991.

Torrance, G. 1971. Generalized Cost-Effectiveness Model for the Evaluation of Health Programs. Dissertation, McMaster University, Hamilton, Ontario.

Torrance, G. et al. 1973. Utility Maximization Model for Program Evaluation: A Demonstration Application. In *Health Status Indexes: Proceedings of a Conference*, ed. R. Berg. Tucson: Hospital Research and Educational Trust.

Tunbridge, R. and Wetherill, J. 1970. Reliability and Cost of Diabetic Diets. *Brit. Med. J.* 2:78.

Tunturi, T. et al. 1979. Cost-Benefit Analysis of Posterior Fusion of the Lumbosacral Spine. *Acta Orthop. Scand.* 50:427.

Urban, N. et al. 1981. The Costs of a Suburban Paramedic Program in Reducing Deaths Due to Cardiac Arrest. *Med. Care* 19:379.

U.S. Bureau of the Budget. 1967. *Report of the Committee on Chronic Kidney Disease.* Washington, D.C.: Government Printing Office.

U.S. Congress, Congressional Budget Office. 1979. *The Effect of PSROs on Health Care Costs: Current Findings and Future Evaluation.* Washington, D.C.: Government Printing Office.

————. 1980. The Impact of PSROs on Health Care Costs: 1980 Update of the CBO Evaluation. Unpublished paper.

U.S. Congress, House, Subcommittee on Oversight and Investigations, Committee on Interstate and Foreign Commerce. 1976. *Cost and Quality of Health Care: Unnecessary Surgery.* Washington, D.C.: Government Printing Office.

U.S. Congress, Office of Technology Assessment. 1976. *Development of Medical Technologies: Opportunity for Assessment* (OTA-H-34). Washington, D.C.: Government Printing Office.

————. 1977. *Policy Implications of Medical Information Systems.* Washington, D.C.: Government Printing Office.

————. 1978*a*. *Assessing the Efficacy and Safety of Medical Technologies* (OTA-H-75). Washington, D.C.: Government Printing Office.

————. 1978*b*. *Policy Implications of the Computed Tomography (CT) Scanner* (OTA-H-72). Washington, D.C.: Government Printing Office.

————. 1979. *A Reivew of Selected Federal Vaccine and Immunization Policies.* Based on Case Studies of Pneumococcal Vaccine (OTA-H-96). Washington, D.C.: Government Printing Office.

————. 1980*a*. *The Implications of Cost-Effectiveness Analysis of Medical Technology* (OTA-H-126). Washington, D.C.: Government Printing Office.

————. 1980*b*. *The Implications of Cost-Effectiveness Analysis of Medical Technology; Background Paper no. 1: Methodological Issues and Literature Review.* (OTA-BP-H-5). Washington, D.C.: Government Printing Office.

————. 1981. *The Implications of Cost-Effectiveness Analysis of Medical Technology; Background Paper no. 2: Case Studies of Medical Technologies.* Washington, D.C.: Government Printing Office.

*U.S. Department of Health and Human Services. 1981. *Health—United States—1980.* DHHS Publication no. (PHS) 81-1232. Washington, D.C.: Government Printing Office.

*U.S. Department of Health, Education, and Welfare, Health Care Financing Administration, Office of Research, Demonstrations, and Statistics. 1979a. *Health Care Financing Research and Demonstration Grants: Current Priority Areas.* DHEW Publication no. HCFA 03001. Washington, D.C.: Government Printing Office.

————. 1979b. *Professional Standards Review Organizations: 1978 Program Evaluations.* Washington, D.C.: Government Printing Office.

*————. 1980. *The National Hospital Rate-Setting Study: A Comparative Review of Nine Prospective Rate-Setting Programs.* DHEW Publication no. HCFA 03061. Washington, D.C.: Government Printing Office.

U.S. Department of Health, Education, and Welfare, Health Services Administration, Office of Planning, Evaluation, and Legislation. 1978. *PSRO: An Initial Evaluation of the Professional Standards Review Organization.* Washington, D.C.: Government Printing Office.

*U.S. Department of Health, Education, and Welfare, National Center for Health Services Research. 1978. *NCHSR Research Priorities.* PHS no. 79-3241. Washington, D.C.: Government Printing Office.

————. 1979. NCHSR-Supported Projects Involving Cost-Effectiveness or Cost-Benefit Analyses. Unpublished list and description of projects prepared for the Office of Technology Assessment, 6 June.

U.S. Department of Health, Education, and Welfare, Office of the Assistant Secretary for Program Coordination, Program Analysis Group on Selected Disease Control Programs, 1966a. Disease Control Programs: Arthritis. Unpublished paper.

————. 1966b. Disease Control Programs: Cancer. Unpubished paper.

————. 1966c. Program Analysis: Maternal and Child Health Care Programs. Unpublished paper.

————. 1967a. Disease Control Programs: Delivery of Health Services for the Poor. Unpublished paper.

————. 1967b. *Disease Control Programs: Kidney Disease: Program Analysis.* PHS Publication no. 1745. Washington, D.C.: Government Printing Office.

————. 1968. Nursing Manpower Programs. Unpublished paper.

*U.S. Department of Health, Education, and Welfare, Public Health Service, 1979. *Healthy People—The Surgeon General's Report on Health Promotion and Disease Prevention.* DHEW Publication no. PHS 79-55071. Washington, D.C.: Government Printing Office.

*————. 1980. *Health—United States—1979.* Washington, D.C.: Government Printing Office.

U.S. General Accounting Office. 1975. *Treatment of Chronic Kidney Failure: Dialysis, Transplant, Costs, and the Need for More Vigorous Efforts.* Washington, D.C.: Government Printing Office.

————. 1979. Problems With Evaluating the Cost-Effectiveness of Professional Standards Review Organizations. Report by the Comptroller General of the United States. Washington, D.C.

Utian, W. 1977. Application of Cost-Effectiveness Analysis to Post-Menopausal Estrogen Therapy. *Front. Horm. Res.* 5:26.

VanPelt, A. and Levy, H. 1974. Cost-Benefit Analysis of Newborn Screening for Metabolic Disorders. *New Engl. J. Med.* 291:1414.

Vehorn, C. et al. 1977. Biomedical Research and Its Impact on Personal Health Care Expenditures, 1930-1975. Unpublished paper. Washington, D.C.: Georgetown University, Public Services Laboratory.

Waaler, H. 1968. Cost-Benefit Analysis of BCG-Vaccination Under Various Epidemiological Situations. *Bull. Int. Un. Tuberc.* 41:42.

Waaler, H. and Piot, M. 1970. Use of an Epidemiological Model for Estimating the Effectiveness of Tuberculosis Control Measures. *Bull. WHO* 43:1.

Wagner, D. et al. 1977. Gains in Mortality From Biomedical Research, 1930-1975: A Macro View. Unpublished paper. Washington, D.C.: Georgetown University, Public Services Laboratory.

Wagner, J. 1981a. The Feasibility of Economic Evaluation of Diagnostic Procedures: The Case of CT Scanning (OTA-BP-H-9(2)). In *The Implications of Cost-Effectiveness Analysis of Medical Technology; Background Paper no. 2: Case Studies of Medical Technologies.* Washington, D.C.: Government Printing Office.

_____. 1981b. *The Implications of Cost-Effectiveness Analysis of Medical Technology; Background Paper no. 5: Assessment of Four Common X-Ray Procedures.* Washington, D.C.: Government Printing Office.

_____. ed. 1979. *Medical Technology.* DHEW Publication no. (PHS) 79-3254. Washington, D.C.: Government Printing Office.

Walker, G. 1976. Primary Health Care in Botswana: A Study in Cost-Effectiveness. *Proc. Roy. Soc. Med.* 69:936.

Walker, G. and Gish, O. 1977. Mobile Health Services: A Study in Cost-Effectiveness. *Med. Care* 15:267.

Walworth, C. et al. 1977. Industrial Hypertension Program in a Rural State. Efficacy and Cost Effectiveness. *JAMA* 237:1942.

*Ward, R. 1975. *The Economics of Health Resources.* Reading, Mass.: Addison-Wesley.

Wardell, W. 1974. Assessment of the Benefits, Risks, and Costs of Medical Programs. In *Benefits and Risks in Medical Care*, ed. D. Taylor. London: White Crescent Press.

*Wardell, W. et al. 1980. Development of New Drugs Originated and Acquired by United States-Owned Pharmaceutical Firms, 1963-1976. *Clin. Pharm. Ther.* 28:270.

*Warner, K. 1978. The Effects of Hospital Cost Containment on the Development and Use of Medical Technology. *Milbank Mem. Fund Q.* 56:187.

*_____. 1979a. The Cost of Capital-Embodied Medical Technology. In *Medical Technology and the Health Care System.* Washington, D.C.: National Academy of Sciences.

_____. 1979b. The Economic Implications of Preventive Health Care. *Soc. Sci. Med.* 13C:227.

_____. 1979c. Epilogue. In *Medical Technology*, ed. J. Wagner, DHEW Publication no. (PHS) 79-3254. Washington, D.C.: Government Printing Office.

Warner, K. and Hutton, R. 1980. Cost-Benefit and Cost-Effectiveness Analysis in Health Care: Growth and Composition of the Literature. *Med. Care* 18:1069.

Watts, C. et al. 1979. Cost Effectiveness Analysis: Some Problems of Implementation. *Med. Care* 17:430.

Watts, M. 1976. The Dollars for Health. *West. J. Med.* 125:219.

Weiler, P. 1974. Cost-Effective Analysis: A Quandary for Geriatric Health Care Systems. *Gerontologist* 14:414.

Weinstein, M. 1979. Economic Evaluation of Medical Procedures and Technologies: Progress, Problems, and Prospects. In *Medical Technology*, ed. J. Wagner.

DHEW Publication no. (PHS) 79-3254. Washington, D.C.: Government Printing Office.

Weinstein, M. and Fineberg, H. 1978. Cost-Effectiveness Analysis for Medical Practices: Appropriate Laboratory Utilization. In *Logic and Economics of Clinical Laboratory Use*, ed. E. Benson and M. Rubin. Amsterdam: Elsevier-North Holland.

Weinstein, M. and Pearlman, L. 1981. Cost-Effectiveness of Automated Multichannel Chemistry Analyzers (OTA-BP-H-9(4)). In *The Implications of Cost-Effectiveness Analysis of Medical Technology; Background Paper no. 2: Case Studies of Medical Technologies*. Washington, D.C.: Government Printing Office.

Weinstein, M. and Stason, W. 1976a. Economic Considerations in the Management of Mild Hypertension. *Ann. N.Y. Acad. Sci.* 304:424.

————. 1976b. *Hypertension: A Policy Perspective*. Cambridge, Mass.: Harvard Univ. Press.

————. 1977a. Allocating Resources: The Case of Hypertension. *Hast. Cent. Rep.* 7:24.

————. 1977b. Foundations of Cost-Effectiveness Analysis for Health and Medical Practices. *New Engl. J. Med.* 296:716.

Weinstein, M. et al. 1977. Coronary Artery Bypass Surgery: Decision and Policy Analysis. In *Costs, Risks, and Benefits of Surgery*, ed. J. Bunker et al. New York: Oxford Univ. Press.

Weisbrod, B. 1961. *The Economics of Public Health: Measuring the Economic Impact of Disease*. Philadelphia: Univ. of Pennsylvania Press.

————. 1971. Costs and Benefits of Medical Research: A Case Study of Poliomyelitis. *J. Polit. Econ.* 79:527.

————. 1975. Research in Economics: A Survey. *Int. J. Health Serv.* 5:643.

Weisbrod, B., et al. 1978. An Alternative to Mental Hospital Treatment. III: Economic Benefit-Cost Analysis. Unpublished paper, Madison, Wisconsin.

Weiss, W. 1971. Routine Sigmoidoscopy Costs and Usefulness. *JAMA* 216:886.

Weissert, W. et al. 1980. Cost-Effectiveness of Homemaker Services for the Chronically Ill. *Inquiry* 17:230.

Welch, L. 1978. Draft Report on PSRO Effectiveness Stirs Commentary. *Hospitals* 52:44.

Welssert, W. et al. 1980. *Effects and Costs of Day Care and Homemaker Services for the Chronically Ill: A Randomized Experiement*. DHEW Publication no. (PHS) 79-3258. Washington, D.C.: Government Printing Office.

Werner, M. et al. 1973. Strategy for Cost-Effective Laboratory Testing. *Hum. Pathol.* 4:17.

White, K. 1976. Planning and Execution, Costs and Benefits of Cross-National Sociomedical Research. In *Cross-National Sociomedical Research*, ed. M. Pflanz and E. Schach. Stuttgart, West Germany: Thiemi.

Willems, J. 1978. Cost-Effectiveness Analysis of Medical Technologies as an Aid to Policymaking. Paper read at the Health Care Technology Evaluation Symposium, Columbia, Missouri, November 6.

*Williams, A. 1972. Cost-Benefit Analysis: Bastard Science? And/Or Incidious [sic] Poison in the Body Politick[sic]? *J. Pub. Econ.* 1:199.

————. 1974. The Cost-Benefit Approach. *Brit. Med. Bull.* 30:252.

Williams, A. and Com, B. 1976. Description versus Valuation in Long-Term Care Data. *Med. Care* 14:148.

Wingert, W. et al. 1975. Effectiveness and Efficiency of Indigenous Health Aides in a Pediatric Outpatient Department. *Amer. J. Pub. Health* 65:849.

Wiseman, J. 1963. Cost-Benefit Analysis and Health Service Policy. *Scot. J. Pol. Econ.* 10:128.

Witte, J. et al. 1975. The Benefits From 10 Years of Measles Immunization in the United States. *Pub. Health Rep.* 90:205.

*Wolf, C. 1978. *A Theory of "Non-Market Failure": Framework for Implementation Analysis.* RAND P-6034. Santa Monica, Calif.: RAND Corp.

Wolfe, H. 1973. Pharmacy: How Cost-Effective Are Generics? *Hospitals* 47:100.

Wortzman, G. and Holgate, R. 1979. Reappraisal of the Cost Effectiveness of Computed Tomography in a Government-Sponsored Health Care System. *Radiology* 130:257.

Wortzman, G. et al. 1975. Cranial Computed Tomography: An Evaluation of Cost-Effectiveness. *Radiology* 117:75.

Wynn, T. 1979. Patient Care Audits Not Cost Effective. *West. J. Med.* 130:467.

Yaffe, R. et al. 1978. Medical Economics Survey-Methods Study: Cost-Effectiveness of Alternative Survey Strategies. *Med. Care* 16:641.

Yates, B. 1977. Cost-Effectiveness Analysis: Using It For Our Own Good. *State Psychol. Assoc. Aff. Newsletter* 8:9.

_____. 1978. Improving the Cost-Effectiveness of Obesity Programs: Three Basic Strategies for Reducing the Cost Per Pound. *Int. J. Obes.* 2:249

_____. 1979a. How To Improve, Rather Than Evaluate, Cost-Effectiveness. *Counsel. Psychol.* 8:72.

_____. 1979b. The Theory and Practice of Cost-Utility, Cost-Effectiveness, and Cost-Benefit Analysis in Behavioral Medicine: Toward Delivering More Care for Less Money. In *A Comprehensive Handbook of Behavioral Medicine*, ed. J. Ferguson and B. Taylor. Englewood Cliffs, N.J.: Spectrum.

Yorio, D. et al. 1972. Cost Comparison of Decentralized Unit Doses and Traditional Pharmacy Services in a 600-Bed Community Hospital. *Amer. J. Hosp. Pharm.* 29:922.

Zapka, J. and Averill, B. 1979. Self Care for Colds: A Cost-Effective Alternative Upper Respiratory Infection Management. *Amer. J. Pub. Health* 69:814.

*Zeckhauser, R. 1975. Procedures for Valuing Lives. *Pub. Pol.* 23:419.

Zeckhauser, R. and Shepard, D. 1976. Where Now for Saving Lives? *Law Contemp. Prob.* 40:5.

Index

in, 36; systemic approach to, 28, 30, 31, 33
Health care costs, 1–26; causes of increasing, 4ff; components, 12; distribution, 1, 3–4; net, 144; magnitude of, 1, 2ff; physician influence on, 36–37; physician interest in containment, 37–40, 176–81; rate of growth, 1, 2, 3, 26; sources of growth, 5
Health Care Financing Administration (HCFA), 30, 31, 34, 190, 191, 201–2
Health care industry, competitive forces in, 32
Health care manpower program, 127
Health care price inflation, 18–21, 41n8
Health Care Technology Act of 1978, 55
Health insurance, 6–7, 10–18, 33, 35. *See also* Blue Cross–Blue Shield; Medicaid; Medicare
Health Maintenance Organizations (HMOs), 15, 27, 33, 180, 204, 208n6, 219 222; and cost-containment, 30, 32, 36; costs of compared with fee-for-service care costs, 36; use of CBA-CEA, 183–84, 185
Health Manpower Bill, 31
Health Planning Amendments of 1979, 55
Health planning organizations, 194–97
Health problem, defining, 63–67, 134–36, 213
Health Resources Administration, 131
Health status indexes, 91–93, 148–49. *See also* Valuation of health benefits
Health Systems Agencies (HSAs), 30–31, 32, 194, 196
Heart transplantation, 73, 190–91
Hellinger, 131
HEW. *See* Department of Health, Education, and Welfare
Hicks, 151, 159, 161
Hill-Burton Act, 25
HMO. *See* Health Maintenance Organizations
Hodgson, 150
Hospital care costs, 12–13, 19, 26
Hospital rate review, 33–34
Hospitals, use of CBA-CEA by, 184–85
Hu, 150
Hudson, 38, 182, 221
Hughes, 33

Human capital. *See* Valuation, of health benefits
Hutton, 131
Hypertension, 54, 72, 140, 150, 153, 156, 159, 164, 187, 217

IBM, 187
Institutional versus home care services, 127
Intermediate outcomes. *See* Benefits and effectiveness, intermediate outcomes
Interpretation. *See* CBA-CEA, presentation and interpretation

Jacobs, 41n8
Johnson administration, 51
Joint production, 74, 139, 141
Joint replacement, 126

Kaiser-Permanente, 30, 183. *See also* Health Maintenance Organizations
Kaplan, 92, 132, 149
Kassirer, 130
Keeler, 40n4
Kennedy administration, 51
Kidney disease, 53, 63, 64, 65, 68–69, 125, 136, 137, 148, 150–51, 152, 156, 165–66, 169n14, 190, 216
Klarman, Herbert, 63, 64, 90, 92, 130, 137, 140, 148, 151, 165
Knox, 85
Kridel, 38, 182, 221

Laboratory tests, 35, 188–89, 224. *See also* Diagnostic procedures
LeSourd, 63, 136, 152, 156, 161, 165
Levy, 152, 166
Lewicki 130, 167
Literature on health care CBA-CEA, 52–53, 56, 61–62, 117–70, 129–32; findings characterized, 167; methodology, 129–32; growth of, 117–21; popular subject areas of noted, 125–27; quality of, 215; readership characterized, 159, 181; shift of emphasis, 215; subject matter, 122–24; technical and conceptual weaknesses, 216–17; unpopular areas noted, 127–29. *See also*

About the Authors

Kenneth E. Warner is a Professor and Chairman of the Department of Health Planning and Administration, School of Public Health, at the University of Michigan. His research has focused on the economics of medical technology and the political economy of disease prevention, with a special emphasis on smoking and health. Dr. Warner has served as a consultant to numerous organizations including the Office of Technology Assessment in Congress and the Office on Smoking and Health and the National Center for Health Services Research in the Department of Health and Human Services. He holds a Ph.D. in economics from Yale University and is a Kellogg National Fellow for 1980-83.

Bryan R. Luce is Director, Office of Research and Demonstrations, Health Care Financing Administration, Department of Health and Human Services. During preparation of this book, he was a Senior Analyst in the Health Program of the Office of Technology Assessment, U.S. Congress, where he directed a project examining national strategies for assessing medical technologies. Dr. Luce's previous research has focused on quality of care issues and cost-effectiveness analysis of disease prevention. He holds an M.B.A. from the University of Massachusetts and a Ph.D. in Health Services Administration from UCLA.